ELLIE

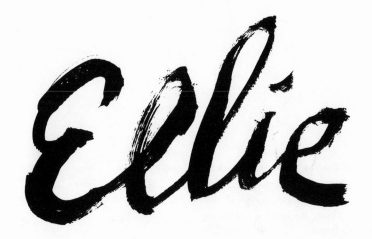

Ellie

A CHILD'S FIGHT AGAINST LEUKEMIA

Jonathan B. Tucker

HOLT, RINEHART and WINSTON   New York

Published by Holt, Rinehart and Winston,
383 Madison Avenue, New York, New York 10017.

Published simultaneously in Canada by Holt, Rinehart and Winston of Canada, Limited.

Library of Congress Cataloging in Publication Data

Tucker, Jonathan B.
  Ellie, a child's fight against leukemia.

  Bibliography: p.
  Includes index.
  1. Leukemia in children—Case studies. 2. Leukemia
in children—Psychological aspects—Case studies.
3. Leukemia in children—Patients—Family relationships—
Case studies   I. Title.
RJ416.L4T83   362.1'989299419   81-7181   AACR2

ISBN: 0-03-057662-8

First Edition

Designer: A. Christopher Simon

Printed in the United States of America

10 9 8 7 6 5 4 3 2 1

ISBN 0-03-057662-8

TO MY COUSIN DAVID BRIN
(1957–1980)
*whose courageous battle against acute
lymphoblastic leukemia inspired this book*

Whether tis nobler in the mind to suffer
The slings and arrows of outrageous fortune
Or to take arms against a sea of troubles
And by opposing end them?

William Shakespeare
Hamlet, Act III, Scene i

Disclaimer

For didactic purposes, this story is a composite of three case histories. All names have been changed. Medical personnel are not intended to represent living individuals but merely illustrate ideas and attitudes. All of the medical, historical, and factual information is, to the best of my knowledge, true, but specific hospitals are mentioned only for background—i.e., not all the events depicted necessarily took place at the institution named.

Although this book is intended to be a fairly representative description of the impact of catastrophic illness on a child and her family, it must be kept in mind that every family is unique and that some parts of the narrative may have limited relevance to other cases and families. It is hoped, however, that the story contains enough universal elements both to be of value to others going through this incredible experience and to increase public understanding and sympathy for the victims of the disease.

Contents

Acknowledgments

I am indebted to many people who provided assistance and background information during the researching and writing of this book. Most of all, I would like to express my deep gratitude to the families who were willing to talk freely and openly about their painful experiences and who have preferred to remain anonymous. Others who provided valuable leads or logistical help were Stuart Schwartz in Los Angeles, Patricia A. Newman and Barbara Blumberg at the Office of Cancer Communications of the National Cancer Institute, Maryanne Bolton at the Children's Hospital of Philadelphia, Grace Monaco of the Candlelighters Organization, and representatives of the American Cancer Society and the Leukemia Society of America.

The following individuals were interviewed in the course of my research: At the Memorial Sloan-Kettering Cancer Center in New York: Denis R. Miller, MD, Peter Steinhertz, MD, Norman L. Straker, MD, Yehuda Nir, MD, Richard J. O'Reilly, MD, Berta Jereb, MD, Brenda Shank, MD, Jimmie C. B. Holland, MD, Michael Tamaroff, Ph.D., and Margaret Adams, MSW. At the Massachusetts General Hospital: John T. Truman, MD, Robert W. Carey, MD, Lois Slovik, MD, and Genevieve Foley, RN. At the Johns Hopkins Oncology Center Bone Marrow Transplant Unit: George W. Santos, MD, Rein Saral, MD, William H. Burns, MD, Lyle Sensenbrenner, MD, Stuart Grossman, MD, David Kessler, MD, John H. Fetting, III, MD, Jacqueline M. Nishimura, RN, Denyse Ledoux, RN, Steven Baust, P.A., Denise E. Carter (transplant coordinator), and Sue

Wright (manager/supervisor, Hemophoresis Center). At the University of Massachusetts at Amherst Infirmary: Paul E. Berman, MD. At Cooley Dickinson Hospital in Northampton, Massachusetts: Jonathan B. Greenberg, MD, and Richard C. Hinckley, MD. At the Children's Hospital of Philadelphia: Audrey E. Evans, MD, Charles S. August, MD, Edith Burkey, P.A., Michelle Lloyd, RN, Arlene Androkites, RN, and Virginia R. Peltz (social worker).

I would also like to thank Kathy Rose and Michael Braffman, MD, for additional insights; Michael A. Fifer, MD, and Jeffrey Rosenstock, MD, for reading the manuscript; Steven Black and Carol Donner for the illustrations; Natalie Chapman, my editor at Holt, for her continuing help and support; and my wife, Karen, for providing superb editorial assistance and tolerating my erratic moods and hours during the writing of this book.

Part I
OUTRAGEOUS FORTUNE

1 Onset

Shortly after noon on Saturday, September 16, 1978, a Suburban Transit bus pulled up in front of the shopping center in Menlo Park, New Jersey, one of the commuter towns in the wide belt of suburbs surrounding New York City. Barbara Murphy, an attractive woman of thirty-two with a distinctively Irish mix of dark hair and blue eyes, stepped down from the bus carrying a small suitcase.

She had come to visit her brother Brian, his wife, Sally, and their two children—six-year-old Beth and four-year-old Ellie. Barbara herself was single and childless, a nurse in the outpatient department of New York Hospital. She was very fond of her nieces and often came to see them on weekends. A few times a year they reciprocated by staying at her apartment on the East Side of Manhattan.

A short time later, a battered white Volvo pulled up to the bus stop. Sally Murphy, a woman of thirty with closely cropped brown hair, green eyes, and a thin, nervous mouth, reached over to open the front door. "Hi, Barb," she said. "Been waiting long?"

"Not five minutes, thanks," Barbara replied, although it had been closer to ten. She got in and turned around to say hello to the children. Immediately she sensed that something was wrong. Ellie had always been a lively and demanding child, a whirlwind of activity, and unusually verbal for her age. But now she seemed lethargic and drained of color, with dark circles under her eyes.

They were driving past rows of suburban houses with trimmed green lawns and station wagons parked in the driveways. A lawn mower droned in the distance, and Barbara caught a whiff of barbecue smoke from someone's backyard. They passed the high school, where children were playing, and a sign reading: YOUTH—MENLO PARK'S PRIDE AND GREATEST ASSET.

Barbara could not stop worrying about Ellie's appearance. "Ellie doesn't look too good to me," she said. "Has she been to the doctor recently?"

"Several times," Sally replied. She went on to describe the series of mysterious fluctuations in Ellie's health over the past two weeks. The child would suddenly develop a fever of 102°, and then almost miraculously her temperature would return to normal the following day. She had also been unusually torpid, taking long naps in the afternoon, and had broken out in a strange rash on her legs that looked like dozens of tiny bug bites. Dr. Brice, the family GP, had said it was probably a low-grade infection, but nothing to worry about; young children were always coming down with colds.

"I took Beth in to see Dr. Brice yesterday for an ear infection, and I had him look at Ellie, too," Sally continued. "She was running a fever again. I told him, 'Look, this is really getting ridiculous. I don't understand why she keeps running these fevers.'"

"So what did he say?" Barbara asked.

"'Oh, she's just a rotten kid.' He was joking, of course."

Sally pulled into the parking lot in front of an A & P. "I've got to do some food shopping," she said. "Would you mind walking home with the kids? I won't be long."

"Sure, I'd love to," Barbara said. "Meet you there."

They all got out, and the children waved good-bye to Sally as she disappeared into the store. Barbara took the two girls by the hand and started to lead them across the street. The light began to flash DON'T WALK, and she told them to hurry.

"I can't," Ellie whined. "My legs hurt."

Thinking she was just being difficult, Barbara picked her up and carried her across the street, setting her down on the other side. They started walking again, and Barbara noticed that Ellie had a stiff-legged, flapping gait as if she were nine months pregnant. The child grimaced with each step, and it was obvious that her legs really were hurting her. "How long has Ellie been walking like that?" Barbara asked Beth.

"Oh, she's been walking funny ever since she fell off her tricycle," Beth said.

Concerned, Barbara picked Ellie up and carried her the rest of the way home. On reaching the house, she took the child inside and laid her down on the kitchen table, telling Beth to run off and play. Then she removed Ellie's overalls, revealing a large, blood-soaked gauze bandage on the child's left knee. Barbara was shocked to notice that Ellie's legs were marble white and mottled with purple bruises and tiny red blood blisters—the "bug bites" that Sally had mentioned.

Barbara was suddenly very scared. Thirteen years before, when she was just starting out on her nursing career, she had worked for a hematologist in a medical group on Staten Island and had seen many children with excessive bruising and the localized skin hemorrhages called petechiae. All of them had serious blood diseases—aplastic anemia, leukemia, and the like—and nearly all had died. Feeling a knot of anxiety tighten in her chest, Barbara picked Ellie up and, with the child resting limply in her arms, carried her into the girls' bedroom and laid her down on the bottom bunk.

Just then the front door opened and Sally came in, carrying two bags of groceries. Barbara helped her carry the bags into the kitchen and put the items away. She knew they had to get Ellie to a doctor, yet she did not want to alarm Sally unnecessarily. There were still many less serious things it could be.

"Ellie was exhausted, so I put her to bed," she said. "She looks very pale to me, and I don't like it at all."

"Oh, she's usually pale," Sally replied, filling the refrigerator.

"Her legs are also terribly bruised, and she can barely walk."

"Yes, I know. She fell off her tricycle the other day and really did it to herself. That kid is so klutzy sometimes." Sally remembered vividly when Ellie had come into the house, crying hysterically, her left knee oozing blood. Sally had bandaged it and told the child to rest for an hour. Later that afternoon, she had looked in on Ellie watching TV and noticed that the bandage was soaked with blood. She had dressed the wound freshly, this time applying pressure until the bleeding finally stopped. It was then that she had noticed the rash and the large black-and-blue marks that Ellie said hurt when she touched them.

"What about her stomach?" Barbara went on. "It's so swollen."

"I mentioned that to Dr. Brice and he said that she seemed a little full in there. He told me to give her an enema. But I don't understand it, because she's been going regularly."

"Have her stools been dark?"

"Yes, how did you know? I guess all children get it. Cindy Lewis was telling me the other day that Jennifer ate something and . . ."

Dark stools could mean that Ellie was bleeding into her stomach or intestines, Barbara thought. That would account for her anemia as well. They had to get her to a doctor fast.

"I'd feel better, personally, if we got Ellie checked out," she said out loud. "Most doctor's offices are closed on Sunday, and if it's a virus or something, why not get it taken care of? Let me call your GP and see if he can examine her today."

"Do you really think it's important enough for him to see her today?"

"Yes, I really do."

"Okay, then. Go ahead and call." She gave Barbara the number of Brice's office, and Barbara went into the next room to make the call, since she preferred that Sally not overhear. The phone rang several times before someone answered.

"Hello, is this Dr. Brice?" Barbara asked.

"No, this is Dr. Johnson, a colleague of his. Dr. Brice is off today and I'm covering for him. What can I do for you?"

"My four-year-old niece, Ellen Murphy, is a patient of Dr. Brice's. She looks severely anemic, with a low-grade fever, fatigue, and suspicious bruising, and I'd like her to have a physical exam and a blood test right away."

"I'm sorry, but it will have to wait until Monday. I've got a cardiac emergency on my hands right now that is going to require my attention all afternoon."

"But it can't wait that long!" Barbara protested. "I'm an RN at New York Hospital with experience in hematology, and I know what I'm talking about. This child is acutely ill and could have a blood disease."

"Look, you could take her to the local hospital emergency room and have the blood drawn there, and they could call me with the results."

"In other words, you can't see her today."

"No, I'm sorry."

"Thank you anyway, doctor."

She hung up, swore under her breath, and went looking for Sally, who was in the living room with Brian. He had just returned from inspecting a neighbor's new sports car. A tall, lanky man of thirty-four with strong, rather handsome features, he had a friendly, easygoing manner that masked a deeper reserve. He noticed the troubled look on his sister's face and asked what was bothering her.

"Ellie looks very anemic and I think she should see a doctor," Barbara explained. "I just called Brice's office but he's not there, and the guy covering for him is busy all afternoon."

Sally shook her head. "Kids never get sick Monday through Friday; it's either a weekend or a holiday. It never fails."

Barbara thought for a minute. "Doesn't your neighbor Pat have a pediatrician in Plainfield that she uses?"

Sally remembered that she did—a certain Dr. Warner.

"Come on, Barbara," Brian protested. "This is really getting out of hand. I don't want to pay for another doctor's appointment. Sally's taken her to see Brice five times already, and he keeps telling her that Ellie has a little bug—nothing to get hysterical about. If she's still sick on Monday we can give him a call."

Barbara's blue eyes lit up with anger. "Brian, Ellie looks severely anemic and I think she should have a blood test. Believe me, I wouldn't insist unless I felt it was important."

Brian shrugged. "All right, Barbara, have it your way. You're the big expert around here. But I still don't think it's necessary."

Barbara turned to Sally and said, "Why don't you get Warner's number from Pat and give him a call?"

Sally did as she was told. Once she had the number, she called Warner's office and spoke to the nurse-receptionist, listing all of Ellie's symptoms. The nurse apparently felt they were serious enough to warrant a physical exam and a blood test, so she made an appointment for them to see Dr. Warner at 2:00 P.M. in the emergency room at Plainfield's Muhlenberg Hospital, which was a twenty-minute drive from the Murphys' house.

Barbara's tension mounted as it neared two o'clock. A gin and tonic helped calm her nerves somewhat. While Ellie slept, Beth and some neighborhood friends played hide-and-seek in the backyard, Sally cleaned the stove, and Brian repaired the screen door. No one but Barbara seemed particularly worried.

Before they prepared to leave for the hospital, Sally decided to give Ellie a bath. She went into the girls' bedroom and woke her, and the child blinked up at her with dazed eyes. Her forehead was hot with fever and her face was flushed except for her lips and gums, which were strangely pale.

"Ellie," Sally said softly. "We have to take you to the hospital to find out why you keep getting these fevers. They're going to give you some tests, but they'll explain everything to you and you'll know exactly what's going on."

"I feel fine," Ellie said, although she was very listless. She really didn't know what a hospital was, except for the time she had been to the emergency room after the accident with the fireplace. She did know that she didn't like doctors at all, with their sharp instruments and lights for peering into her body. "Do I have to go to the hospital?" she asked.

"Yes, sweetheart," Sally replied. "Aunt Barbara thinks it's a good idea, and she's a nurse so she should know. But first you need a bath. We have to make you nice and clean for the doctor."

Sally took her into the bathroom and ran the water while she helped Ellie undress. As she pulled off the child's shirt, she noticed a new bruise just below the wing of Ellie's left shoulder blade. Strange, she thought. The bruise had not been there that morning, and as far as she knew Ellie had not fallen all day. She would have to ask Barbara about that. . . .

Sally stared at the bruise as Ellie bathed, and wondered what it meant. Was there something beyond the fever, something more serious, that was causing all this? She remembered reading once in a women's magazine about bruising being common in children with leukemia. It was the only thing she knew about the disease, other than that it was a death sentence. Everyone who got leukemia on the soap operas she watched always died after a few agonizing weeks. A chill ran down her spine. "Oh, my God," she murmured to herself. "Is that what Barbara thinks?"

As soon as Ellie was dried and dressed, Sally hurried into the living room, where Barbara was nursing a drink. Sally leaned over and whispered in her ear, "It couldn't be leukemia, could it?"

Barbara looked up. "What makes you think that?"

"Because Ellie has more bruises on her than she did this morning."

"Let's wait and see what the doctor has to say," Barbara replied quickly.

Sally nodded, but the fact that Barbara had not denied her suspicion terrified her. In a daze, she told Beth to go over to the Lewises' house to play while they were at the hospital.

"Can I come to the hospital, too?" Beth asked, tugging insistently on her mother's skirt.

"I'm sorry, Beth, you're too young."

"How come Ellie gets to go and I don't?"

"Because Ellie's sick and has to see the doctor, that's why. You can play with Jennifer until we get back. Please be a good girl, okay?"

Beth scowled, her tears welling up. It just wasn't fair.

Several minutes later, the whole family got into the car. The first stop was the Lewises'. Beth looked sad and abandoned as she got out, but when she saw Jennifer waving from the doorway, she cheered up and ran off without a backward glance.

2 Examination

The emergency room was crowded and confusing, filled with the mingled sounds of conversation, babies crying, and doctors being paged. Pushing Ellie in a stroller, Sally followed Barbara and Brian up to the reception desk, fighting the nausea that gnawed at her insides. The triage nurse took down some basic information, recorded their Blue Cross number, and told them to wait in one of the rows of contoured plastic chairs.

Sally sat down obediently and lit a cigarette with shaking fingers. She had always had a mild phobia of hospitals. Whenever she went to visit a sick friend or relative, she would become faint and queasy, panicking at the thought of this vast building filled with the ill and dying. The cool, dispassionate atmosphere of the emergency room only heightened her feeling of helplessness. She looked at Ellie's chalky complexion and burning forehead, refusing to believe it was anything serious—most likely just a bad case of the flu.

To Ellie, the hospital looked strange and smelled funny. It was so big, with gleaming corridors, stairways, elevators, doors—a place to get lost in. More sick people than she had ever imagined existed were passing in and out through the automatic doors, many with casts and crutches or in wheelchairs. She clung tightly to her mother's arm, afraid of needles and pain and the doctor's probing.

Brian was annoyed by the wait, looking around him at the other children in the room and comparing their appearance with Ellie's. She really didn't look so bad, he thought, angry at his sister for having dragged them to the hospital to waste the better part of a Saturday afternoon. Barbara, meanwhile, considered the diagnostic possibilities and hoped that her suspicion was wrong.

Finally their name was called. Sally picked up Ellie in her arms and they went to the reception desk, where Dr. Warner was waiting to meet them. He was a tall man of about fifty, with a lean, ascetic face tempered by gentle brown eyes. "Is this Ellen Murphy?" he asked.

"Yes," Sally replied. "I'm the mother, and this is my husband, Brian, and my sister-in-law, Barbara, who's a nurse at New York Hospital. She's the one who urged us to have Ellie examined today. My neighbor Pat Bradley recommended you, since our GP wasn't in."

"I see. I'm glad to meet you," Warner said. "Now if you'll just follow me . . ." He led them past the reception desk and into one of the small examining rooms that lined the corridor beyond.

Closing the door behind him, he gestured the Murphys into chairs; Ellie sat on her mother's lap. Warner looked over the form the triage nurse had given him. "I see that Ellen has a problem with recurrent fever, pallor, and bruising," he said. "How long has this been going on?"

"About two weeks," Sally answered. "She's been sick before, but never like this. She gets a high fever and it seems to go away for a while, but then it comes back, higher than ever."

"Has she had all the usual childhood infections?" Warner asked. "Mumps, measles, German measles, chicken pox?"

"All but the chicken pox," Sally said. "She was vaccinated for mumps and polio."

"Has she ever been hospitalized for any reason?"

"This past June she was playing and had an accident and we brought her here to be treated. She had seven stitches in her scalp, but no concussion."

"I see. All right, let me examine her and see what's what." He opened his black bag and took out an electronic thermometer, about the size of a pocket calculator with a long probe attached by a flexible wire. Placing a clean plastic tip on the probe, he told Ellie to open her mouth wide. She did so reluctantly, and he slipped it under her tongue.

Usually Ellie was very uncooperative at the doctor's office; as much as she trusted the doctor's ability to make her well, she disliked the bodily intrusions and constantly feared pain. But this one seemed gentle, and anyway she was too tired to resist.

The digital readout began to climb rapidly until a beep sounded, and Warner withdrew the probe.

"What's her temperature, doctor?" Sally asked.

"It's 102. Did you give her any aspirin before you came?"

"Yes, two. They were children's aspirin, though," she added hopefully.

Warner nodded. He took the child's pulse and blood pressure, jotting the values down on the form. "Ellie, will you do me a favor?" he said. "Would you get undressed down to your underwear? I want to do a little examination."

Ellie was embarrassed, but she stood up and, with her mother's help, began undressing listlessly. Sally folded her clothes and held them in her lap. Warner lifted the child up onto the examining table and placed his stethoscope on her back. "Okay, big breath through your mouth. Good." The child's lungs were clear and aerated well. "Now I want to listen to your heart. You can breathe normally for this." The child's heart rate was elevated—160 beats per minute—and there was a murmur. These symptoms were most likely due to her anemia, which was making her heart work harder to oxygenate her tissues.

Next Warner examined Ellie's head, shining a bright light into her ears. Her eardrums were normal, with clear landmarks. "Very good," he said. "Okay, how about if we turn out the light and open the door a crack, and you look at the blue star on the wall." There was a star painted on the opposite wall in phosphorescent blue so that it glowed in the dark. While Ellie stared at the star, Warner picked up an ophthalmoscope from the electrically powered wall unit and peered through it at Ellie's eyes. Her pupils were of equal size and constricted rapidly in the light. Then he got closer and looked through each pupil at the optic disk, the pink spot at the back of the eye formed by nerve fibers converging from the retina into the optic nerve. If there had been bleeding inside Ellie's head or a tumor of some kind, it would have displaced some of the cerebrospinal fluid cushioning her brain and spinal cord, thereby increasing the pressure of the fluid within the rigid skull. Since the optic disks were extensions of the brain, the increased pressure would have caused them to swell with fluid and bulge forward, a phenomenon known as papilledema. But Ellie's optic disks looked sharp, indicating that the pressure inside her cranium was normal. Clearly the source of her problems lay elsewhere.

"That was wonderful, Ellie," Warner said, turning the room lights back on. "You did that very well." Ellie's eyes were watering and green spots floated over her field of vision. Before she had time to recover fully, the doctor told her to open her mouth wide while he held down her tongue with a flat wooden stick and looked at the back of her throat with a flashlight. "Open wider," he said. Ellie gagged, inhaling the doctor's minty breath. Warner noted that her throat was somewhat inflamed, but not seriously.

Next he tested her strength, asking her to squeeze his index fingers as hard as she could. "Now I'm going to give your knee a little tap," he told Ellie, and took out his rubber hammer to test her deep-tendon reflexes. When Ellie saw the hammer poised near her knee, she began to cry. "Please don't hit me," she begged. "My knee hurts."

Warner stopped and examined her legs, frowning at the bruises and petechiae. "How did you get these?" he asked. The question was directed more toward Sally than Ellie.

"I first noticed them after she fell off her tricycle last week," Sally said. "But then more kept appearing, along with a couple of red dots that I thought at first were bug bites. But then they spread all over her legs. That bruise on her back wasn't there this morning, and I'm pretty sure she didn't fall down today."

Warner cleared his throat. "Mrs. Murphy, has Ellie had any problems recently with nosebleeds, or cuts that fail to clot?"

With a chill, Sally told him about the scraped knee that hadn't stopped bleeding. For some reason she had forgotten to mention it. Warner's clairvoyance, the accuracy of his probing, frightened her. Was he leading up to what she feared?

If Warner suspected something, he did not let on. He merely said that it was important that Ellie not get any more aspirin, since that would worsen her bleeding problem. He recommended Tylenol instead. "Could you lie down on your back now?" he asked Ellie, continuing his examination. "I want to feel your tummy."

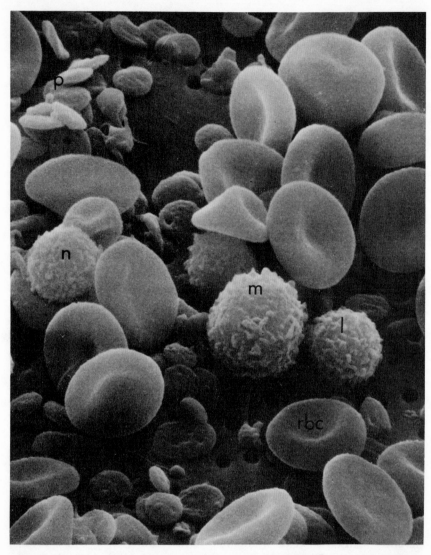

Cells from normal human blood are viewed with a scanning electron microscope, which uses a beam of electrons to generate a detailed three-dimensional image. The following cell types can be seen in this micrograph: platelets (p), red blood cells (rbc), and three types of white blood cells: a lymphocyte (l), a monocyte (m), and a neutrophil or poly (n). The other two types of white cells (eosinophils and basophils) are not present in the field. *Photo courtesy of Bruce Wetzel, Edwina W. Westbrook, and Harry Shaefer of the National Cancer Institute, NIH.*

The child obeyed, and he gently palpated her swollen abdomen. As he had suspected, both her liver and spleen were enlarged below the rib cage, and the lymph nodes in her neck, armpits, and groin were swollen to nearly twice their normal size.

The pieces were beginning to fit together in Warner's mind: a two-week history of lethargy and recurrent fever; pallor, rapid pulse, and a heart murmur due to severe anemia; bruising, petechiae, and slow clotting; bone pain, an enlarged liver and spleen, and swollen lymph nodes. These signs and symptoms were consistent with several possible diagnoses: a serious bacterial infection, rheumatic fever, acute leukemia (of which there were several types), aplastic anemia (a total failure of the bone marrow to produce new blood cells), thrombocytopenia (a severe shortage of platelets, which were essential for the normal clotting of the blood), infectious mononucleosis (a viral infection that affected white cells), or neuroblastoma (a cancer that invaded the bone marrow). To narrow down this list of possibilities, he would have to do a blood test and, if warranted, a bone-marrow exam.

"I'm going to do a blood test now," he told the Murphys. "No needle this time," he reassured Ellie. "Just a little finger-stick."

He held her hand firmly and wiped her middle finger with a ball of cotton soaked in alcohol. Ellie inhaled the strange odor of sickness and began to cry. She was afraid that when the doctor made a hole in her skin, all of her blood would leak out and she would die.

Before Ellie had a chance to squirm away, Warner removed a small metal tine from its sterile package and jabbed it suddenly into her fingertip. Ellie cried out, but Warner was already squeezing a large drop of blood from the tiny cut. He sucked up some of the drop into a thin glass capillary tube and also placed small drops on four glass slides. By rubbing the edge of one slide across the surface of another, he spread the drops into thin, even smears of blood.

Sally hugged Ellie to console her and then helped her dress. When she had finished, Warner told them that he would personally deliver the smears and the blood sample to the hematology lab for immediate processing. It would take about fifteen minutes to get the results; when they were ready, he would call the Murphys to the reception desk. As Sally watched Dr. Warner walk away down the corridor, slides in hand, it seemed to her as if the future of their family was contained in those pale streaks of Ellie's blood.

In the hematology lab, a technician began processing the blood sample immediately, as Dr. Warner had instructed. She diluted the contents of the capillary tube in a larger volume of saline solution and then took the pink mixture over to the Coulter counter, a desktop machine with a console and an oscilloscope screen. This device would electronically count the number of red cells and white cells in the blood sample, a laborious and time-consuming process by hand. The counter worked by passing a stream of blood cells in single file through a narrow slit between two electrodes. As

13

each cell passed through the slit, it momentarily interrupted the current flow between the electrodes, generating an impulse.

The technician pressed a button on the console and the diluted blood was pumped up through a tube into the machine and diverted into two glass chambers. In one chamber the red cells were counted; in the other a chemical destroyed the red cells so that only the much less numerous white cells remained to be counted.

The machine took just a minute to go through its entire cycle. A spatter of green peaks appeared on the screen; then, with a whirring clatter, the device printed out a series of numbers on a special card: the white-cell count, the red-cell count, the hemoglobin content of the blood, and the hematocrit: the percentage of the blood volume occupied by red cells.

A separate run had to be done to determine the platelet count. First the red cells and white cells were allowed to settle out of a small sample of blood, leaving only the lighter platelets suspended in the clear plasma on top. A precise amount of this plasma was then diluted and injected into the machine.

Warner had also ordered a differential white count: a tabulation of the relative numbers of the various types of white cells in the blood. To do this, Ellie's blood smears were immersed for three minutes in a navy-blue dye known as Wright's stain, washed well with distilled water, and air-dried. The technician chose the clearest of the slides she had made and placed it under her microscope. Using the low-power, 100-fold magnification, she focused until a dense carpet of cells came into view.

Most of the field was covered with red cells, looking like round cherry lozenges with a dimple on each side. Occasionally there was a cluster of tiny blue granules—platelets—but they were few and far between, not scattered throughout the field as would be seen in a normal smear. Also distributed sparsely among the throng of red cells were the white cells, each about twice the size of the surrounding red cells. They were normally transparent, but the dye had stained them a pale blue and their nuclei dark purple.

The technician proceeded to count 100 white cells at random, using a desktop tabulator to record the number of each cell type. Several different types of white cells were always present in a normal blood smear: the polys (ravenous devourers of bacteria, with a snaking, multilobed nucleus and a densely granulated cytoplasm), the lymphocytes (makers of antibodies and coordinators of the immune response, with a large, round nucleus and a thin rim of clear blue cytoplasm), the monocytes (large amoeboid scavenger cells, engulfing bacteria, fungi, and cellular debris), the eosinophils and basophils (rare and enigmatic white cells associated with allergic reactions), and immature polys known as "stabs" or "bands."

14

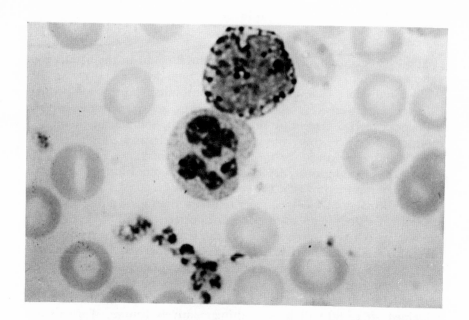

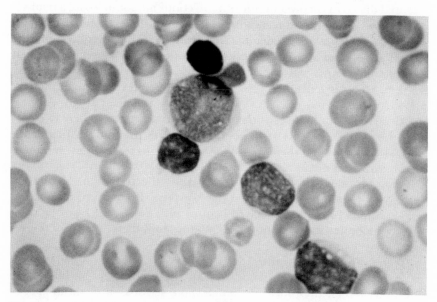

Blood smears from a healthy child *(top)* and from a child with leukemia *(bottom)* are shown for comparison. In the normal smear, the field is dominated by red blood cells with occasional white cells scattered among them. In the leukemic smear, there is a dramatic increase in the number of white cells. Closer examination of these cells would reveal that they have abnormal features characteristic of leukemic blasts. *Photos courtesy of Dr. Denis Miller, Memorial Sloan-Kettering Cancer Center.*

The technician tabulated Ellie's differential count in the blanks provided on the card and gave it to an orderly, who delivered the card to Dr. Warner in the doctors' lounge. Scanning the results, Warner could see that Ellie's counts were very abnormal. She was severely anemic, with a hematocrit of 18.5 percent (normally 44 percent) and a hemoglobin of 6 (normally 14). Her white count was markedly elevated: 28,300 cells per cubic millimeter instead of the normal mean of 7,500. Moreover, her platelet count was seriously depleted: 27,000 per cubic millimeter instead of the normal minimum of 250,000.

Ellie's differential was even more ominous than her counts. Instead of the normal ratio of 65 percent polys to 25 percent lymphocytes (with the rarer white-cell types accounting for the remainder), Ellie had only 10 percent polys and 88 percent lymphocytes. Moreover, all of her lymphocytes were "atypical": grossly abnormal in appearance.

Together with Ellie's physical signs and symptoms, these results supported a tentative diagnosis of acute leukemia. But significant doubt remained—it could still be something relatively benign. Warner's differential diagnosis had yet to rule out infectious mononucleosis, a relatively harmless viral infection of white blood cells. Like acute leukemia, it could give rise to fever, anemia, enlargement of the liver, spleen, and lymph nodes, and atypical lymphocytes in the blood. The difference was that mononucleosis was a self-limiting disease that eventually burned itself out, whereas leukemia, if left untreated, would continue to produce a flood of abnormal cells that would rapidly kill the patient. A bone-marrow exam would be essential to discriminate between these two possibilities: leukemic cells invaded the bone marrow and displaced the normal cells growing there, but lymphocytes infected with the mononucleosis virus did not.

A few minutes later, Warner appeared at the reception desk in the emergency room and beckoned to the Murphys. Brian and Sally walked over to him, while Barbara stayed behind with Ellie.

"Her blood tests were abnormal," Warner told them, "but I'm not yet sure of the diagnosis."

"Do you think it's serious?" Sally asked nervously.

"It's too early to say. It could be something relatively harmless, like infectious mono, or something much more serious—a blood disease of some kind. Ellie should definitely have some more tests, including a bone-marrow aspiration, which will involve sucking out a bit of bone marrow from her hip under local anesthesia so that the marrow cells can be examined under a microscope. The test is painful, but only for a few seconds. It's absolutely necessary for the diagnosis and really quite harmless."

"Why does it have to be done?" Brian asked, eager to spare Ellie any more discomfort.

Warner went on to describe the bone marrow as a spongy tissue inside the ribs, sternum, pelvis, and long bones that functions like a factory for the blood, producing the red cells that carry oxygen, the white cells that fight off infections, and the platelets that clot the blood. Because blood cells survive in circulation for only a few days to a few weeks, they have to be replaced continually by new cells grown in the bone marrow. "When we find abnormal cells in the peripheral blood," Dr. Warner concluded, "it often makes sense to go back to their source in the marrow to find out why. Unfortunately, we don't have the facilities here to do a thorough analysis of the marrow. For that you'll have to take her to a specialized hospital, such as Memorial Sloan-Kettering in New York."

Warner offered to call a hematologist at Memorial, Dr. Roger T. Nelson, to whom he had referred other patients in the past. The Murphys agreed, and Warner left them to make the call, saying he would return in a few minutes.

The Murphys waited in silence, each absorbed in thought. Sally felt shrouded in layers of numbness; she had accepted that Ellie had something serious but could not grasp what it meant. Brian, on the other hand, was convinced that a mistake had been made. Warner was just a small-town pediatrician—what could he know about serious blood diseases? No, they would go to Memorial and the experts would look Ellie over, and she would have something, but it wouldn't be serious.

After a few minutes, Warner returned with the news that he had reached Dr. Nelson, who would meet them on the fifth floor of Memorial Hospital at 7:00 P.M. The Murphys thanked him and then left for home, controlling their emotions in front of Ellie for fear of frightening her even more. The child looked up at her mother's drawn face and asked, "Mommy, am I going to be all right?"

"Yes, honey, you're going to be fine, but tonight we have to take you to see another doctor—a specialist in blood—who works in a hospital right near where Aunt Barbara lives." Sally still felt dazed and disbelieving. What made it so unreal was that Ellie looked normal—she didn't look as though she had a serious illness.

When they got back to the house, Sally went into the master bedroom and shut the door behind her. She started to pack a small bag for the hospital and then broke down in tears. Striving to pull herself together, she dried her eyes with a tissue and picked up the bedside phone to call her closest friend, Cindy Lewis.

She and Cindy had met in 1975, a year after the Murphys had moved to

Menlo Park from Queens. For a moment Sally thought back to those happy, hectic days. She and Brian had been married in 1970, she for the first time, he for the second, and two years later Beth was born. Although Beth had been conceived accidentally, Ellie was a planned child. By the time they moved into their shingled, one-story house in the spring of 1974, Ellie was already two months old.

After about a year, feeling bored and isolated at home, Sally had joined the Junior Women's Club. There she had met Cindy, and the two of them had risen quickly to positions of authority: Sally was now president and Cindy treasurer. Sally relished the opportunity to socialize with other women her age and to organize and attend the monthly luncheon meetings to which interesting outside speakers were invited. In addition, there were the bridge games, bake sales, and white elephants for worthy causes. Sally and Cindy had worked together to plan such events and had become increasingly close. With a third neighborhood mother, Pat Bradley, they had also organized a play group for their children. Each mother was responsible for watching their collective offspring one day a week, giving the other two time to go shopping or to enjoy an all-too-brief escape from the incessant demands of home and family.

Sally dialed Cindy's number and waited while the phone rang several times. She was about to hang up when Cindy answered, out of breath. "Hi, Sally. I just got in the door this very minute."

"I'm glad I reached you."

"Have you found a speaker for next Tuesday's luncheon meeting?"

"Cindy, I have some bad news," Sally said. "We took Ellie to Pat's pediatrician and he did some blood tests and told us that Ellie may have something seriously wrong with her blood. So we're all in a state of shock. We're taking her to Memorial Sloan-Kettering tonight so they can do some additional tests and try to determine what's going on."

Cindy was stunned by the news and astonished at Sally's apparent calm. Sally didn't even sound upset. "Are you sure it's serious?" she asked.

"That's what the doctor said, but I still can't believe it. Anyway, since Ellie might be in the hospital for a while, I'm canceling everything, including the luncheon meeting and the play group. I'm terribly sorry to leave you in the lurch, but—"

"My God, Sally, please don't worry about anything like that!" Cindy exclaimed, amazed that Sally would be preoccupied with trivial details at such a moment of crisis. "Is there anything I can do?"

"Well, Cindy, I'd be very grateful if Beth could stay with you overnight while we take Ellie to the hospital. Brian can pick her up in the morning."

"Beth can stay here as long as she likes," Cindy said warmly. "We'd love to have her."

"Thanks, Cindy."

"It's nothing. God, this is so terribly unfair—it's just rotten. I want you to know that I'll always be here whenever you need me. Please keep me posted about Ellie—just call when you get a chance. Be strong, Sally."

"Thanks. Everything will be all right, I just know it." Sally hung up the phone with shaking fingers. She felt completely out of touch. Her body was there but her mind was removed, disconnected, suspended between terror and denial. When she went into the kitchen, she looked so drained that Barbara reached into her pocketbook for her pillbox. "Here, take a Valium," she said. "It will calm you down a bit."

Sally started to refuse, since she never took tranquilizers, but Barbara insisted and she finally agreed to take half a tablet. She washed it down with some water and then went into the girls' room to pack some of Ellie's clothes. Ellie watched her, a fearful look in her eyes. She seemed to understand that she was going away for a while, since she said good-bye to her stuffed animals and insisted on bringing Polly, her favorite doll.

At 6:00 P.M. Brian put the stroller in the trunk of the car and they left for New York. As they drove past the rows of suburban houses and trimmed lawns, Sally suddenly felt that the town's reassuring order and cozy domesticity were hollow and unreal, a big lie. Nothing was certain; disaster could strike at any time, whether in the shape of a speeding car or the no less terrifying form of an invisible, deranged cell. The drone of a distant lawn mower seemed no longer soothing but menacing, like the buzz of a wasp.

Leaving Menlo Park, they passed through a succession of towns, each slightly more urbanized than the last. The lawns shrank into plots, the large houses into two-family dwellings and condominiums. Massive high-tension towers marched resolutely across the landscape, dwarfing the cars swarming along the highway.

An anxious silence reigned in the car. Brian was obviously preoccupied, and a few times the car began to drift away from the lane markers. Barbara, alarmed, told her brother to keep his eyes on the road. Sally absently stroked her sleeping child's soft hair. She felt groggy; the Valium was probably taking effect.

They turned off onto the New Jersey Turnpike, driving past miles of reclaimed marsh and once-fertile farmland now filled with sprawling warehouses at which dozens of trailer-trucks were moored like boats in a harbor. The warehouses were soon succeeded by vast chemical plants and oil refineries: snaking landscapes of pipes and tanks and cracking towers, emitting steam, smoke, and flame from innumerable vents and stacks.

They passed Newark Airport; a jet took off over their heads, trailing sooty black exhaust. To the east, the tips of the Empire State Building and the World Trade Center towers loomed over the heights of Jersey City like immense crystalline growths. Several minutes later, they crossed a bridge and the jagged skyline of Manhattan rose up before them against the roseate evening sky. Then they spiraled down into the mouth of the Lincoln Tunnel, emerging into the light again in the heart of the city.

The Saturday-evening traffic was dense, and it took Brian half an hour to traverse the width of the island and head uptown to the East Sixties. After circling for some time, he finally found a parking space three blocks from the main entrance of Memorial Hospital, on York Avenue and Sixty-eighth Street. The hospital was a sleek, modern high rise, not much different from the luxury apartment houses surrounding it.

They took an escalator up to the main floor, where a receptionist directed them down a corridor to the elevators. White-coated staff people hurried past, with an occasional patient providing a jarring note of reality: a man in a bathrobe with a bandage over one eye, a woman with indelible red lines on her face as a guide for radiation treatments, a man with a cavity the size of an orange in the side of his head, where a tumor had presumably been removed. Sally felt as if they were entering an eerie and frightening new world, as remote from everyday experience as the surface of the moon.

3 Diagnosis

As the Murphys emerged from the elevator on M-5, the pediatrics floor, two printed signs on the opposite wall caught Brian's eye. The first, posted near the weighing station, read: "Remove all prostheses before being weighed." The second, next to the glass-walled nurses' station, was equally ominous: "To all families: If your child has been exposed to any communicable disease (e.g., measles, chicken pox) or has a rash of any kind, please let us know before coming or as soon as you arrive to prevent exposure to other children."

Brian went up to the nurses' station and peered inside, waiting for a few minutes before a nurse caught sight of him and came over. She informed him that Dr. Nelson was seeing a patient but would be back soon.

They sat down on some chairs in the hallway and waited, fearful and uncomfortable. A child cried in a distant room. A girl of eleven or twelve walked past, pushing a wheeled metal pole laden with intravenous bottles, her face pale beneath the colorful scarf wrapped around her bald head. A few minutes later a mother brought a little boy, also bald, down the corridor in a wheelchair. He wore sneakers with little Mickey Mouse dolls on the toes that amused Ellie. Some time later a Puerto Rican boy of about sixteen came down the hall in a wheelchair pushed by his brother. One of his legs had been amputated above the knee, and he was bald and unnaturally bloated by chemotherapy.

Sally avoided the boy's eyes, which were full of pain and smoldering anger, feeling a strong urge to flee such unbearable sights. Then she noticed Ellie's stiff, scared glance and explained quickly that the boy's leg had been sick so that the doctors had to remove it, replacing it with a new leg made of plastic that he could walk on. "Don't worry, Ellie," she said. "That won't happen to you." Wiping the cold sweat off her brow, she glanced over at Brian, who was slumped back in his chair in exhaustion, his eyes closed. Barbara also looked anxious and depressed.

Finally Dr. Nelson emerged from the nurses' station to greet them. Sally liked his appearance and manner. The chief of pediatric hematology-oncology was a stocky man of about forty-five with strongly cut features and dark brown eyes that, behind wire-rimmed glasses, conveyed equal measures of compassion and authority. His dark hair, graying at the temples, was neatly combed, and his shirt, tie, and white coat all looked freshly pressed.

He shook their hands warmly. "I'm so glad you could bring her in right away," he said, and invited the family to be present during the bone-marrow aspiration to give Ellie moral support. Barbara agreed, and after some hesitation Sally decided to join her, afraid that Ellie might feel her parents were abandoning her. But Brian chose to wait outside; he could not bear the thought of witnessing his child's pain.

A nurse came to assist Dr. Nelson with the procedure, and Ellie was brought into a treatment room and placed face-down on the examining table. Barbara helped the nurse pull down the child's pants and underwear, holding her down while she cried and squirmed. Ellie was terrified that they were going to do something to her behind her back. As Dr. Nelson got near her, she screamed, "Get away from me, you dummy! I hate you!"

While the nurse opened up a sterile bone-marrow kit and spread out the instruments, Nelson pulled on a pair of surgical gloves. "I'm not going to lie to you, Ellie," he said. "This is going to hurt for a few seconds. I'm sorry, but we have to do this test to find out what's wrong with you and how to make you better. You can scream and yell as much as you need to, but please try not to move. If you hold still, it will all be over a lot sooner."

Sally held tightly to Ellie's hand while the nurse held up a small vial of local anesthetic so that Nelson could fill a hypodermic syringe with the clear fluid. "Remember when you go to the dentist, Ellie, and he gives you a shot before he fills a cavity so it won't hurt so much?" Nelson said. "Well,

I'm going to do the same thing for you. You'll feel a little sting, and then it will get numb back here."

When the nurse had cleaned the skin over Ellie's right hipbone with antibacterial soap and swabbed it with Betadine, Nelson slowly injected the local anesthetic into the skin and muscle. Ellie flinched and began to cry louder: the needle stung like a big bee. "Mommy, Mommy!" she cried, furious that her parents, her supposed protectors, were doing nothing while this stranger tortured her. Sally stroked her child's arm, murmuring, "I'm here, Ellie, Mommy's here," but she felt like an accomplice to her child's pain. Meanwhile Brian paced restlessly outside the door of the treatment room, wincing at Ellie's screams.

Nelson waited a few minutes for the anesthetic to take effect and then picked up an aspiration needle from the surgical tray. It was a hollow needle with a removable metal stylet inside to prevent the needle from bending or becoming clogged when it entered the bone. Nelson pushed it through skin, fat, and muscle and then penetrated the hard outer layer of the pelvic bone and the soft marrow within. Ellie screamed—the anesthetic had not gone that deep. Sally could not bear to watch any longer; feeling queasy, she averted her eyes.

Nelson quickly slid the metal stylet out of the aspiration needle and attached a disposable plastic syringe to the open end. "Ellie, please bear with me," he said. "It will be over in a minute."

He pulled back the plunger, but nothing came. "Damn!" he muttered under his breath as he disconnected the syringe from the needle, replaced the stylet, and redirected the needle within the marrow space. Then he reattached the syringe and tried again. On the third try he managed to suck a small quantity of red marrow into the syringe. As he did so, Ellie screamed again, digging her fingernails deep into her mother's palm.

"Okay, Ellie, from now on it's all bandages and tape," Nelson said with a sigh of relief. Working quickly, he removed the needle and syringe and placed a single drop of marrow onto each of six glass slides. These he immediately made into smears, while the nurse bandaged the puncture site.

"It's all done, Ellie," he said. "You're a very brave little girl, you know that?"

But Ellie was crying too hard to hear him.

Nelson took the marrow smears directly to the small hematology lab on the floor, where he soaked the slides in Wright-Giemsa stain for three minutes and then rinsed them on a rack with distilled water. When the smears had dried, he covered them with thin glass cover slips, selected the

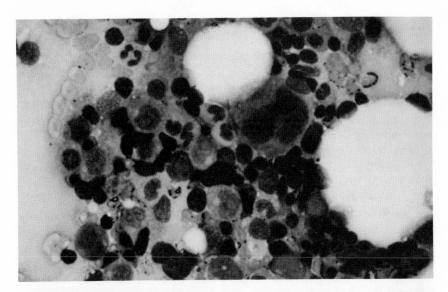

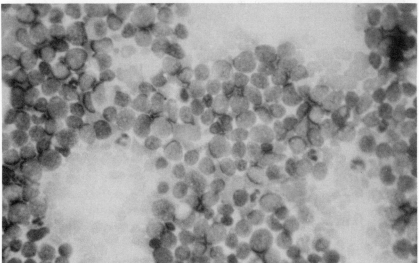

Bone-marrow specimens from a healthy child *(top)* and from a child with leukemia *(bottom)* are shown for comparison. The normal marrow contains a diversity of precursor cells in different stages of maturation, which give rise to red cells, white cells, and platelets. The clear areas are accumulations of fat, which constitutes about two thirds of the marrow in its healthy state. In the leukemic marrow, the uniform leukemic blasts not only have displaced the blood-forming elements but have infiltrated the fatty marrow as well, so that the normal structure of the tissue is completely obliterated. It is clear that such a bone marrow cannot be producing the various types of blood cells. *Photos courtesy of Dr. Denis Miller, Memorial Sloan-Kettering Cancer Center* (top), *and Dr. Jeffrey Rosenstock, Children's Hospital of Philadelphia* (bottom).

best slide, and sat down at one of the microscopes to examine it, using the low-power objective.

He saw immediately that something was very wrong. Normal bone marrow contains clusters of blood cells in various stages of maturation, interspersed among the large fat globules that constitute two thirds of the marrow in its healthy state. But in Ellie's smear there were virtually no healthy precursor cells belonging to any of the blood-cell lines. Instead the field was filled with large, abnormal white cells, all of them monotonously identical. Nelson recognized them as leukemic cells, or "blasts."

To get a closer look, he picked up the small plastic squirt-bottle on the bench beside him and squeezed a drop of clear mineral oil onto the center of the cover slip. Then he rotated the 400-fold magnification objective into position. The drop of oil bridged the narrow gap between the lens and the slide, greatly improving resolution.

Nelson refocused. Now a single cluster of leukemic blasts filled the microscope field. They were larger and more oval than normal lymphocytes, about three times the size of a red cell, with large purple nuclei and a blue rim of cytoplasm speckled with vacuoles (tiny air bubbles). The bizarrely convoluted nuclei had a coarse, grainy appearance and contained bluish spots called nucleoli: sites of intense gene activity and the hallmark of an immature, proliferating cell.

Although dozens of these blasts could fit comfortably on the dot of a typewritten *i*, Nelson knew they were an insidious enemy that could kill as surely as a bullet if left unchallenged. It would take all of the resources of modern medicine to destroy them before they colonized and overwhelmed Ellie's body from within.

The next step was to determine what type of leukemia Ellie had. Nelson knew that of the twenty-five hundred American children who develop leukemia each year, more than 80 percent have acute lymphoblastic leukemia (ALL), affecting the precursor cells that give rise to lymphocytes. Another 18 percent have acute myeloblastic leukemia (AML), affecting the bone-marrow cells destined to mature into polys and monocytes. The remaining 2 percent of stricken children suffer from rare forms of the disease such as erythroleukemia, affecting the precursors of red blood cells (erythrocytes) in the bone marrow. A few children also develop chronic myelocytic leukemia (CML), in which the leukemic polys or monocytes are mature and functional but continue to multiply, so that there are simply too many of them.

Ellie's leukemia appeared to Nelson to be ALL, although special stains and a sophisticated battery of tests on the extracted marrow would have to be done before the diagnosis was verified and further refined. Routinely nowadays, marrow specimens from a single patient were sent off in mailers to twenty experts around the country for detailed analysis. But there was no avoiding the basic fact: Ellen Murphy had leukemia. Feeling a lump form in his throat, Nelson packed up the slides and headed back to the waiting area to tell the family the diagnosis. Although he tried to maintain his clinical distance at such moments, he could not help identifying somewhat with the parents' agony. After all, he had two teenage children of his own.

The Murphys were waiting restlessly when Nelson arrived. Ellie was playing with her doll, the pain of the bone-marrow exam apparently forgotten. Her parents and aunt seemed surprised that the results of the test had been obtained so quickly.

Nelson wanted to tell them the news in a quiet place where they would not be disturbed, and he finally decided on the nurses' lounge. He asked the parents to follow him down the hall, leaving the child behind with her aunt.

Fortunately the lounge was empty, and they sat down in some armchairs surrounding a coffee table. The Murphys sat poised on the edge of their chairs, their faces open and expectant.

Nelson cleared his throat. "I'm afraid I have some bad news," he said gently. "Your daughter has acute lymphoblastic leukemia, or A-L-L. It's the most common type of childhood leukemia, and fortunately the most treatable."

Sally flinched as if she had been struck across the face. Her mouth opened, her arm rising instinctively as if to ward off the blow. Brian felt as if he were falling into a black pit; the room was collapsing; he had no air. He struggled to control his tears and failed: Ellie, his precious little girl, was going to die.

"Is there any hope?" Sally asked faintly.

"Yes, definitely," Nelson replied. "Since Ellie is young and has ALL rather than some other type of leukemia, chances are good that we can get her into a remission in which she can enjoy years of good life. But there is no certain cure. It's very important for you to understand that."

"But Ellie's only four," Brian said hoarsely. "Even in a few years she'll still be a little girl."

"Perhaps in a few years we'll have a definitive cure," Nelson said. "Until then, we have effective treatments that allow us to buy time."

Brian stood up and began to pace the rug. "This is ridiculous," he muttered suddenly. "There must be some mistake."

"I'm sorry, Mr. Murphy. The bone-marrow smear was unusually clear."

"No, it's impossible!" Brian shouted, his despair suddenly transformed into frustrated rage. "Your test has to be wrong. Ellie cannot have any goddamn cancer. Are you trying to tell me that a few fevers and some bruises on her legs are cancer? I don't believe it."

Nelson had seen the same horrified denial many times before, whenever he made the diagnosis of a dread disease. Just as the body would expel a graft of incompatible tissue, so the mind rejected an intolerable idea. The Murphys were fighting it, as any parents would.

"Mr. Murphy, I understand how you feel," Nelson said. "I only wish you were right."

"I just can't see any connection between what's been happening to Ellie and cancer of the blood."

"Let me explain a little about the disease," the doctor replied, "and then maybe it will make a bit more sense. Although it's true that leukemia is often called 'cancer of the blood,' in fact that is somewhat of a misnomer. It's more accurate to think of it as a cancer of the tissues that produce blood cells. The disease begins when, for reasons we don't fully understand, abnormal white cells known as blasts spring up in the lymph glands—such as the lymph nodes and spleen. These cells have stopped maturing at an early stage and hence are incapable of fighting infection. Nonetheless, they continue to multiply out of control, invading the bone marrow, where they crowd out the healthy precursor cells and suppress their growth—sort of like weeds choking a vegetable garden. Soon the entire marrow space is packed with blasts. When this happens, they spill over into the bloodstream, which carries them to every part of the body. Since we can't just reach into the blood and marrow and pick out the bad cells, we have to kill them off with chemicals and radiation, much as you would use a herbicide to eliminate those weeds from the vegetable garden."

Brian still seemed puzzled. "But how could the leukemia cause those bruises on her legs?"

"The reason is that Ellie's bone marrow has stopped making normal blood cells of any kind, including platelets, which are the tiny bodies that clot the blood and plug leaks in the walls of tiny blood vessels, or capillaries. Without enough platelets, there is spontaneous bleeding from the capillaries in the skin, nose, and gastrointestinal tract, which causes bruising, blood blisters, nosebleeds, and bloody stools."

So that was why Ellie's scraped knee wouldn't stop bleeding, and why her stools were so dark, Sally thought. As much as she wanted to believe her husband, she knew, with growing terror, that the doctor was right.

But Brian was still fighting. "Why would the leukemia make her so tired? Are you sure it's not just a vitamin deficiency or something?"

"Her fatigue is due to the fact that her bone marrow isn't producing

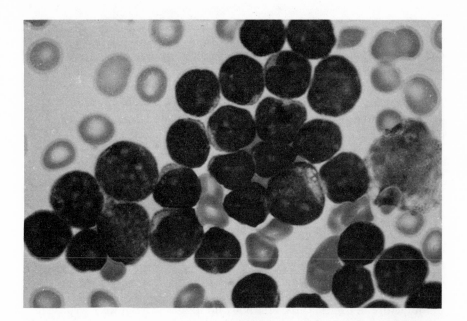

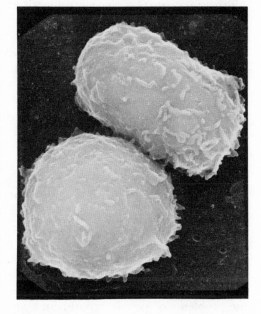

Leukemic blasts from a bone-marrow specimen are shown here in two complementary views: one taken with a light microscope at high magnification *(top)*, and the other taken with a scanning electron microscope *(right)*. The light micrograph provides a view of the interior of the cells, showing the large, coarsely grained nucleus with the abnormal light spots known as nucleoli, indicative of intense gene activity. (Normal lymphocytes differ in appearance from leukemic ones only in that they are slightly smaller and have a round nucleus and no nucleoli.) The scanning electron micrograph, magnified 8,250 X, provides a view of the surface of leukemic cells, which are covered with short projections called microvilli. *The light micrograph was provided by Dr. Jeffrey Rosenstock of the Children's Hospital of Philadelphia; the scanning electron micrograph was prepared by Dr. Etienne DeHarven and Ms. Lina Lampen at the Sloan-Kettering Institute in New York.*

enough red cells, so that insufficient oxygen is being carried in the blood to her tissues," Nelson explained patiently. "That's why she's so pale, weak, and short of breath. Her heart also has to work harder, pumping the blood faster to make up for the lack of oxygen. It's true that such symptoms can be due to anemia, which in young children is often caused by an iron deficiency. But leukemia can produce the same effects."

"What about the pain in her knee and her swollen belly?" Brian pursued. "How could they be caused by a blood disease?"

"Her bone pain is due to the expanding marrow space, which is packed with leukemic blasts, and also to bleeding beneath the sensitive membrane that sheathes the bone. Also, some blasts have been carried in the bloodstream throughout Ellie's body to her liver and spleen. They have continued to multiply there, causing these organs to swell massively and distend her abdomen. If the disease were left untreated, the leukemic cells would invade every part of her body, including her brain."

Finally Brian understood. Ellie's blood factory had been subverted to the manufacture of useless cells. Her body no longer worked well because her blood was not supplying it with what it needed.

Brian sat down, his resistance exhausted for the moment. "So where do we go from here?" he asked with a sigh.

"We're going to take care of it," Nelson replied immediately. "I'd like to start Ellie on treatment tomorrow, since the disease has a rapid clinical course. It's important to begin therapy as soon as possible."

Brian shook his head—it was all happening so fast!

"Fortunately a patient was discharged earlier today, so a bed is free," Nelson continued. "Let's get Ellie set up in a room, and then a member of the house staff will do an admitting history and physical. After that's done with, I'll talk with you some more about the plan of treatment."

When Brian and Sally returned to the waiting area, Barbara could tell from their faces what had happened. Having suspected leukemia all along, she was less surprised by the diagnosis than by Brian's red eyes. It was the first time she could remember him crying.

Brian had always been emotionally detached. He was very likable and outgoing and could talk your ear off with jokes and wisecracks, but as soon as you tried to probe beneath that ebullient surface he became uncomfortable and backed off. Few things seemed to touch him; he was off in his own little world, approaching life with a careless optimism that seemed blind to the problems of people around him. In that way he and Sally were at opposite extremes: he felt that nothing bad could happen, and she constantly anticipated disaster. Barbara remembered several occasions when a crawling child had been about to knock over a lamp or plummet down a stairway and Sally had shouted at Brian to do something, but he hadn't budged. When the anticipated tragedy did not take place, he always said, "Nothing happened, did it?" Nevertheless, it was clear to Barbara that the diagnosis had shaken him. It was the first real crisis in his life, and it was bringing out emotions that he did not usually allow himself to feel.

4 Admission

The duty nurse led the Murphys down the corridor to Ellie's room, circumnavigating an IV team with a blood cart and a nurse distributing medications. In darkened rooms, children were sleeping or watching TV, many with a mother present and a few with a father. In every case, a metal tree hung with bottles fed plastic tubes into the patients' arms. Outside one room, two mothers were sitting on a bench, talking. They looked up and stared at Sally intently for a moment as she passed, and then returned to their conversation.

Ellie had been assigned to 524, a semiprivate room. When the Murphys arrived, a curtain had been drawn across the other side of the room. From behind it came the murmur of voices; an examination of some kind was underway. The duty nurse fastened a name bracelet onto Ellie's wrist, and Sally helped the child change into some hospital pajamas and climb into bed. Ellie was tired but obviously excited and apprehensive about her strange new environment.

A short time after, Bill Robbins came in to examine Ellie and do an admitting history on both her and her parents. Although each patient on the floor had a member of the senior medical staff as his doctor of record, ultimately responsible for his care, it was the residents—young medical-school graduates in their second or third year of hospital training—who conducted the day-to-day and hour-to-hour management of the patients. Most of the specific decisions concerning a patient's care were made by the admitting resident, since he or she was expected to know the most about that child. The residents each took care of five or six patients and were also on call every third night, so that they had to know enough about the other patients to handle routine care and occasional crises when the "primary" resident was off duty. While on call, a resident spent the entire night on the floor, sleeping on the cot in the house staff lounge. Since nights on a pediatric cancer ward were almost always eventful, more than a few hours of undisturbed sleep was a rare commodity.

Robbins was a tall, soft-spoken young man of twenty-six who had graduated from Cornell Medical School and done his internship at New York Hospital, just across the street from Memorial. As a junior resident, he was training for a specialty practice in pediatrics and was doing a two-month rotation in pediatric oncology at the Cancer Center: first a month on the fifth floor inpatient unit, and then a month in the Children's Day Hospital on the seventeenth floor.

M-5 was very hard on residents because they came for a limited rotation and had to adapt to its intense pressures in a very short time. For someone like Robbins, who did not plan to select oncology as his field of specialization, it was overwhelming. He had been warned that oncology was a demanding rotation, but he had been unprepared for the emotional stresses of working with cancer-stricken children and their families. Knowing that he had to put in his time before moving on made establishing relationships with patients and families difficult on both sides.

Robbins introduced himself to the Murphys and told them that he would be taking care of Ellie and that if they had any questions, however trivial, he would be happy to answer them. He then proceeded to take a careful medical history. Sally told him that Ellie had been a seven-pound, five-ounce product of a full-term gestation with a normal spontaneous vaginal delivery, a normal neonatal course, and normal developmental milestones. The child's immunizations were up to date and she was not on any medications. She had no allergies. Robbins asked about the incidence of chronic illness on both sides of the family: the history was positive for heart disease, cancer (Ellie's maternal grandfather had died of lung cancer), stroke, hypertension, and hay fever, and negative for leukemia, diabetes mellitus, seizures, and asthma. Then they discussed the major medical events of Ellie's life, including childhood infections, the accident in June with an artificial fireplace, and the presenting symptoms of her leukemia.

Robbins also spoke to Barbara at length, reflecting how fortunate it was that she had arrived on the scene in time to recognize Ellie's symptoms, since it was clear that the child's parents had been actively denying the possibility that she might be seriously ill.

After completing the history, Robbins made accurate measurements of the size of Ellie's liver, spleen, lymph nodes, and head circumference, along with her height, weight, and vital signs: temperature, pulse, blood pressure, respirations. Then he drew a few cc's of blood from Ellie's arm for repeat blood-cell counts, blood chemistries, and bacterial cultures. Ellie cried, but Robbins cheered her up quickly by letting her play with his penlight.

A few minutes later, Dr. Nelson appeared, accompanied by Dr. Laura

Fein, a fellow in pediatric oncology. The two halves of M-5 were covered by separate medical teams, each made up of an attending physician, a fellow, and three residents. Nelson, one of the attendings, was on active duty on M-5 for only a month at a time, but he continued to see all of his outpatients in the clinic even when he was not attending. Like most senior staff physicians at Memorial, Nelson was also intensively involved in clinical research.

Dr. Fein, a striking dark-haired woman, was six months pregnant and wore a maternity dress under her white coat. She had completed her two years of residency in pediatrics and was now in the midst of a two-year fellowship program that would enable her to specialize in the treatment of children with cancer. Although the majority of the cases on M-5 were leukemics, there were also children with rare malignancies not seen in the adult population, such as neuroblastoma, Ewing's sarcoma, Wilms's tumor, Burkitt's lymphoma, retinoblastoma, and others. Fein loved her work and was determined not to begin her maternity leave until the last possible moment, even though she had already suffered two miscarriages due to viral infections contracted on the floor. Compassionate but very pragmatic and down-to-earth, she had a dry sense of humor that contributed to her popularity among interns and residents.

Dr. Nelson asked Dr. Fein to examine Ellie while he took Brian and Sally somewhere to talk. The nurses' lounge was now occupied, so they went into an empty examining room. Nelson's philosophy was that parents should know as much about the situation as he did. It was better for both sides that way. He presented the facts with as much optimism as they allowed, never destroying hope but not creating false hope. It was important at the outset to dispel any idea that miracles could happen, so that parents would be able to participate directly and realistically in decisions regarding their child's care. If he started telling white lies, he might forget where he had left off. With the parents aware of what he was thinking, he was free to think out loud.

"What will the treatment involve?" Brian asked.

"First we'll use a combination of three strong drugs to kill off most of Ellie's leukemic cells," Nelson replied. "That should get her into a remission and relieve her symptoms. When her marrow is free of blasts, the healthy blood-forming tissue will have room to grow again and her blood counts should begin to rise toward normal, protecting her against infection and bleeding. She should feel much better and may even return to full activity. Once she's in remission, she'll need additional therapy to prevent the disease from spreading to her central nervous system. Then we'll put her on an oral drug regimen that she can take at home, while continuing her normal activities. If she's still in remission after two years, we'll take her off the drugs entirely."

"Don't those drugs have bad side effects?" Sally asked.

"Yes, but most children make it through without too much difficulty because their tissues are remarkably resilient. All of our leukemic patients lose their hair temporarily while on chemotherapy, although it does grow back. They may also have nausea, vomiting, diarrhea, and low blood counts, and it's important to keep a close watch on the liver and the lining of the bladder. If a major toxicity problem develops—say, if the bone marrow is so depressed that the white count drops below 1,000 and there is great risk of infection—then we will lower the dosage of the chemotherapy or stop it completely until the situation improves."

"What are Ellie's chances?" Brian asked. He wanted to know some percentages, something solid to hang his hopes on.

"Let's get her into remission first, and then we can start talking about long-term survival," Nelson replied.

"You mean you can't say how long you expect her to live?" Brian asked.

Nelson hesitated. "I'd say her chances of getting into remission are excellent, better than ninety-five percent. The hard part will be maintaining that remission. Her age and sex are definitely in her favor, statistically, although her high white count and enlarged liver and spleen put her in the average-risk category, which means she has about a sixty-five percent chance of surviving five years or more. Practically speaking, a continuous first remission that lasts more than five years is generally considered a cure, meaning that the chances of a relapse are extremely small."

There was a pause. Then Sally spoke, in a quavering voice. "What if the chemotherapy doesn't work and the disease comes back?" she asked. "What then?"

"If she does relapse, chances are good that we can get her into a second remission. Second and subsequent remissions tend to be shorter and more difficult to achieve, so our goal is to keep a child in first remission for as long as possible, ideally forever. After a child relapses the chances for a cure are very small, so if there's a compatible donor we suggest doing a bone-marrow transplant. The transplant offers real hope of a cure, but if the graft fails, death is almost inevitable. So we're hoping that Ellie will respond well to the drug regimen and that a transplant won't be necessary."

Nelson reached into the pocket of his white coat and took out a folded piece of paper. "The only way we can get progress now in treating leukemia is by learning as much as we possibly can about the biology of the disease," he went on. "For this reason, all leukemia patients treated here are asked to participate voluntarily in a national research program, run by a consortium of pediatric cancer centers known as the Children's Cancer Study Group. This group draws up research protocols that aim to combine the best of current therapies with the most promising new drugs and regimens. By participating, you will not only give Ellie the best therapy current knowledge permits, but also improve the chances for children who develop leukemia in the future. Of course, we need your permission to go ahead."

He handed the folded paper to Brian. "This is an informed-consent waiver for you to sign. Please read it carefully, and feel free to ask any questions."

Brian nodded and looked over the form with Sally. It was titled "Consent for the Use of Investigational Drugs and Experimental Chemotherapy," and read:

> The regulations of the Food and Drug Administration and this hospital require your informed consent for the administration of the following drugs in your participation in an investigation of the treatment of acute lympho-blastic leukemia. It is understood that the therapy to be employed will use a single mode of inducing remission of the disease and choose one of six modes of maintaining remission. It is similarly understood that both the therapies to be employed in induction and in remission are, to the best of our knowledge, at least as efficacious as the best current procedures available for the treatment of this disorder. . . .

The rest of the form itemized the drugs to be used in the protocol and enumerated their possible side effects in excruciating detail. Depending on which "arm" of the protocol Ellie was assigned to by a computer, she would either receive the three drugs conventionally used to maintain a remission, or an additional drug as well. Although it was hoped that the added drug might prove more effective than conventional therapy, there was always the risk that it might have toxic and even lethal side effects.

Brian could not argue with the principles of clinical research, but he had a hard time fitting his child into that picture. "How experimental is this thing?" he asked. "I don't want my child to be some kind of guinea pig."

"The protocol is experimental only to the extent that the children are randomly assigned to one regimen or another," Nelson explained. "I can't tell you which arm is the best treatment—we're doing the study to find that out—but we feel that for any of the six possible maintenance regimens to which a child could be assigned, the therapy we've designed is potentially the best available. We will not in any way risk Ellie to try something less effective; we're simply getting more sophisticated in the effective ways that we're treating the disease."

"What if you find out that the regimen Ellie is on isn't the most effective or has bad side effects?" Brian asked. "Would it then be possible to switch her to another one?"

"Yes. Every three months, doctors from each of the twenty-eight cancer centers using this protocol meet to discuss their latest findings. As soon as the statistics indicate that one arm of the protocol isn't doing as well as the others, it is stopped and the children are put on one of the better regimens. Basically everything that goes on in a cancer center like this is research, and we learn an enormous amount from each patient. There's a positive side to that: you get either the best proven therapy, or an experimental one that we think might be even better. As long as the treatment of leukemia can be improved, clinical studies will be necessary."

"What kinds of questions are you trying to answer?" Brian asked.

"Our basic goal is to tailor the intensity of the therapy to the severity of the disease, which varies from patient to patient. The questions we're asking at the moment are: How can we reduce the toxicity of therapy in good-risk patients? How can we lessen the rate of central-nervous-system involvement and prolong survival in poor-risk patients? Can we do away with radiation therapy in some patients? Can we do away with more intensive maintenance therapy in other patients? How long should therapy be continued? What is the role of testicular therapy in boys? Do girls need less treatment than boys? Why do black children with ALL do significantly worse than white children with the disease, even if they're treated at the same centers? That kind of thing."

Brian nodded. Those questions needed answering, and anyway, what choice did they really have? Initially he had thought that by putting Ellie on a research protocol, they would be sacrificing her welfare for the sake of future patients with the disease. But now that he realized they weren't offering Ellie a treatment that they knew was inferior, he felt better about it. For all the painful trade-offs of the therapy, it still offered hope. He took out his pen and glanced at Sally, who nodded weakly. With an unsteady hand, he signed the form and returned it to Nelson.

"Will we ever be able to breathe easily again?" Sally asked quietly.

"We all keep hoping for a breakthrough," Nelson replied, "but in the meantime we're doing our best to keep children alive and in remission until research shows us the way to a real cure. Even without understanding what causes leukemia, we've made real strides toward controlling it. Just fifteen years ago, childhood leukemia was considered a hopeless disease. Now we treat every child as a potential long-term survivor. Indeed, many children with ALL are surviving five or more years after diagnosis and may well be cured; a few are now in their twenties, married, and with children of their own. But there are no guarantees. If you have any more questions, I'll be happy to answer them when I see you tomorrow.''

He got up and left the room, leaving the Murphys alone with their grief.

5 Protocol

After leaving the Murphys, Nelson went to the nurses' station to enroll Ellie in the protocol study. Talking to the child's parents had made him think back to his years as a medical student in the early 1960s, when he'd had to sit down with the family and tell them that for certain their leukemic child would be dead in a matter of weeks or months. Since then, a quiet revolution had taken place in the treatment of leukemia and other childhood cancers. Nelson had seen the gradual improvement during his years as a house officer, a fellow, a member of the junior medical staff, and finally now, as a middle-aged member of the senior staff. What a relief that in his professional lifetime he could now tell parents, "There's better than a fifty-fifty chance of long-term survival, and perhaps even cure."

Looking back, it was amazing how fast the field had evolved. The existence of leukemia as a distinct disease was not even recognized until the mid-nineteenth century. Before then, its protean symptoms were usually confused with pneumonia, influenza, diabetes, or other forms of cancer. Then in 1845, in one of those strange coincidences of insight that mark the history of science and medicine, two complete descriptions of the disease were published independently and almost simultaneously in Scotland and Germany.

The October 1, 1845, issue of the *Edinburgh Medical and Surgical Journal* featured a pair of articles under the title "Two Cases of Disease and Enlargement of the Spleen, in Which Death Took Place from the Presence of Purulent Matter in the Blood." The first case, presented by David Craigie, an Edinburgh physician, was of a patient with an enlarged liver and spleen who at autopsy was found to have large quantities of "pus and lymph cells" in his blood.

It is unlikely that Craigie would have recognized the significance of this observation had not his colleague John Hughes Bennett, a professor of medicine at Edinburgh, come across a nearly identical case. This second patient, a man of twenty-eight, complained of increasing fatigue for twenty months and a growing tumor in the left side of his abdomen for seven months. He died soon after admission to the hospital, and at autopsy Bennett found that the patient's liver and spleen were massively enlarged and that some of his lymph nodes, normally the size of lima beans, had swollen as large as hen's eggs. Material resembling thick pus could be squeezed from the cut ends of many veins, and examination of the patient's blood under a microscope revealed the presence of large numbers of white cells. The striking similarity between this case and that of Craigie suggested that a new medical phenomenon had been uncovered. Through consultation, Craigie and Bennett concluded that the presence of excessive numbers of white cells in the blood was due to a chronic infection of the spleen, which had leaked large quantities of pus into the bloodstream. Neither physician suspected that the cause might be a disorder of white-cell production in the blood-forming tissues.

One month after the publication of the Edinburgh cases, a pathology professor in Berlin by the name of Rudolf Virchow published a similar case, interpreting it in a strikingly different way. Virchow's patient was a fifty-year-old female cook who suffered from an enlarged spleen. After her death, the German pathologist observed that her blood was pink because of the greatly elevated number of white cells. He determined that this situation bore no resemblance to a local inflammation that had spread to the blood, as Craigie and Bennett had proposed, and concluded instead that his patient had died of a previously unknown disease. In 1847 he proposed to name the new illness "Weisses Blut," meaning white blood; the Greek form, "leukemia," was subsequently adopted. Virchow is generally credited with the discovery of the disease since he was the first to recognize that leukemia is not an inflammatory response to infection but rather a disorder of white-cell production: an uncontrolled proliferation of abnormal cells similar to cancer.

Although Virchow's pioneering work led to the rapid characterization of the different types of leukemia in adults, it was not until after the turn of the century that the disease was routinely diagnosed in children. Before 1948, childhood leukemia, like the adult forms of the disease, was a virtual death sentence. Infections and hemorrhaging accounted for 80 percent of fatalities; the rest were due to the late complications of the disease. Many exotic and desperate remedies were attempted, such as massive blood transfusions, exposure to cyclotron radiation, and injections of radioactive isotopes, gold salts, and even Vitamin B, but none proved effective. Because the disease was considered incurable, many doctors were reluctant to embark on a hazardous or unpleasant course of therapy merely to secure a short postponement of the inevitable. Treatments were therefore designed to make the child as comfortable as possible while awaiting death, without attempting the heroic measures that might prolong life but render it unbearable.

The first glimmer of hope came in 1947. Researchers at Lederle Laboratories in New Jersey developed a new drug, aminopterin, whose chemical structure closely resembled that of folic acid: a vitamin required and actively taken up by frequently dividing cells, particularly cancer cells. Because the drug molecule was biologically inactive, it served as a molecular counterfeit, fooling leukemic cells into accepting it instead of folic acid. It then blocked the action of the natural vitamin, causing the leukemic cells to starve to death. In studies on leukemic mice, the drug was found to induce remissions of the disease.

Encouraged by these findings, Dr. Sidney Farber, the director of the Children's Research Foundation in Boston, decided to test the new drug in the clinic. In November 1947 he obtained a vial of the yellow aminopterin powder from Lederle and administered the experimental drug to sixteen children dying of acute leukemia. By the following spring, the results were impressive: ten of the children had responded favorably to the drug, and a few even regained their strength enough to leave the hospital in a remission, indicating that large numbers of leukemic cells had been killed.

Tragically, all of the children soon relapsed and died, but the median survival time had been extended from three months to eight. This improvement was of a magnitude never before achieved with any leukemia therapy. The fact that a single drug was capable of inducing remissions of this previously intractable disease created a burst of enthusiasm and excitement among workers in the field. The April 26, 1948, issue of *Newsweek* quoted Farber as saying, "It is the most wonderful hope we have, and we now know that with this drug, and with other chemical agents, we are working in the right direction." Farber went so far as to predict that it would be possible to devise curative treatments for leukemia without knowledge of the disease's actual cause.

From that moment on, remission became the goal toward which all treatment was directed. In the words of Dr. William Dameshek, himself a leader in the field of leukemia therapy, the mood among pediatric oncologists changed virtually overnight from one of "compassionate fatalism" to one of "aggressive optimism." Rather than merely providing palliation while awaiting death, doctors began to strive to achieve long remissions, no matter what extreme measures might be required.

Farber's partial success with aminopterin stimulated the search for other, more effective drugs with which to battle leukemia. In the early 1950s, the newly founded National Cancer Institute in Bethesda, Maryland, began to invest heavily in chemotherapy research, sponsoring a nationwide program of drug development and screening. Eventually the NCI was testing thirty-five thousand chemicals a year, both novel molecules created in the synthetic chemist's flask and natural substances extracted from plants, fungi, bacteria, and even mammalian cells.

By the mid-1960s, several new drugs had been developed that were capable of inducing temporary remissions of childhood leukemia. Methotrexate, a close chemical relative of aminopterin, was found to be less toxic to the bone marrow. Vincristine, an extract of the periwinkle plant, a tropical herb, was discovered serendipitously in 1958. The juice of this plant had been described in the medicinal folklore of many countries as being valuable in treating diabetes. Careful studies revealed, however, that while the extracts were useless against diabetes, they did decrease the normal white-cell count of experimental animals. Vincristine was subsequently shown to inhibit leukemia in animals and to produce clinical remissions in children with the disease.

A similar sequence of events led to the use of prednisone, a synthetic relative of cortisone and the other steroid hormones secreted by the adrenal glands. Prednisone was known to suppress inflammation by destroying lymphocytes, and so it was tested in children with acute leukemia. It frequently brought about rapid remissions with fewer side effects than other drugs.

A third category of chemotherapeutic agents arousing interest in the 1960s interfered specifically with the metabolism of leukemic cells. Although leukemic blasts divide more slowly than normal cells, they do so continually rather than intermittently. As a result, the leukemic cells are more vulnerable to the action of antimetabolite drugs (such as cytosine arabinoside, 6-mercaptopurine, and adriamycin) which block the replication of the DNA molecules in the cell nucleus, thereby preventing the leukemic cells from multiplying. Increased knowledge of the nutritional requirements of leukemic cells also led to the development of new medications. For example, it was found that leukemic cells, unlike normal cells, are unable to manufacture the amino acid L-asparagine and hence must obtain it from outside sources. Once this fact had been discovered, researchers treated leukemic patients with L-asparaginase, the enzyme that destroys the needed amino acid, and were able to induce remission in many cases.

The excitement that followed each of these discoveries soon gave way to disillusionment. Doctors found that the remissions they achieved, however dramatic, were always short-lived. Sooner or later the leukemia recurred, no longer responded to the chemotherapy, and killed the patient.

The problem seemed to be that during drug treatment, a few leukemic cells underwent genetic alterations that enabled them to become resistant to the action of the drug and survive in spite of it. As a result, even though the most effective chemotherapeutic agent might destroy 99,999 out of every 100,000 leukemic cells, this was not enough, since the few survivors, continuing to divide, could repopulate the patient's body with an entire new series of leukemic cells. Indeed, laboratory experiments showed that leukemia could be induced in a healthy mouse by the transplantation of a single leukemic blast!

Another closely related problem was toxicity. The long-sought "magic bullet" that could eradicate leukemia without harming healthy tissues remained elusive, largely because of the apparent lack of major biochemical differences between leukemic cells and their normal counterparts. All known drugs capable of killing leukemic blasts (usually by inhibiting cell division) damaged normal tissues as well, in particular rapidly growing ones such as the skin, the hair follicles, the bone marrow, and the linings of the mouth and the gastrointestinal tract. The quantity of a drug that could be administered was therefore limited by its toxic effects on healthy tissues, and the dose required to eradicate every last leukemic cell was usually sufficient to kill the patient first.

A few intrepid researchers pointed the way out of this depressing deadlock. They proposed to administer two or more antileukemic drugs in combination that would attack the leukemic cells through different mechanisms and at separate phases of the cell cycle. Their rationale was that the chances of leukemic cells becoming resistant to multiple agents were much less than with a single agent. Moreover, if the drugs chosen had side effects that differed and were not necessarily additive, the total amount of toxicity produced by a multiple-drug regimen would be less than that caused by high doses of a single drug.

This approach, known as combination chemotherapy, was not an entirely new idea; it had been implemented in 1947 to treat tuberculosis. At that time it was found that although the antibiotic streptomycin killed 9,999 bacilli out of 10,000, it was not sufficient to cure TB. A second drug, known as PAS, was also ineffective by itself, but combined the two drugs were able to bring about cures. The reason was that bacilli resistant to one drug or the other were very unlikely to be resistant to both.

In much the same way, investigators found that a combination of two antileukemic drugs, vincristine and prednisone, was much more effective in inducing remissions than large doses of either drug by itself. While vincristine alone induced remission in 47 percent of patients and prednisone in 57 percent, together they induced remission in 84 percent of the patient population.

At first, the various antileukemic drugs were combined in a haphazard fashion. Nobody knew which combinations would produce the best results with the least toxicity, or what dosages or sequences would be the most effective. Each individual researcher was groping in the dark, and there was an obvious need for controlled clinical studies to determine the best possible treatment program. The problem was that any one pediatric cancer center had too few leukemic patients to obtain statistically valid data about the relative effectiveness of two competing drug regimens, at least within a reasonable length of time. In a remarkable cooperative effort to solve this problem, clinical investigators at several cancer centers across the United States banded together in 1957 to form a research consortium known as Acute Leukemia Group B, combining their resources and patient populations to evaluate new combination-chemotherapy regimens.

The members of the cooperative group all agreed to adhere strictly to an experimental protocol: an elaborate set of instructions drawn up by the group that specified all drugs, dosages, modes of administration, and a precise day-by-day schedule for giving the various drugs. The protocol was like a battle plan, with each move plotted out in advance. Patients were assigned randomly to either the best available chemotherapy regimen or a modified regimen that the expert members of the cooperative group believed would prove even more successful in inducing or maintaining remission.

Since all of the cancer centers belonging to the group used the exact same treatments, their results could be pooled: extensive data on each patient enrolled in the study were recorded on standardized flow-sheets and sent to a central computer-processing facility for analysis. In this way, as much data could be collected in one year as a single cancer center could have accumulated in a decade. When sufficient information had been obtained to judge one regimen significantly better than the other (usually after two or three years), the study was terminated and the more effective arm of the protocol was adopted in all subsequent studies. The cooperative group held regular meetings to discuss the latest developments in therapy, to draw up new protocols, and to update, evaluate, or discontinue existing ones. The results of the studies were also published in established medical journals.

Over the next fifteen years, two other national cooperative groups were formed for the purpose of research on leukemia and other childhood cancers: the Children's Cancer Study Group (CCSG) and the pediatric section of the Southwestern Oncology Group (SWOG). Each of these groups drew up its own research protocols. In addition, two major pediatric cancer centers, the St. Jude Children's Research Hospital in

Memphis and the City of Hope Medical Center in Southern California, managed to attract enough patients to do their own independent clinical studies without the need for collaborators.

With the evolution of the protocol and the emergence of the nationwide study groups, it became possible to attack childhood leukemia on a broad front. The newest anticancer drugs were provided to the cooperative groups free of charge by the National Cancer Institute, before these drugs had been approved by the FDA and released for general use. The protocol studies revealed that many drugs were more effective at certain dosages or combinations, or if given intermittently rather than continuously. Increased knowledge of the kinetics of leukemic-cell proliferation enabled specialists to design drug regimens that eliminated leukemic cells at different phases of the cell cycle. It was also discovered that the use of a wide variety of drugs prevented the development of resistance: one set could be used to induce remission, a second set to reinforce it, and a third set to maintain it.

A major step forward was made in 1967, when Donald Pinkel and his coworkers at the St. Jude Children's Research Hospital developed the prophylactic use of radiation to the skull, and chemotherapy injected into the spinal fluid, to kill off leukemic cells infiltrating into the brain and spinal cord. This therapeutic innovation proved to be crucial in preventing the spread of leukemia to the central nervous system—an often fatal complication of ALL—and was largely responsible for the later achievement of cures.

The protocol studies were at best a long, painful process. There were no sudden breakthroughs, no headline-making achievements by a few celebrated names. Rather it was a labor of thousands of unheralded, dedicated physicians, a matter of hundreds of small victories and disillusionments, of retaining what worked and rejecting what did not. Each question took two or three years to answer, and at times the pace of progress seemed to crawl. Even worse, some of the experimental treatments inevitably gave rise to severe side effects, making the children sicker than they were before. But there was basically no choice. As long as the fundamental causes of leukemia remained obscure, physicians could only grope in the dark, using this systematic method of trial and error to find the best way to treat the disease. Much of the success of the protocol studies also depended on the willingness of parents to risk exposing their child to severe side effects in the hope of prolonging his or her life.

It was not until the early 1970s that the huge quantity of time, sweat, and money invested in the protocol studies began to pay off in a major way. Much like the weary hiker who has trudged for hours through dense forest and suddenly finds himself in an open field, so did leukemia specialists come to the realization that more than half of the children in their care suffering from ALL were surviving five years or more in continuous first remission. The picture was not as bright for childhood AML, the less common form of the disease. These leukemic blasts were not as sensitive to the available drugs, so that the average survival time was only about one year. Nevertheless, tremendous strides had been made since 1960, when nearly every leukemic child was dead in a matter of months.

The next challenge was to explain why about half of the children with ALL who received the standard therapy did well, remaining in first remission for five years or more after diagnosis, whereas the other half relapsed and died. No one had clearly explained the difference between these two groups. What were the various factors present at diagnosis that could be used to predict how a given child would respond to treatment?

With solid tumors, prognosis had long been predicted by means of staging systems that graded the extent of a cancer's spread. Since leukemias were almost always widespread at the time of diagnosis, however, some other criteria had to be found. The first prognostic factor to be identified was age: young children with ALL did significantly better than either infants or older children and adolescents. Girls also tended to do better than boys. Moreover, it was found that the degree of maturation of the leukemic blasts, as reflected by the presence or absence of specific immunological markers on the surface of the cells, could have a significant influence on the clinical course of the disease.

The first systematic attempt to determine the relative contribution made by different pretreatment factors to the prognosis of ALL was a Children's Cancer Study Group protocol study done between 1972 and 1975, involving 936 children newly diagnosed with the disease. In addition to such obvious criteria as age, sex, and race, the investigators recorded each child's white count at diagnosis, the degree of enlargement of the liver and spleen, the presence or absence of central-nervous-system involvement, and specific characteristics of the leukemic blasts, including size, shape, and surface markers. After three years, the length of the first remission in these children was correlated retrospectively with the various criteria in order to determine which factors were the most critical. Age and white-cell count at diagnosis turned out to be the most important variables.

On the basis of this study, it became possible to subdivide children with ALL into three basic prognostic groups. "Low-risk" patients were between the ages of three and six, inclusive, at diagnosis and had a white count of less than 10,000 per cubic millimeter. This group, comprising 29 percent of the study population, had an 85 to 95 percent chance of being alive and in first remission five years after diagnosis, and many of them came off treatment and were apparently cured.

"Average-risk" children were of two sorts: those who had a white count of less than 50,000 but were younger than three or older than six; and those who were in the three-to-six age bracket but had a white count of between 10,000 and 50,000. The average-risk group comprised the majority (54 percent) of the study population, and 65 percent of these children were in first remission five years after diagnosis.

Finally, "high-risk" children had a white count of greater than 50,000 at diagnosis, regardless of age. The median survival of this group, which made up 17 percent of the study population, was only two years.

It was therefore clear that ALL was not a single disease but rather had at least three subtypes with strikingly different outlooks. By doing a number of diagnostic tests on a patient's blood and bone marrow, a physician could now predict with some degree of accuracy how well or how poorly a child would be expected to do on the standard therapy. Since large numbers of children with the good prognostic types of ALL were now living for several years after diagnosis, and of these about half appeared to be permanently cured, there was a new concern about the long-term effects of intensive chemotherapy and radiation and its impact on these children's future well-being. An intensive research effort was therefore begun to determine precisely the toxic effects of treatment and to find ways of minimizing them.

Another drawback of the otherwise successful protocols was their complexity and expense. The average cost of the first year of treatment was about $10,000 for an uncomplicated case of ALL and as much as $50,000 for a child with AML. Clearly, there was still a need for a treatment that was not only safe and effective, but simple and cheap enough so that children throughout the world could benefit from it.

A first step in this direction was made in March 1978, when the Children's Cancer Study Group implemented three new protocols designed to be more closely tailored to the treatment needs of the three different subtypes of ALL. Low-risk children were assigned to Protocol 161, which provided less intensive treatment so as to reduce the toxic side-effects of therapy without decreasing the number of long-term remissions and apparent cures. Average-risk patients were assigned to Protocol 162, which provided a modified treatment regimen to improve survival without increasing toxicity. High-risk patients were put on Protocol 163, whose aim was to intensify therapy in an attempt to improve survival. Each of these protocols branched off into six different maintenance regimens, to which the children would be assigned randomly by computer.

Now Nelson walked to the nurses' station to enroll Ellie in the protocol study. He entered the glass-walled enclosure and went over to the row of loose-leaf binders arranged in a cubbyhole along one wall. Selecting the one labeled "CCSG Leukemia Protocols," he flipped to Protocol 162, for average-risk patients. The single-spaced typed pages specified every detail of therapy, including what was to be done in the event of major complications or side effects.

Nelson filled out a registration form for Ellie, along with a front-end report form that listed all the tests that would have to be done before Ellie was randomly assigned to a particular maintenance regimen. Nelson scanned the list, noting that the front-end studies were becoming ever more sophisticated. The new tests were part of the continuing effort to characterize each child's leukemia more precisely at the outset, so that the intensity of the treatment could be even more closely matched to the aggressiveness of the disease:

1. History and detailed physical exam
2. Complete blood counts with differential and platelet count
3. Bone-marrow aspiration

    a. Cell-surface markers (T, B, "null")
    b. Terminal transferase
    c. DNA-RNA cytofluorometry
    d. Monoclonal antibody studies
    e. T-cell suppressor function test
    f. B-cell function test
    g. Glucocorticoid receptors
    h. Chromosomal abnormalities
    i. Colony-forming units
    j. Influence of thymic factors on leukemic-cell differentiation

4. Blood chemistries, electrolytes
5. HLA typing
6. Varicella titers
7. Serum immunoglobulins
8. Immune complexes
9. 5 cc's of serum frozen for future use
10. Urinalysis (IVP to be done if serum creatine elevated)
11. Lumbar puncture [spinal tap]

    a. Cell count
    b. Cytology
    c. Protein
    d. Sugar
    e. Culture

12. Chest X-ray, PA and lateral, for extent of anterior mediastinal involvement
13. Wrist X-ray, for determination of bone age
14. Assessment of pubertal status

It was Nelson's job to transcribe the lab values, therapies, complications, supportive treatments, and side effects of each of his patients onto standardized flow-sheets, which were mailed four times a year to CCSG's central operations office in Los Angeles. There the patient files were computerized and continually updated. Nelson often found the voluminous paperwork associated with the protocol studies tedious, but he knew he was doing his part to further progress in the field. And every step forward, however modest, would be reflected directly in the lives of the children in his care.

Nelson had no doubts about the significance of his work. In spite of the rarity of leukemia, it was second only to accidents as a killer of children between the ages of two and fifteen. Hence the successful treatment of the disease had a major impact: whereas the most common cancers usually struck in late-middle or old age, a young child saved from leukemia might have six decades or more of productive life ahead of him or her. Moreover, the prolonged illness and death of a child was a great tragedy that encompassed the entire family, making it of paramount importance to avert such an ordeal.

Nelson was also aware that the careful study of leukemia could provide valuable insights into the causes, mechanisms, and treatments of other, more common types of cancer. Although leukemia was rare compared to the solid tumors of the lung, breast, skin, and colon that claimed the majority of the 400,000 cancer victims in the United States each year, it was the cancer most amenable to systematic study both in the laboratory and in the clinic. Thus the medical importance of leukemia had always been disproportionate to its actual incidence.

Leukemia was, by its very nature, a generalized, systemic cancer. For this reason it served as an excellent model for the treatment of the advanced stages of more "conventional" malignant cancers, in which cells shed from the primary tumor spread in the bloodstream throughout the body, lodging in other organs and giving rise to secondary tumors. This process, called metastasis, could result in the patient's death even if the primary tumor was removed surgically or destroyed with radiation. Localized methods were therefore inadequate for the treatment of advanced cancer; the task required systemic methods, such as chemotherapy, which could seek out and kill the metastasized cancer cells throughout the body. Combination chemotherapy had been developed initially to treat patients with leukemia and had subsequently been applied to patients with solid tumors; the same was true of supportive therapies such as specialized blood transfusions and intravenous feeding. Because one in every four Americans was expected to develop some form of cancer in his or her lifetime, progress in understanding and treating leukemia, in spite of its rarity, had significance for millions of people.

There were other advantages to studying leukemia as a key to the enduring enigmas of cancer. Because the disease affected a fluid tissue—the blood—its clinical course and response to therapy in both patients and laboratory animals could be monitored at frequent intervals simply by taking blood samples. This approach was clearly much more convenient, safe, and accurate than taking multiple X-rays to follow the growth or regression of a tumor. In addition, whereas most solid tumors grew slowly, leukemia was a rapidly progressing disease, making it possible to assess quickly the effectiveness of a particular drug or therapeutic regimen.

For these reasons, more was known about leukemia than about any other type of cancer. Thousands of scientific papers about the disease were published every year, and cancer specialists who worked on solid tumors were careful to keep up with the latest developments on the leukemia front. Indeed, the problems encountered in the systemic treatment of leukemia were indicative of the general directions in which cancer research as a whole was headed.

6 Sally

The house staff room was cluttered but comfortable, with a white Formica desk and four swivel chairs, a set of open shelves containing patients' charts, and a bookcase crammed with medical books. A microscope stood on a table in one corner, with a few scattered blood smears beside it. On one wall hung a long illuminated screen for viewing X-rays; on the other, a bulletin board displaying an anatomical drawing of the major superficial veins of the body, a useful aid when inserting IV's. There were also several diagrams illustrating the latest protocols in use for the various childhood cancers, from Wilms's tumor and neuroblastoma to osteogenic sarcoma and the leukemias. Each diagram consisted of a horizontal time-line marked off in days, with dozens of bars and vertical arrows of different sizes above it, representing the administration of various drugs and radiation.

Robbins was seated at the desk reading Ellie's chart and filling out an order sheet. He saw Nelson enter the room and nodded to him. "What's the latest on the new leukemic?" he asked.

"Ellen Murphy? I've looked at her marrow slides and it's ALL," Nelson replied. "Because her white count is over 25,000 she should go on Protocol 162. That is, unless her front-end studies turn up some additional factors justifying a more aggressive approach. We should have the results of the studies in a day or two. Until then, you should start a standard induction, giving vincristine tonight."

Nelson went on to describe what Robbins should do for Ellie that night. "She should get 140 cc's of packed red cells for her anemia, and four units of platelets tomorrow," he said. "Your main job at the moment is to keep her well hydrated."

Robbins nodded. He knew the importance of keeping a leukemic child well flushed with fluids during chemotherapy. Ellie had a large volume of leukemic cells in her body—about two trillion of them, or approximately a quart—which they were aiming to wipe out with high doses of vincristine and prednisone. Destroying millions of leukemic cells in a short time would release large quantities of DNA and RNA molecules from the dying cells, and these molecules would be broken down in the liver to uric acid. If Ellie wasn't given large volumes of fluids to dilute the uric acid in her urine, the chemical would crystallize out in her kidney tubules, blocking them and causing kidney shutdown. To avoid that disastrous result, Robbins would give Ellie large amounts of intravenous saline along with pills of allopurinol, a drug that inhibited the formation of uric acid. If all went well, Ellie would be able to safely excrete the excess uric acid in her urine.

Robbins conferred with Nelson about some of his other patients, and then he went off to start Ellie's IV. An intravenous line had to be kept running almost the entire time a leukemic child was in the hospital, both to maintain adequate hydration and to administer chemotherapy, antibiotics, transfusions, and emergency medications. Robbins had learned early in his month on M-5 that his relationship with young patients and their families revolved around his ability to "stick well"—to get the IV flowing on the first try. Special skill was required to locate a child's tiny veins, and often as many as ten sticks were required before a vein could be found. More important still was to avoid "blowing" a vein, causing it to collapse and leak blood and fluid into the surrounding tissue to form a painful swelling, or hematoma. The problem was that a child had only a finite number of superficial veins. After a month of hospitalization, the veins in the arms were usually exhausted, and IV's had to be attached to vessels in the legs, scalp, or even big toe. In the worst cases, they had to call a surgeon in to do a "cut-down": an incision made under local anesthesia, usually in the wrist, to find a deep vein through which a catheter might be threaded. When a child had a low white count and hence was in danger of infection, cutdowns were to be avoided at all cost because they multiplied the risk.

For this reason, Robbins tried to find a superficial vein whenever possible, even if it meant making repeated sticks. The child would cry and scream, and the parents would get upset and extremely protective. Robbins would never forget one father who became so angry after an unsuccessful attempt to start an IV that he stepped forward and kicked Robbins in the shin.

On his way to Ellie's room, Robbins enlisted the help of Sue Kramer, RN. Like most of the nurses on M-5, Sue was young—twenty-three. There was a high turnover rate in the nursing staff because of the debilitating nature of the work. People who couldn't take the stress left very quickly; those who remained found ways of dealing with it, as well as rewards in doing something difficult and useful.

Sue had been on M-5 for nearly two years, having come to Memorial immediately after receiving her nursing degree from a college upstate. She had arrived with great expectations because of the hospital's reputation as one of the leading pediatric cancer centers in the world. It had come as a brutal shock for her when many children did not do as well as she had hoped. During her first year, she had become very involved with a twelve-year-old boy with AML, staying overtime almost every day to care for him. It got to the point where she was confusing the mother's role with her own. Although she was committed to the child, she began to resent him and his mother for draining her emotionally, and this made her less effective as a nurse. When the boy finally died, she went to his funeral and knew at that point that she was totally burnt out.

After a three-week vacation, she returned to the floor with a more realistic sense of what she could do for the children and how much was beyond her control. Sue realized that her purpose was to help the children enhance their living and, if it came to that, to ease their dying. She became close to all of them without becoming too close to any one.

She also found it essential to her sanity to maintain a separate life outside the hospital. The other nurses made fun of her because she took vacations every three or four months, just for a few days or a week, to visit with friends and regain her strength. Friends would ask her, "How can you keep doing that depressing work?" She had seriously considered leaving M-5 to work in general pediatrics, where the patients usually did well, but each time she returned to M-5 the remarkable emotional and physical resilience of the children would reassure her.

The work was rewarding and draining at the same time. The aggressiveness of the therapy was hard to take, even for the nurses. It was particularly difficult to help a child heal from surgery, only to have him or her begin chemotherapy; the suffering caused by the drugs seemed so unfair after the child had already been through so much. When Sue left the ward at 4:00 P.M. to go out into the world, it was as if she were descending from another planet. On the bus there would be people hassling each other over a seat, and she would stand there thinking, "You don't understand—you just don't know the things I know."

Sue helped Robbins wheel the IV cart into Ellie's room. They were going to start a special kind of IV known as a heparin lock, which could be turned off and reused at a later time. A heparin lock was used routinely whenever a patient required access to a vein at regular intervals for chemotherapy, antibiotics, fluids, or blood products. The device consisted of a regular butterfly needle attached to several inches of plastic tubing with a rubber plug on the end. The tubing would be filled with a solution of heparin anticoagulant in order to keep the needle open when fluids were not being infused, and the tubing simply taped to Ellie's arm. Whenever access to the vein was needed, an IV could be needled in through the plug adapter. When the heparin lock was not in use, it had to be flushed with heparin solution every six hours to prevent it from clotting off, but it could remain in place for as long as four days. The advantages of the system were many: the kids got stuck less often, they had more mobility, and their veins did not collapse as fast.

Robbins removed the needle and tubing from its sterile pack and then drew up a few cc's of heparin solution into a hypodermic. He then stuck the hypodermic into the rubber plug adapter and injected the clear fluid into the tubing, filling it.

Barbara held Ellie down while Robbins prepared to start the IV. Brian and Sally had gone downstairs to the cafeteria for a quick cup of coffee, and Sue was relieved to see that Barbara helped dispel what must have been Ellie's worst fear—abandonment.

Even so, as Robbins approached the bed, the child spewed out an astonishing repertoire of protests for a four-year-old. "Get away from me! I hate you! Leave me alone!" she howled.

"Come on, Ellie," Robbins said, exasperated. "I'm going to put a little needle in your arm, just like a little butterfly. We have to make you better by giving you some medicine. If we can't give it to you, you won't get better."

"I don't want any medicine! I have to go to the bathroom!"

"Just hold on a minute until I—"

"Not that arm!" Ellie insisted. When Robbins pointed to the other arm, she said, "Not that arm, either."

Robbins shook his head. Kids were amazingly ingenious when it came to delaying tactics. "I think I'll stay with this one," he said, tying off Ellie's right arm with a piece of rubber tubing.

"Ouch, that's tight!" Ellie exclaimed.

"That guy's your friend," Robbins said soothingly. "It means the needle goes in faster."

Robbins had no trouble finding a vein, since Ellie was a new patient. Grasping the two plastic wings of the fine butterfly needle, he slid it into one of the larger blue veins on the underside of Ellie's forearm. He aspirated slightly with the syringe to check for blood return, and injected two cc's of heparin solution into the vein to flush the needle. He then taped the heparin lock securely to Ellie's arm. Sue Kramer handed him the bag of packed red cells, which had arrived from the blood bank, and he connected it to the heparin lock to begin the transfusion.

Ellie continued to cry for a while until, exhausted, she dozed off. When the Murphys returned, they let Sue assure them that Ellie would be asleep for a while. Barbara insisted that they go back to her apartment for supper, since she lived only a few blocks away on Sixty-eighth Street and Second Avenue. Sally was very tense and felt it would help to leave the oppressive atmosphere of the hospital for a while.

They stopped at a deli on First Avenue to pick up some sandwiches. Sally was too queasy to eat, so she stood outside while the others went in and ordered. While she was waiting, utterly numb and drained, a bearded man with ragged clothes and wild eyes stumbled toward her, carrying a large cane. As he passed the deli, he suddenly lunged at Sally with his cane, but she was in such a daze that she did not even flinch. The worst had already happened; nothing else could faze her.

As soon as they got to the apartment, Barbara called her brother Jim in St. Louis. Brian got on the phone and, weeping, told him the news. Then Sally called her sister, Lynn, in Chicago. Lynn was extremely upset and asked if Sally wanted her to fly immediately to New York. Sally said no, but that she might be of help later on, when Ellie was out of the hospital. Finally Sally called Cindy Lewis. Cindy was shocked: the whole thing was too horrible to believe. She had read about childhood leukemia in magazines, but she had never considered the possibility of it happening to anyone she knew, let alone her best friend's daughter.

Groping for something positive to say that might assuage Sally's grief, Cindy offered, "Well, Ellie could have been hit by a car and killed instantly. That would have been worse."

There was a pause, and then Sally said in a strained voice, "No, Cindy, that would have been easier. Because then that's it. If she's going to die, why

worked the needle through the muscles of the child's lower back and slid it slowly between the spines of her lumbar vertebrae, while her body shook with sobs. Leaving the needle embedded in her back, Robbins carefully withdrew the stylet. A moment later clear spinal fluid began to drip from the open end of the needle. Moving quickly, Robbins attached a graduated plastic cylinder to the needle and held the tube vertical. The spinal fluid rose slowly in the cylinder like mercury in a thermometer, revealing the pressure of the fluid bathing the brain and spinal cord. "Her opening pressure is normal, and it looks nice and clear," Robbins said.

That was a good sign, since it meant that the leukemia had not invaded Ellie's central nervous system in a major way. If it had, it would have displaced some of the cerebrospinal fluid, raising the pressure within the closed reservoir. In addition, the presence of large numbers of leukemic cells would have made the fluid somewhat turbid.

Robbins drained the spinal fluid from the column into the four specimen tubes, so that a microscopic examination of the fluid could be done along with various chemical analyses and cultures. He then quickly removed the needle and bandaged the puncture site. "She should be okay now," he told Barbara. He checked the IV to make sure it was flowing smoothly and left the room.

Brian and Sally came back in and tried to cheer Ellie up, but she was silent and withdrawn, clutching Polly close. "My arm hurts," she whined. "I don't want this needle."

Several minutes later Robbins returned, carrying a bottle filled with a clear solution, which he plugged into Ellie's IV set. "This is vincristine, one of the drugs Ellie will be getting to put her into remission," Robbins explained. "We give vincristine once a week because it kills only leukemic cells that have started to divide. Since the blasts do not all divide at once, we hope that each time the drug is administered, we're wiping out a new set of leukemic cells. Ellie will also be getting prednisone pills every day and L-asparaginase injections three times a week until she's in remission."

Vincristine was administered in a precise dose proportional to the surface area of Ellie's body, since an overdose could be life threatening. Robbins checked again to make sure the IV needle was well into the vein and that the solution was flowing slowly. If, by accident, the IV blew and the drug infiltrated into the surrounding tissue, it would severely damage both skin and muscle, causing ulcers much like third-degree burns.

Ellie's supper was brought in along with her medication, and Sue Kramer crushed the tablets of prednisone and allopurinol into her applesauce. Sally tried to spoon the mixture into Ellie's mouth, but the child hated the taste and kept spitting it up. Sally resolved to teach her to swallow pills, so that her frequent medications would be less of an ordeal for both of them.

Around 10:00 P.M. Brian and Barbara got up to go: Brian to drive back to New Jersey and Barbara to return to her apartment, since she had to be at work early the next morning. Sally walked them to the elevators and returned to the room. When she arrived, she saw to her horror that Ellie had pulled out her IV. The sheets were stained with blood and the fluid from the IV bottle was dripping into a puddle on the floor. Ellie was crying—she had thought that her mother was leaving and had tried to climb out of bed to find her.

Somehow Sally found the presence of mind to shut off the IV. Then, still in shock, she ran out into the corridor to find help. She finally located Sue, who in turn paged Robbins. Ten minutes later the resident appeared, carrying an IV kit and a set of cloth arm restraints. He looked exhausted, and the night was just beginning. "I'm afraid we'll have to restrain her," he said, shaking his head while Sue Kramer mopped up the spilled drug. "She just can't afford to ruin any more veins."

While Sally held her squirming child, Robbins restarted the IV in Ellie's other arm, trying to explain to her the importance of her cooperation. Then he fastened the Velcro restraints to her wrists and tied the free ends to the sidebars of the bed. Ellie struggled furiously against her bonds. "Let me go!" she screamed. "I'll be good!"

Robbins tried again. "Look, Ellie, I know it's scary and you don't like it, but it's important for you to get the IV. If you promise not to pull the needle out again, I'll untie you. But you have to promise."

Ellie nodded through her tears, and Robbins undid the restraints. It was hard for him to understand Ellie's mentality. He had often tried to put himself back in time and remember how he had perceived the world as a child, but it was impossible. Kids were kids. Their thinking was concrete and primary, and their responses were much less inhibited. Sick children reacted to the pain and the loneliness. If they hurt, they cried, and if they were happy, they laughed. If they didn't like you, they said mean and nasty things, but they forgot quickly. They experienced and reacted, without analyzing, and they certainly did not know what it meant to die. Their fears were more concrete: separation from their parents, or the loss of some body part.

Before Robbins left, he told Sally to keep a close watch on Ellie, but once the child understood that they were not just torturing her, she slowly became more cooperative and left the IV alone. Finally she dozed off, and Sally went out into the corridor for some fresh air. She felt unable to cry; she was still numb and detached, unwilling to accept the situation. Could Ellie really be here in this strange hospital, the victim of a horrible disease?

Sally

There were four other mothers sitting together at the other end of the corridor. They obviously knew one another and were chatting nonstop. Although they glanced at Sally curiously, she avoided them; she was bitterly unhappy and did not feel like discussing Ellie with strangers. Instead, she walked back to Ellie's room, washed up in the small sink, and lay down on the cot that had been set out for her.

But sleep would not come, even after the lights in the corridor had dimmed. The illuminated nurses' station cast a muted glow into a corner of the room, highlighting the stuffed giraffe that Barbara had bought for Ellie. Sally got up and stood beside the bed, looking down at her daughter's pale face, luminous in the half-light from the hall. Ellie was sleeping soundly, her mouth open, her eyelids trembling with dreams.

Why Ellie? Sally asked herself. In a way, because Ellie was the younger, she was the more precious. What had they done to cause this? Perhaps it was some combination of her own and Brian's genes—after all, hadn't her father died of lung cancer? Or maybe it was something she had eaten or some medicine she had taken during her pregnancy. Why hadn't she stopped smoking when she was pregnant with Ellie? She knew that she had not received any X-rays at that time, but Ellie was in the habit of sitting too close to their color TV. Didn't it emit some kind of radiation? She shouldn't have let Ellie sit so close.

And why hadn't she recognized the symptoms sooner? If Barbara hadn't been there, they still would not have realized. How could they have been so blind? Wasn't it a mother's duty to protect her children from such awful things?

With a twinge, she remembered back to Ellie's accident in June, only four months earlier. Ellie had always been clumsy, constantly bumping into things and falling down. But nothing really serious had happened until the accident. Brian's parents had given them a wrought-iron artificial fireplace that Sally had not really wanted but had kept to be polite. When they had finished converting the basement into a playroom and a guest room, they had put the fireplace down there.

That day in June, Ellie and Beth were playing downstairs. Ellie decided to get a book down from the top of the fireplace and climbed up on her tricycle to reach for it. Suddenly she lost her balance, grabbed wildly for a handhold, and brought the whole massive fireplace crashing down on top of her. She lay pinned under it, dazed and screaming, while Beth tried in vain to lift it up and release her.

Hearing Ellie's screams, Sally rushed downstairs and saw her bloody child. Paralyzed by the horrible sight, she was unable to react until Brian arrived a few moments later, lifted the fireplace off Ellie, and picked her up in his arms. The child's hair was matted with blood and her face was bruised and swollen, making her features almost unrecognizable. Suddenly she vomited, and Brian feared that she might have suffered a concussion, or worse.

They ran with her out to the car and rushed to the Muhlenberg Hospital emergency room, where Ellie's head was stitched up and several X-rays were taken. Although the doctors could find no evidence of a concussion or skull fracture, she was badly bruised and very frightened.

Now Sally began to fear that the accident had set off some kind of physiological reaction in Ellie's body that could have triggered the leukemia. Perhaps the stress of the accident had lowered her resistance to the disease. Hadn't some adults she knew developed cancer not long after some traumatic event in their lives, like the death of a spouse or the loss of a job? If only she had refused to accept that damn fireplace! What a fool she had been! She had gotten rid of it quickly enough after the accident, donating it to a garage sale sponsored by the Junior Women's Club. Her anger and guilt over Ellie's leukemia now attached itself to the image of the hated fireplace, moving over and over through her mind.

The cot was hard and uncomfortable, her head ached, and her mind spun feverishly on, unable to rest. She had always prided herself on being in control of her life, and now here, suddenly, was something she could do absolutely nothing about. The more she thought about it, the angrier she became. What kind of God would take an innocent child? Why had He let her survive the accident, only to get leukemia? Was He testing them, or was He merely remote and uncaring? It would be wonderful to have great faith, she thought, to be able to go to church and bow down at the altar and say, "I'm putting Ellie in your hands, God. Thy will be done." But she didn't have that kind of faith, had not had it even back in Catholic girls' school in Chicago. She only hoped there was some purpose to their suffering.

Whatever happened, the essential thing was for her to be strong for Ellie and be there when the child needed her. Ellie had to face months of painful and terrifying treatments, and she needed parents she could rely on to alleviate her fears. Sally remembered the look of fear that had come into Ellie's eyes when she saw the boy with the amputated leg, no doubt thinking the same thing would be done to her. Clearly the child's fantasies were even more threatening than the actual ordeal before her.

Sally realized that for Ellie's sake, she could not afford to lose control over her emotions. She would have to do whatever the doctors told her and pretend that everything was going fine. They would live one day at a time, savoring its joys and enduring its hardships. But she just couldn't let Ellie see how scared she really was.

7 Doctor Doll

Sally was awakened at six-thirty the following morning. She blinked her eyes and looked around, unsure for a moment of where she was. Then she saw a nurse looking down at her and realized that she was on the cot in Ellie's room. Hearing the sound of her child's voice, she sat up. "What's happening?" she asked.

"We have to weigh her and take vital signs," the nurse explained.

Sally was furious. "You woke both of us just to weigh her? Why can't this wait until a more reasonable hour?"

The nurse explained that the hospital shifts changed early in the morning, and that certain things had to be done before the night shift left. Sally shrugged, still angry. She did not want to risk alienating the nursing staff, for fear they would not take optimal care of Ellie. Although she knew that care would never be withheld, she was concerned that it might not come as quickly. It was becoming clear to her already that the hospital was run largely for the convenience of the staff, not the patients.

Because Ellie's legs were too sore for her to put her full weight on them, the nurse weighed Sally alone and then again with Ellie in her arms, subtracting to obtain the child's weight. She also took Ellie's vital signs and changed her IV bottle. Then Ellie and Sally went back to sleep for an hour, until breakfast was served and Sally folded up the cot in anticipation of doctors' rounds.

A few minutes after nine, Dr. Nelson appeared at the door along with Dr. Fein, the three residents rotating through M-5 that month, including Robbins, and two medical students from Cornell and Columbia. The white-coated group filed into the room and took positions around the bed, watching while Nelson examined Ellie. He checked her eyes, ears, and throat and carefully inspected her mouth for any sign of bleeding gums or sores. Turning to Sally, he asked, "Has she been eating?"

"Nothing at all," she replied. "This morning she put a piece of toast in her mouth and you would have thought she was eating poison."

"Any vomiting?"

"Just dry heaves."

"Well, keep trying to feed her," Nelson said. "Otherwise she seems to be doing well." He smiled at Ellie, who scowled in return, and then he and his entourage went out in the hall to discuss the case. Sally was annoyed that they were using her daughter as a teaching tool; she felt that their privacy was being violated.

Ellie was watching "Sesame Street" on TV when Jan Stevens, the play therapist, came into the room with a tray full of rubber dolls, syringes, IV bottles, tubes, and Band-Aids. As soon as Ellie saw the IV bottles she began to scream, "No needles, no needles!"

Jan put down her equipment on a side table and went over to comfort Ellie. "You won't be getting any needles now, Ellie," she said. "We're going to play hospital. This time you can pretend to be the doctor and give all the shots."

The hospital was such a bad place for children to be, Jan thought, even though Memorial tried to make it as pleasant as possible. There was the pain of getting repeatedly pricked and probed, the disruption of being awakened several times during the night, the loneliness and all the fears that a child's active mind conjured up from the strange smells, sounds, and sights of the hospital. Perceived through the distorting filter of a child's imagination, the scent of antiseptic became a whiff of poison gas, a blood-pressure cuff an instrument of torture, and a group of white-coated doctors making rounds a team of executioners.

Jan brought her tray over to the bed, sat down on the edge, and filled a syringe with water. Next she injected it into a girl-puppet's arm, making crying noises and offering reassurance that it would only hurt for a minute. She seemed well rehearsed at acting out both parts. "Do you want to play now, Ellie?" she asked.

Ellie nodded hesitantly, and stopped crying.

"See all the dolls we have here? We have a nurse doll, a doctor doll, some grown-up dolls, and a little boy and girl. Which do you want?"

"The doctor."

"Okay," the therapist said, and handed her the rubber doll. The doctor was dressed in a white coat, with a mirror strapped to his forehead and a stethoscope around his neck. "Now, we have some syringes and IV's and some play blood. What would you like?"

"A needle."

"All right, here you are." She took out a plastic disposable syringe with a cut-off needle and filled it with water from a jar. "Tell me about your patient," she said. "Is this guy sick? Does he need a shot?"

Ellie nodded.

"What's wrong with him?"

"His blood is bad."

"That's right, Ellie. He has some bad cells in his blood. The medicine is going to get rid of the bad cells, but it might make him feel sick at the same time. Here, give him a shot."

Ellie took the syringe and jabbed it hard into the doctor doll's back.

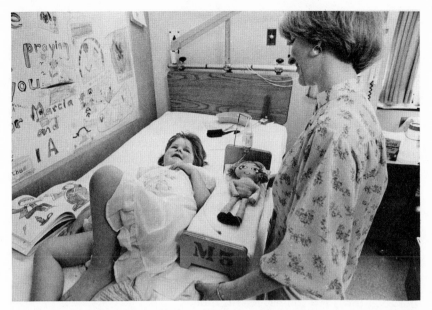

Play therapy on the pediatric inpatient floor at Memorial Hospital helps a leukemic child adjust to painful procedures by having her play the role of "doctor" on a doll. Here, under the guidance of a play therapist, the child has started an IV on the doll as a way of working out her fear of needles. *Photo courtesy of the Memorial Sloan-Kettering Cancer Center.*

"Are you giving him a spinal tap? What does he think about that?"

"It hurts."

"I guess he doesn't like that very much, does he?"

"No."

"What happens next?"

"Bandage."

"Okay, here you are." The therapist handed Ellie a box of Band-Aids, and the child busily applied eight of them to the doll's back.

"IV," Ellie said with a malicious grin, not waiting to be prompted.

"An IV, too? Boy, I bet he thought it was bad enough just to get a shot in the back, and now he has to get an IV, too. I bet he's not so happy about that. Why does he need an IV?"

"To get his medicine."

"What's the medicine for?"

"To make him better."

"That's right, Ellie. An IV's a good way to get medicine. Okay, here's your butterfly needle. What else do you need to start an IV?"

"A bottle, silly!"

Jan could not help laughing. "We can't do much without that, can we? Boy, Ellie, you sure have learned a lot about what happens in the hospital."

The therapist took a small IV bottle filled with water and hung it from the metal tree beside the bed, next to the real IV bottle that was draining into Ellie's arm. She connected the plastic tube from the play bottle to a blunt, cut-off needle, which she let Ellie stick into the doll's arm. While the child jabbed with the needle, Jan held the doll and pretended to talk for it. "I don't want an IV," she whined. "It's gonna hurt. Ouch! I don't like needles. I'm scared of them."

Ellie poked the needle into the doctor doll's head.

"Why did you do that, Ellie?" Jan asked.

"Because he's bad."

"No, Ellie, he isn't bad. It's not his fault that there's something wrong with his blood. It just happened, that's all. Because of his illness, which is serious, there will be times when he feels very good and times when he won't feel so good. If he gets his medicines, chances are that we can make the good times last longer. Right, Ellie?"

The child nodded solemnly.

"Good. I have to go now, but I'll come back and see you real soon. Bye-bye, now."

"Bye," Ellie said and waved, and Sally thanked Jan for having come.

Ellie spent much of the day watching TV and playing with her toys in bed, except when she had to go down to Radiology or Special Procedures for tests. Most of the time she was irritable and listless, and her attention span was short. Sally entertained her for brief intervals doing puzzles, stringing beads, or reading books out loud, but soon her supply of ideas ran out. At about three o'clock, when Ellie was feeling somewhat stronger, Sally put her in a wheelchair and took her down the long corridor to the playroom. Normally it would have thrilled her, since it had everything she loved: dozens of dolls, games, puzzles, oversized stuffed animals, and a large tank of water with rubber ducks and model boats floating in it. But Ellie was constantly afraid, and nothing really appealed to her. She avoided the other children and clung tightly to her mother's hand.

For Bill Robbins, the day passed without major crises, which was just as well because he had caught only a few hours of sleep the night before. One child had spiked a high fever, another had developed a severe nosebleed, a third's IV had infiltrated, and so on all night long. Throughout the afternoon, reports kept coming in from the nurses and test results from the lab, and Robbins had to modify the treatment of his patients accordingly. Most of his responses were straightforward: if a patient had a low blood

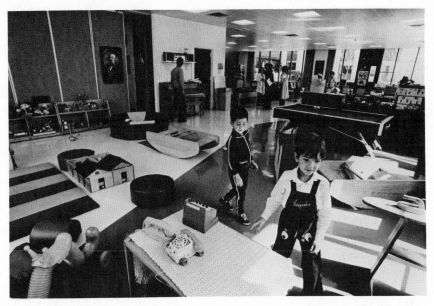

Playroom on the pediatrics inpatient floor of Memorial Hospital provides opportunities for children with cancer to interact. *Photo courtesy of the American Cancer Society.*

count, he ordered a transfusion; if there was a suspicious sound in a patient's chest, he ordered an X-ray. Although he was very busy, he made sure to look in on Ellie three times during the day.

At four-thirty Robbins went down to Radiology with Dr. Fein to review all of the X-rays that had been taken of his patients. Then he went to the pathology lab to watch the autopsy of a child who had died during the night. After that, he sat down and read over his patients' charts, trying to figure out what medications they would be needing and keeping track of the data on file cards. Finally at five-fifteen there were chart rounds, when the medical team went over the results of all the lab tests, X-rays, and consultations by specialists that had been ordered during the day, reviewing each case in some detail. Before Robbins left for home, utterly exhausted, he signed out his patients to Sarah Cooper, the resident on call that night.

The residents on M-5 used the "RICH MAN" sign-out system, with each letter of the mnemonic representing an area in which problems might arise: *R*espiratory, *I*nfectious, *C*ardiovascular, *H*ematologic, *M*etabolic, *A*limentary, and *N*eurologic. Sarah was used to this shorthand, and her ears were attuned to hearing a capsule summary under each heading. For example, summarizing the status of one of his patients, Robbins said, "John Kelly is a four-year-old with ALL. Respiratory: he has pneumonia, on penicillin. Infectious: he's undergoing a bacteriological work-up for his pneumonia. Cardiovascular: he has congestive heart failure, on digitalis. Hematologic: his counts are in the chart, and he's receiving transfusions of packed red cells and platelets. Metabolic: he's getting normal saline IV fortified with potassium. Alimentary: diet as tolerated. Neurologic: has had seizures from his brain metastases and is on phenobarbital. Tonight you should . . ." Robbins then went on to list the tests and procedures needed for that patient.

Sarah Cooper took notes and Robbins went through the RICH MAN sequence for all eight of his patients, including Ellie. Sarah would do another round with the fellow at 9:00 P.M. and then, most likely, the activity would continue well into the night. She hoped she would get at least a few hours of sleep.

8 Brian

At ten past eight Monday morning, September 18, Brian Murphy left the house in Menlo Park to drive to New York. He had slept poorly and was still bleary eyed as he climbed into his car. Beth was staying at the Lewises', since Cindy had kindly offered to look after her until Brian's parents returned from Connecticut, most likely on Wednesday.

Brian had considered taking an unpaid leave of absence from his job as a sales representative for a medical-equipment company in Newark to spend more time with Ellie, but they just could not afford it. On top of the mortgage and living expenses, they now had additional transportation, food, and medical costs to deal with. Luckily, Brian's group insurance plan at work would cover most of Ellie's hospital costs, and the government underwrote much of the experimental chemotherapy. In addition, the insurance covered the bone-marrow tests, since they were considered a surgical procedure, and Memorial did not charge for blood tests. But there were dozens of tests that were not covered, including the matching and checking of blood for transfusion. Those alone could add up to a lot of money, especially now that Ellie had begun receiving frequent transfusions. So leaving work just would not make sense. Brian did make a lot of sales calls in Manhattan, however, so he would have numerous opportunities to visit Ellie at the hospital.

At nine-thirty that morning, in fact, he was scheduled to give a demonstration of his company's new adjustable-grade treadmill at the Institute for Rehabilitation Medicine in the East Thirties, after which he planned to drive up to Memorial. As he backed his station wagon out of the driveway, he wondered how he would find the strength to go through with his presentation.

He followed the familiar road to Route 1, letting his mind take him there unthinkingly, by pure force of habit. But as he drove along the highway, looking out at the chemical plants that bordered the road on both sides, he began to wonder whether Ellie's leukemia might have been caused by some pollutant in the air or water. Those refineries certainly didn't help, with all the garbage they were pouring into the atmosphere. On hot summer days, when the wind blew the right way, he could smell the gasoline distillation fumes in their backyard. Maybe Ellie's illness could have been avoided if they had stayed in Queens instead of moving to New Jersey when she was just an infant. Didn't the state have one of the highest cancer rates in the country? Their dream of a house in the suburbs may have turned into a nightmare.

The cars were stacked up outside the Lincoln Tunnel, and Brian began to ruminate obsessively about pollution. The heat shimmered up off the car tops, and the air was thick with exhaust. He rolled up his window but the sickening smell permeated the car. His mind wandering, he began to spell the word "leukemia" backwards, visualizing the letters one by one. . . . A I M E K U E L . . . He repeated the strange word over and over like an alchemist's incantation, as if by some magical process the inverted word might somehow reverse the disease and make Ellie well again.

Brian finally emerged from the tunnel at Forty-second Street. Passing through Times Square, he looked out at the human detritus of society: whores, pimps, bums, junkies, dope dealers, pornographers. A three-card monte player was attempting to con passersby, until a cop approached and he picked up his cards and fled. It angered Brian that these people were alive and thriving while his little girl, who had never harmed a soul, was dying. Why the hell were all these evil people making it, he wondered, when so many good people were dying? It seemed as if there was something very wrong with the world, a vast conspiracy to replace all things good, pure, and beautiful with those corrupt, degraded, and perverse. He slammed his fist down hard on the empty seat beside him.

The light changed and he continued across town through the dense traffic, feeling grief stricken and alone. Parking not far from the Institute, he took an elevator up to the lecture room. The physical therapist who would be conducting the demonstration was waiting for him, obviously annoyed. "You're late," she said. "It's almost time."

He made some excuse about the traffic and helped her set up the treadmill. She was talking, but he could not concentrate. He excused himself and walked over to the window overlooking the East River and gazed down at the sparkling light. An oil barge steamed by, and helicopters darted like dragonflies among the gleaming office towers.

Brian mused that he might never again be able to take Ellie to Atlantic City, to take a walk along the boardwalk or build sand castles on the beach. The tears began to roll silently and uncontrollably down his cheeks. He wasn't sure he could go through with the demonstration.

Behind him, he heard the murmur of the audience entering: physical therapists in white uniforms and administrators in business suits. He would just have to pull himself together. He wiped his eyes, blew his nose, and, convincing himself to be strong, returned to the treadmill.

"Is everything all right?" the therapist asked, with just a hint of feeling, looking him over curiously.

"Yes, thanks. Just tired, that's all. Had a bad night."

Somehow he made it through the demonstration, although his mind was elsewhere; the machine was familiar and the questions mercifully brief. Still preoccupied, he went down to his car and drove to the hospital.

M-5 was more lively than it had been the previous day, but not by much. A few wan-looking children were walking in the corridor with their mothers, who pushed IV poles laden with clinking bottles. Brian spotted Dr. Nelson talking to another set of parents outside their child's room. There was an ISOLATION sign on the door and piles of disposable surgical masks and gowns stacked nearby.

Nelson caught sight of Brian and beckoned him over. "Mr. Murphy, I'd like you to meet the Gordons. They're neighbors of yours—they live in Metuchen."

Mr. Gordon, a balding man with glasses, extended his hand, his friendly smile in sharp contrast to the weary look in his eyes. He explained that his eight-year-old son, Billy, had AML, the "bad" type of childhood leukemia.

Grateful to find someone who understood, Brian told them about Ellie. Mr. Gordon nodded. "If your child is newly diagnosed, the word *leukemia* is still a devastating thing. Once your child has been in remission for a while, though, you learn to live with it. When they're well, they're really well."

Mrs. Gordon, a petite woman with a perpetual half-smile, added, "Every day I wake up grateful that Billy is still here with us. And I know he's going to be with us for many, many more days."

Mr. Gordon mentioned the monthly meetings for parents that Dr. Nelson held at the hospital and suggested that they car-pool together from New Jersey. When Brian asked about the purpose of the group, he replied, "It's a place where we can share the problems we experience and express the feelings that are hard to let out to people who don't really know what it's like. By meeting together, we feel a little less isolated." Brian thought car-pooling to the meeting was a great idea, and they parted a bit more cheerfully.

When Brian entered Ellie's room, the child was watching cartoons on the TV suspended above her bed. Her lunch was sitting on a tray, untouched, and she looked fragile and pale; an IV was feeding a yellowish solution of platelet concentrate into her arm. Sally sat in an armchair nearby, working on a needlepoint, and seemed surprised and pleased to see her husband.

Brian plopped down in a chair across from the bed. He wanted to talk with Sally about his feelings, but he was inhibited with Ellie present. Communicating emotions had always been difficult for him, and now he was protecting very vulnerable areas within himself. Oppressed by the silence, Brian mentioned that he had met some other parents from New Jersey in the hall, and that perhaps Sally might want to talk to them.

"No, thanks," she said firmly but quietly. "I don't want to hear what they have to say, and I don't want to discuss Ellie with strangers."

Brian was annoyed by her reaction, but he also understood it. Better not to become too involved with other people's problems; they had enough of their own. He mentioned that he had called several of their close friends from Queens and Menlo Park, all of whom had said they wanted to visit Ellie in the hospital. Then he began to talk about his misgivings concerning their move from the city to New Jersey, close to such a heavy concentration of chemical plants and refineries. Sally brought up her own theories about the disease, and for several minutes they ruminated over what had gone wrong and what they could have done to prevent it.

This depressing conversation was interrupted by the arrival of Dr. Nelson, who brought them out into the corridor to tell them the results of the morning's blood tests. Thanks to the red-cell transfusions, he said, Ellie's anemia was improving. Her hematocrit had climbed from 18.5 at admission to 30 and had now stabilized at that level. Her platelets were still under 20,000—the threshold below which spontaneous bleeding could occur—and he planned to give her eight additional units of platelet concentrate in an attempt to raise her count and provide more of a margin of safety. Nonetheless, the transfused platelets would only survive in her bloodstream for seventy-two hours, so that if her marrow was not producing its own platelets, her count would soon plummet again.

The Murphys were beginning to get a feel for the normal values of the various blood components, so that they could hear a string of blood counts and have a fair picture of how Ellie was doing. As a result, their hopes and fears now focused on her platelet count or on the percentage of blasts in her differential. Laboratory values were the language of modern medicine, bewildering to the uninitiated but strangely comforting to those who became familiar with them. The numbers gave both the doctors and parents a sense of precision and control, creating the illusion of order and reason in what was really an anarchic disease.

"Did you like the Gordons?" Nelson asked Brian. "They're very special people, real veterans who have been through a lot. I think it's very useful for parents of leukemic children to exchange experiences and concerns—that's why the parents' group is so important."

"The Gordons were encouraging in a way," Brian said. "I got the impression that their son Billy is doing well. Is he in remission?"

Nelson seemed surprised. "Billy was in remission for six months, but he relapsed a week ago. We've been trying our best to induce a second remission, but so far his disease has proved resistant. The drugs that are used to treat AML are much more toxic to the healthy bone marrow than those used for ALL, so Billy's counts are now very low. We've put him in protective isolation to prevent him from getting a serious infection, and with intensive therapy we hope to get him back into remission."

"My God, I had no idea. . . ." Brian murmured. "They never said a thing about that." He shook his head. "Christ, I hope he makes it." Accepting the fact that Ellie had leukemia was one thing; confronting all the ramifications of the disease was still another. Brian refused to believe that a hard-earned remission might not last—it was just too much reality. Clearly the Gordons were denying it, too.

"Do you have any questions?" Nelson said. "Even if you're bothered by something that seems minor or ridiculous, please don't hesitate to ask."

There was a pause before Sally spoke. "Dr. Nelson, what I'd really like to know is why my daughter got this disease, when there is no family history of it."

Nelson scratched his head. "That's the one question I was hoping you wouldn't ask," he said, "since I don't know the answer myself. First of all, childhood leukemia is a very rare disease. There are only twenty-four hundred cases in this country per year under age fifteen. That's an incidence of about one in every twenty thousand kids, or one in every fifty elementary schools. In most cases of leukemia, no cause or predisposition is found. There are also several different types of leukemia, so it's possible that each form of the disease is triggered by a different agent or combination of agents."

"I read something once about a leukemia virus," Brian said. "Is there anything to that?"

"That's been a popular theory for years, but lately it has fallen into disrepute. A link between viruses and human leukemia would not be entirely surprising, since it's known that leukemia in cats, birds, and mice is caused by specific viruses that can be transmitted from one individual to another. Moreover, viruslike particles have in fact been found, if very rarely, in the blood and tissues of human leukemia patients. What's lacking is proof of causation: the viruses could well have appeared in the patient after the leukemia was induced. To date, no one has succeeded in demonstrating that crucial point."

"But could the disease be catching?" Sally asked nervously. "Every time my legs ache, I'm convinced that I'm coming down with it, too."

"I wouldn't worry about that, Mrs. Murphy," Nelson replied. "Even if viruses do turn out to cause leukemia, there's no evidence of contagion or transmissibility. The frequency of leukemia among mothers and nontwin siblings of leukemic children is no greater than among the population at large. That's why leukemic children should be allowed to mingle and play with healthy children, at no risk to their young friends."

"What about heredity?" Sally asked. "Could that play a role?"

"Perhaps, but probably not in the way you mean. Genetic damage, such as chromosome breakage, may be involved, but when most people think of heredity they think of physical traits that are passed on from one generation to the next. Leukemia does not seem to be an inherited disease. In fact, there are only seven families in the world in which there are more than three first-degree relatives who've had any form of leukemia, and in every case it's AML. There's never been a family in which three first-degree relatives have developed ALL.

"We do see cases of two siblings with ALL, though. One pattern is identical twins: one twin develops ALL, and then the other twin comes down with the disease within a few months' time. Yet nonidentical twins have no greater chance of developing leukemia if the other twin does than the general population. What does this mean? The discrepancy between identical and nonidentical twins suggests that the cause is not primarily heredity but external factors. Identical twins have a shared blood supply in the womb, so perhaps in identical twins that develop ALL, the disease is caused before birth.

"Another bit of evidence suggests that ALL is not inherited. In the seven AML families I mentioned, all of the relatives developed the disease when they hit a certain age, such as fifteen, nineteen, or fifty. This suggests that there is a true genetic predisposition to the disease. But the sibling pairs who develop ALL tend to get the disease close together in time, regardless of their respective ages, which suggests that an external cause is responsible. For example, we've had a case here of two siblings, one three years old and the other seven years old, who both developed ALL within six months. Biologically these two ages are very different, which tells me that the cause was an external event, and that they shared the common source."

"But what could that external event be? Could chemical pollution be responsible?" Brian asked, remembering the fuming chemical plants along the New Jersey Turnpike.

"Chemicals have been linked to some types of leukemia, but not to ALL," Nelson replied. "For example, a study of chemical workers in Italy who were exposed to benzene, an organic solvent, showed that they had a high incidence of AML, and industrial workers exposed to the heavy metal chromium have a high incidence of CML. But no chemical has yet been linked to ALL. The same is true of radiation. Among the survivors of the atomic bombing of Hiroshima, there was a very high incidence of AML and CML, with the highest incidence in people who were closest to ground zero when the bomb was dropped, and the lowest in people who were farthest away. But we haven't found a persuasive association between radiation and ALL."

"Weren't there a lot of childhood-leukemia cases in Rutherford, New Jersey, a few years ago?" Brian asked. "I remember reading about that in the paper."

"Yes, in 1976 the Rutherford cluster was investigated. Several cases of leukemia were reported in the town over a two-year period, five of them in children who attended a local elementary school. The state public-health people came in and did an extensive investigation, analyzing the air and water and even digging up the schoolyard, but they were unable to come up with any environmental factors that might have caused the disease. Since then, careful analysis of the Rutherford cluster suggests that the actual types of leukemia involved were quite different, and the interaction patterns diffuse, so it may have been a statistical fluke. There are other clusters that are more convincing, though. After a decade of careful analysis, we seem to have found three communities where something actually happened in terms of a statistically significant clustering of ALL cases in time and space. The rest of the reported clusters are apparently just random events. Because the disease is so rare to begin with, it's hard to know when a cluster is real. Some good studies suggest that clustering exists; other equally reputable ones indicate it does not."

By now, Brian and Sally were utterly confused. "So you're saying that you really don't know what causes the disease?"

"Yes. The cause or causes of childhood leukemia remain a great mystery. It's most likely a result of a complex interaction between environmental factors and individual vulnerabilities. Internal events may make somebody susceptible to one of a number of external events. But whether the internal events are genetic or immunological in any one individual, you can't predict. Many people suspect that the immune system is at fault, but in fact people with immune disorders do not get ALL, although they do get tumors of the lymphatic system. And if you look at the past histories of children with ALL, they have no higher frequency of infections than healthy children, contrary to what you would predict if their immune system was somehow defective. Another problem is that we don't know the latency period for leukemia: the time between the causative event and the appearance of the disease. Did the causative event occur one week before the kid came in, six months before, or during pregnancy? In adults, chemically induced cancers can take years to develop.

"So I'm afraid I can't convey much more than the current mystery that surrounds this subject. Still, there's hope to be found in the fact that thousands of research scientists are devoting their careers to finding out the answers."

"I have one more question, although it may sound a little foolish," Sally said.

"That's all right, please go ahead."

"Ellie had a bad accident four months before she was diagnosed and had several stitches in her scalp. Do you think that could have somehow triggered the disease?"

"No," Nelson replied firmly. "Young children are constantly falling down and bruising themselves, with no serious ill effects. What's more likely is that Ellie's undiagnosed leukemia made her weak and poorly coordinated, increasing the chances of an accident. Whatever the cause of leukemia turns out to be someday, it's important for you to realize that there was nothing you consciously did or failed to do that caused the disease. You should try to accept that, and not torture yourself with feelings of guilt or responsibility. That doesn't do anyone any good, least of all Ellie. There's one positive thing you could be doing, though, and that's donating blood for her, so that you won't be charged for so many of the blood products she needs. You could also ask your friends and relatives to do the same, having the blood credited to Ellie's account here. I would also encourage you to come to the parents' group meeting next Tuesday evening. I think you'll find it of value. I'll look in on Ellie again later today, just to make sure everything is fine."

After the doctor had left, Brian stayed with Ellie while Sally went to lunch. He had brought a new animal puzzle for her, and they worked on it together for a while. But Ellie quickly became nauseated and irritable. Impatient with the toy, she flung the pieces across the floor and began to cry. Brian felt angry at her for not appreciating his gift. It was so hard loving Ellie, knowing that they might lose her!

By the time Sally returned, Brian was restless and decided to go donate blood on Ellie's behalf. Never having given before, he dreaded the idea, but knowing what Ellie was going through and how stoically she was taking it, he was determined to do the same.

He took the elevator down to street level and walked the two blocks to the New York Blood Center on East Sixty-seventh Street. At the center, a receptionist greeted him and filled out a basic information form, stipulating that the blood be credited to Ellie's account. She then sent Brian into the next room, where a nurse asked him for a brief medical history, took his vital signs, and gave him some preliminary blood tests. From there Brian went on to the donation area: two rows of reclining contoured chairs. He lay down on one, smiling nervously at the man across from him who had just finished donating and was holding his right arm vertical to stop the bleeding.

Brian rolled up his right sleeve and looked away as the nurse inserted the needle. After the initial sharp pain, it was surprisingly tolerable, just a dull pressure in his arm. Looking down, he felt queasy at the sight of his dark red blood draining into a plastic bag that was being agitated back and forth by a machine. He lay back and stared up at the neon ceiling lamps, convinced that they were growing fainter. . . .

Fifteen minutes later it was over, although it had felt like hours. When he stood up from the chair, his shirt was glued to his back with sweat. He swayed, momentarily dizzy, and the nurse insisted on taking him by the arm and leading him into the lounge. A few other donors were there already, sipping coffee and orange Tang, eating stale cookies, and putting BE NICE TO ME, I GAVE BLOOD TODAY stickers on their lapels.

"You seem very nervous," the nurse said to Brian. "Is this your first time?"

"Yes," he replied. "I've never given before. I've always been terrified of it."

She looked at him curiously. "Then why are you here? What made you change your mind?"

"My daughter . . . has leukemia," he replied, suddenly feeling his composure crack open and the pain break through. He broke down in great racking sobs. Everyone in the room turned around and stared.

"Sit down and rest," the nurse said gently. "You've been through a lot."

She brought him a cup of coffee and a packet of Lorna Doones. Trying to ignore the curious faces of the other donors, Brian sipped the warm liquid and dried his face with a napkin, still feeling acutely embarrassed. When he had regained his composure, he waited until the other donors had left and then got up and went out into the street.

He hesitated outside the blood center, wondering if he should go back to the hospital. Guilt tugged at him, but then the despair and hopelessness returned, and he shook his head. Everything would turn out all right, he told himself. Ellie was in highly competent hands, and thinking about it constantly and getting depressed did not accomplish anything. He had to keep on living.

On his way to the car, he stopped at a phone booth and called the room, telling Sally that he was due back at the office in Newark for the remainder of the afternoon.

9 Coping

Over the next few days, the Murphys continued to adjust to the wrenching changes in their lives. Ellie's induction chemotherapy was proceeding as planned: she was receiving prednisone tablets daily, intravenous vincristine once a week, and L-asparaginase injected into her buttocks three times a week. The drugs seemed to be working well, with relatively few side effects other than nausea, vomiting, and diarrhea. Ellie's white count dropped dramatically from more than 28,000 on September 16 to 7,100 on September 19. There was also a marked decrease in swelling of her liver, spleen, and lymph nodes, although her legs continued to hurt.

The staff on M-5 made a real effort to make life as enjoyable as possible for the children. Every Monday there was a bingo game in the playroom, complete with a guaranteed prize for everyone, and for those children who had appetites, cookies were served on Tuesdays and pizza on Wednesdays. Sally also appreciated the cheerfulness and smiles of the elderly volunteers who walked around the floor handing out lollipops and games. Overall, the children seemed to be coping beautifully; whenever she saw someone who really looked depressed, it was probably a visitor.

Sally threw herself into every aspect of Ellie's care. She began to familiarize herself with routine procedures—giving sponge baths, helping Ellie with the bedpan, holding her while blood tests were done or an IV was started, changing her dressings—so that she could be of real assistance to the nurses. Her initial instinct was to do everything for Ellie, including cutting up all of the child's food and feeding her, but the nurses discouraged her from treating Ellie as if she were totally helpless. It was important to treat her as normally as possible, since otherwise she would regress and develop severe behavior problems.

Sally also became obsessed with the details of the disease and treatment, insisting on an explanation for every procedure and laboratory test. When the doctors' answers made her anxious, she would vacillate for a time between the fear of knowing and the fear of not knowing. Nearly always her urgent need to be informed would win out. At least if the danger was defined, she could muster her emotional resources to deal with it. Both she and Brian also tried to glean information, as positive as possible, from diverse sources. Brian clipped articles on new cancer treatments from newspapers, magazines, and even medical journals that friends referred him to, bringing them in to show the doctors in a desperate search for a miracle cure that might have been overlooked. Sally had heard about the importance of nutrition and vitamins to a child's health, and she wanted to supplement Ellie's diet in the best possible way. Both of them were disappointed and annoyed when Nelson and the other doctors treated their suggestions condescendingly, dismissing the articles Brian had collected without even reading them. It angered the Murphys that the doctors often seemed so caught up in their protocols and statistics that they failed to see the human beings involved.

Since Ellie panicked whenever she was left alone in her room, even when Sally left for a few minutes to go to the bathroom or make a phone call, it soon became apparent that someone the child could trust would have to be with her during every waking minute. Because Brian was usually not around during the day, Barbara would walk across the street from New York Hospital to Memorial Sloan-Kettering and relieve Sally during meals and major procedures, such as bone marrows or spinal taps. Barbara's visits were invaluable, bringing new ideas and energy to Ellie and respite to Sally. During these one-hour escapes, Sally would walk back to Barbara's apartment for a shower or a nap, or go just around the corner for a cup of coffee.

In spite of Barbara's participation in painful procedures and the fact that she wore a white nurse's uniform, Ellie never lost trust in her aunt, even as she hated and feared the doctors. It got to a point where Nelson would ask Barbara to palpate Ellie's liver and spleen, since the child screamed when he tried to get near her. Although Ellie's constant combativeness was wearing on both her family and the staff, Barbara thought that her fighting back meant that she still had some of her usual spunk. If she ever stopped fighting completely, Barbara thought, she would be preparing to die.

It was hard on Barbara, both physically and emotionally, to spend so much time with Ellie and work a full day as a nurse as well. Although

		9/16	9/18	9/19	9/23	9/26
	1. DATE	9/16	9/18	9/19	9/23	9/26
	2. Course	IND	IND	IND	IND	IND
	3. Days on (phase)	0	2	3	7	10
	4. Hosp or outpt (h or o)	H	H	H	H	H
Hemogram	5. HGB / HCT	6.1/18	8.3/25	8.5/25	10.6/30	10.2/29
	6. Platelet x 10^3	27	108	86	20	19
	7. WBC x 10^3	28.1	13.8	7.1	3.3	3.4
	8. Granulocytes (%)	3	13	26	9	
	9. Lymph/Atyp (%)	74	87	70	88	93
	10. Monocytes (%)			3	3	7
	11. Eosin/Baso (%)	3		1		
	12. Blast - Malig (%)	20				
	13. ANC					
Marrow	14. Erythroid (%)	1				
	15. Granulocyte (%)	2				
	16. Lymphoid (%)					
	17. Monocyte (%)					
	18. Blast - Malig (%)	97				
	19. Other					
	20. Cellularity	1				
	21. Megakaryocyte (%)					
	22. Marrow Rating	3				
Lab	23. BUN (mgm %)	33				
	24. Uric Acid	5.3				
	25. SGOT/SGPT	27/20				
	26. Alk. Phosphatase	94				
	27. Chest X-ray	Normal				
	28. Mediastinal Mass					
Physical	29. Weight (kg)	13.92			13.2	
	30. Height (cm)	94			94	
	31. Liver	2		2	2	
	32. Spleen	2		2	1	
	33. Lymph nodes	2		1	1	
	34. Kidney	0		0	0	
	35. Testes	0		0	0	
	36. Bone Pain	2		1	1	
	37. B / P	112/82	120/80			
Infect	38. Temperature	37.8	37	37	37	
	39. Site	0		0	0	
	40. Organism					
CNS	41. CSF: OP / CP	180				
	42. Total WBC/RBC	neg				
	43. Leukemic Blasts	0				
	44. Protein (mg/dl)	8				
	45. Sugar (mg/dl)	67				
	46.					
Toxicity	47. CNS/Neurologic	0				0/1+
	48. G I	0				1+
	49. Pancreas	0				0
	50. Liver	0				0
	51. Renal	0				0
	52. Hematologic	0				0
	53. Heart	0				0
	54. Lung	0				0
	55. Bone	0				0
Therapy	56. Meter^2	0.6			0.6	
	57. Prednisone	25	25	25	25	25
	58. Vincristine	0.9			0.9	
	59. L-asparaginase			3600		3600
	60.					
	61.					
	62.					
	63.					
	64.					
	65.					
	66. I T					
	67. Bactrim/Septra					
	68. Allopurinol	50 TID	50	50	50	50
	69. XRT					
	70. Antibiotics					
Blood Products	71. R B C Transfusion	140		140		
	72. Platelet		4 units		4 units	
	73.					
	74.					

NAME MURPHY, ELLEN

STUDY I.D. No. 162

PHASE INDUCTION

SIGNED Roger T. Nelson, MD

PRINCIPAL INVESTIGATOR R. NELSON, M.D.

REMARKS

9/19, 9/21, 9/24, 9/26 =
L-ASP 3600 IM

9/26 - Discharge
abd cramps

↓ DTR

SUBMIT ORIGINAL FLOWSHEET ONLY, NOT PHOTOCOPY

Page 1

Standardized flow-sheets distributed by the Children's Cancer Study Group are used to record patients' signs, symptoms, laboratory data, side effects, complications, and therapies.

Barbara did not admit it to Sally, she did not really think Ellie was going to make it. She had worked with several leukemic children in the past, and none had survived more than a year or two. Admittedly, that had been a few years ago, and a lot had happened since then, but sometimes after a particularly hard day, Barbara felt that if Ellie was going to die it would be better for all of them if it happened sooner rather than later. Why did any of them need to go through this agony if she was just going to relapse in another six months and die?

Brian's parents finally returned from Connecticut on Wednesday, September 20. As Barbara had predicted, as soon as they heard about Ellie they insisted on coming immediately to Menlo Park to look after Beth and help in any other way they could. Once the grandparents had settled in, Brian was able to drive directly from his office to the hospital in the evening and stay with Ellie while Sally went back to Barbara's apartment for longer breaks. Brian usually left the hospital around 10:00 P.M. and made his forty-five-minute commute back to New Jersey, only to wake at six the next morning to go to work. The routine was exhausting, and he began to feel increasingly weary and preoccupied at the office. Many times during the day he found himself staring off into space, thinking of Ellie, and repeatedly on the verge of tears. His work suffered badly; he was making fewer sales and hence earning fewer commissions at a time when the family needed the money more than ever.

Finally he felt compelled to tell a few of his coworkers, in confidence, about his daughter's illness. In spite of their promises of discretion, word soon spread to the entire office, and Brian was deluged with words of condolence and sympathy. Yet at the same time, people seemed to avoid him, averting their eyes when they passed him in the corridor. Others said foolish, clumsy things. One salesman he knew only slightly came up to him and said, "I heard about your daughter. I thought they had a cure for leukemia by now. Are you sure they can't cure it?"

Brian merely smiled politely and said, "Would that were the case."

It was almost funny: some people were convinced that leukemia was hopeless, a death sentence, while others considered it as mild and curable as the common cold. The thing that upset Brian the most was that when people heard about Ellie's leukemia, they almost invariably asked if he had other children. What the hell difference did that make? he wanted to shout at them. Ellie was unique and irreplaceable, and even if they had ten children, none of them would be another Ellie.

People were so frightened by disease, by tragedy of any kind. Perhaps they were afraid that the same thing would happen to them or to their children, as if Brian's misfortune were somehow contagious. They were all so awkward and false. Brian spent much of the day feeling very alone.

In great contrast, many of the Murphys' good friends and relatives made a moving effort to help out. Dozens of familiar faces from Queens and Menlo Park converged on Ellie's hospital room during visiting hours, bearing dolls, games, and toys. Cindy Lewis mobilized the Junior Women's Club to run a blood drive, and several dozen pints of blood were donated in Ellie's name at local hospitals.

In addition, Brian's great-aunt Maude and several second cousins whom he had not met more than five times in his life organized a raffle of homemade handcrafts to raise money to help pay for Ellie's medical expenses. The Murphys knew nothing of their efforts until they received a check in the mail for nearly $500, along with an explanatory note. Not needing the money immediately, they opened a bank account in Ellie's name.

Then there was Ellie's godmother, Pauline, whose long-term interest in faith healing had intensified when Ellie became ill. She had organized a group of acolytes who would meet twice weekly to gather in a circle, squeeze hands, and concentrate hard on sending "positive energy" to Ellie. Brian found the whole thing rather silly, but he knew that it certainly wouldn't do her any harm.

Even Beth's first-grade class got into the act, making dozens of get-well cards for Ellie.

The Murphys were grateful for such gestures of support, but they could not help feeling that few people really understood what they were going through. Friends were curious about what had happened and asked certain questions, but Sally really could not impart to them the impact of knowing that her child might die. She was alone with that thought. She tried to put it in the back of her mind, but it was always lurking there.

Even worse, she and Brian were finding it increasingly difficult to communicate. Most of the time they only saw each other coming and going at the hospital, and there was simply no time to recognize or respond to the other person's needs. When they did talk, it was always about the disease, which was constantly on their minds. Their own goals and aspirations were put on the back burner, and as a result resentments built up. All too often their stored-up anger was vented on each other.

Most marriages never had to weather a crisis like this, but certainly such traumas brought out either the best or the worst in a relationship. While things had been going smoothly, it had been possible to coast along without confronting fundamental problems that had always existed in their marriage. But suddenly, with Ellie's leukemia, all the difficulties began jumping out at them.

Instead of uniting them, the disease had begun to accentuate their fundamentally different styles of coping and relating. Sally was confronting the crisis head-on and being too hard on herself, whereas Brian was running away from it. Initially the disease had touched him deeply and brought out a variety of emotions, but they had been too painful and threatening and he had quickly pushed them back down again and tried to ignore them.

Sally realized that Brian loved Ellie and had to work to support the family, yet she resented the fact that she was so much more involved than he was in Ellie's care. She suspected that he came to the hospital less often than he could have because he could not bear the idea that Ellie might not survive. Perhaps by avoiding the illness, he was trying to make it go away. Brian, on the other hand, resented Sally's total absorption in Ellie's care. It just wasn't normal for a mother to be with a child all day and all night. As a result, he was left at home with all the responsibilities and the housework, deprived of physical contact with his wife, emotional support, and a normal family life.

By Sunday, September 24, Ellie's white count had dropped to 3,100. She had eaten poorly all week, and that morning she began to retch violently and suffer from diarrhea and abdominal cramps. The drugs were also having an effect on her appearance: the vincristine was causing her hair to fall out whenever Sally combed it, and the prednisone was making her face and body swell with fluid. Ellie's platelet count, which had risen briefly in response to multiple transfusions, had fallen back to 20,000, and her bone marrow was not yet producing new platelets on its own. Due to her low platelet count, Ellie had some bleeding in her gastrointestinal tract, resulting in black, tarry stools.

In spite of these setbacks, Sally continued to maintain a calm, controlled exterior, locking away her emotions in some deep psychic cabinet. The only times she talked about her feelings were when Barbara questioned her directly. Barbara was both amazed and worried by her sister-in-law's stoicism. She herself was taking Valium quite often these days, but whenever she offered Sally one she got the same reply: "No, thanks, I don't need a tranquilizer, I'm fine."

Barbara would shrug and say, "Well, I'm taking one. I don't know about you, but all this is making me very nervous."

Sally began to worry about her own lack of emotion, however, and on Monday morning she discussed it with Helen Davis, a social worker on M-5. "I would have thought I'd be hysterical in this situation," she confided, "but in fact I've been moving from day to day like a zombie, without feeling much of anything. Is it normal to react like this?"

"People really can't know how they will act in a crisis until they're actually confronted with it," Davis replied. "You're coping, Sally. It's just that people cope in different ways. What you're dealing with in a disease like leukemia, even if Ellie does well, is grief and loss. The disease involves the loss of previous functioning, of the belief in one's invulnerability. A lot of the sense of freedom and confidence and the assumptions of what life will be like must now change. There's also a physical loss, since the treatment physically changes the child. In order for you to go on as a family, you have to acknowledge that loss, and then rechannel in new ways some of the energy that was attached to the lost things."

"I just get so angry sometimes," Sally said. "But since nobody knows what caused the leukemia, there's no one to be angry at. So it just stays bottled up inside."

"First, you have to allow that anger to be expressed—to open up the abscess," Helen said. "But then, after expressing it, you need to be able to say, 'Okay, I'm angry. What am I going to do about it?' Just being angry isn't helpful. In fact, that sense of helplessness often makes people lash out and blame those close to them. You have to channel that anger in a way that can be useful toward the future. You know that you have to take care of Ellie now, but you should also get involved in things that make you feel good, that are self-gratifying and esteem building."

"I suppose so. It's just hard to think about anything else when I'm not getting much support from Brian."

Helen nodded. "This is a very stressful time on a marriage. I've found that it's unusual for two people to see the situation the same way. In almost every case, one parent is an optimist and the other is a pessimist, and each person clings to his or her way of looking at things—I don't think I've ever seen a pessimist become an optimist overnight, or vice versa. The problem is that people expect tragedy to unite them automatically, and that just doesn't happen. It's not easy to accommodate oneself to the moods of another person. Every couple going through a crisis like this feels that they're unique and that their marriage is in trouble because they're divided by the illness. That's why the parents' group is so useful. The more experienced parents in the group have been living with the disease for years, and they can reassure new parents that they are not freaks for feeling the way they do, and that it is indeed possible to survive this ordeal."

Sally nodded. "Thank you, Helen. That makes me feel a lot better."

"Good. I hope I'll be seeing you at the group meeting tomorrow."

That night, Sally was reading to Ellie from a children's book while a bag of platelets dripped into her arm. Suddenly Sally noticed Ellie begin to tremble, then shake uncontrollably. The child's face swelled up and her eyes became wide with fear. "Mommy!" she gasped, "I can't breathe!"

Terrified, Sally ran into the hall and grabbed a nurse, who immediately paged Dr. Robbins. He rushed in, shut off the IV, and gave Ellie a quick injection of Benadryl, an antihistamine that blocks allergic reactions. Almost immediately the child's body relaxed and she began to breathe normally again.

"It was a platelet reaction," Robbins explained, obviously relieved that the drug had worked. "An allergic reaction to the donor's blood. It happens sometimes when there are a lot of transfusions."

The resident tried to reassure Sally that no harm was done, and that from now on Ellie would be premedicated with Benadryl and Tylenol before receiving her transfusions. Nevertheless, Sally was profoundly shaken. It was her first inkling of the terrible things that could go wrong.

10 Parents' Group

Tuesday evening, Brian drove into the city from Newark, dreading the search for a parking space near the hospital, which usually consumed the better part of a half hour. To his amazement, there was an open space directly across the street from the main entrance. This struck him as a good omen and, suddenly optimistic about Ellie's chances, he took the elevator up to M-5 to pick Sally up for the parents' group meeting. Although Sally had been reluctant to go to the meeting, fearing horror stories told by other parents, Brian had successfully convinced her to join him.

The group met in a conference room on the main floor. Brian and Sally were ten minutes early and served themselves coffee from a large percolator that had already been set up. They sat down at the long table and watched as other parents arrived: three couples and two mothers alone, in total. Some of them nodded to one another and a few even seemed cheerful. The Gordons did not appear, and Brian guessed that they were spending time with Billy.

At precisely seven-thirty Dr. Nelson appeared, accompanied by Dr. Fein and Helen Davis. Nelson nodded to the Murphys with a friendly smile as he sat down at the table, and the murmur of conversation died out. Helen Davis began the meeting by asking all the parents to introduce themselves for the benefit of the newcomers, mentioning their child's name, age, diagnosis, and when the illness began. This was obviously a painful task for many of the parents, and they presented the information in subdued tones. Nearly all of their children were being treated as outpatients, and some had been in remission for months or even years.

Davis then asked the Murphys how they felt about coming to the group for the first time. Sally said she had been anxious about discussing the illness and feared the shock and pain of hearing about children who had relapsed or were not doing well. She wondered if it was a good idea to dwell on such things, but Brian had finally convinced her to come and see what the group was all about. Brian said that his main motivation for coming was that he felt increasingly alienated from his friends and needed the support of people who truly understood what he was going through.

Davis elaborated to the group, explaining that the Murphys were still learning to cope with the situation, their child having been so recently diagnosed. It was no surprise that everything still seemed overwhelming to them. The social worker then opened up the meeting to discussion.

Mr. Stein, whose sixteen-year-old son Mark had recently returned to the hospital with a relapse of his ALL, said that he often felt burdened by guilt when signing consent forms for experimental chemotherapy or surgical procedures. Since the relapse, he often questioned whether the treatment was worthwhile and was angry at the medical staff for causing his son what he felt was unnecessary discomfort.

"Last week one of the new residents came in and really messed up Mark's spinal tap," he complained. "The boy is so good natured that they think they can practice on him with impunity, since he doesn't scream and holler like the younger kids. This resident tried four times to do the tap, twice without the numbing medicine. The pain must have been terrible—I could see the tears in Mark's eyes. He was bleeding, and once the patient bleeds the tap is worthless, but still this resident kept poking. Sometimes I get the feeling that the purpose of this place is to train house staff and conduct clinical research, instead of caring for patients."

"Four tries for a spinal tap is inexcusable," Nelson replied, clearly upset. "I'll see to it that from now on residents practice on cadavers, not patients. In general, if there is ever a conflict between research or teaching and patient care, the rule is that the patient has to take precedence. In most cases, the two go hand in hand. Patients benefit from protocol studies in two ways. First, the new knowledge research provides enables us to improve our best therapies for the disease, and second, clinical research requires very careful monitoring of the patient and hence results in better care."

Mrs. Jeffries, whose daughter Robin, ten, had ALL in remission, described the anxiety she felt when Robin's maintenance chemotherapy was discontinued briefly because her white count was too low. "We were terrified that with the chemotherapy gone, even temporarily, the leukemia might come back," she said.

Nelson nodded. "The inevitable ups and downs of maintenance are understandably stressful, but the chances of the disease returning during a time the child is off medication are extremely low. As always, it's a question of balancing risks. When the absolute poly count in the peripheral blood drops below 1,000, the risk of developing a life-threatening infection if the chemotherapy continues is very real—and of much greater concern than the very small risk of relapse when the drugs are temporarily stopped. We just give the bone marrow a chance to recover from the chemotherapy enough so that the child is out of danger, and then start up the medicine again."

Mrs. Jeffries nodded wearily. "The hardest part is the uncertainty. If I only knew what was going to happen, I could prepare myself. Robin's been in continuous first remission for two years, and they say the chances of a relapse drop off rapidly after five. But they can't make any promises, so there's always that small kernel of doubt in the back of my mind. Of course, I don't think about it all the time—I couldn't maintain my sanity if I did. But sometimes I won't let her go out and play with other children or do anything because I'm afraid something will happen. . . ."

"What exactly are you afraid of, Mrs. Jeffries?" Davis asked.

"Well, that she'll catch a bad infection, or fall down and her platelets will be low and she'll bleed. . . ."

"In other words, that she might die?" Helen pursued.

"Well, I try not to think of it that bluntly," Mrs. Jeffries said quickly. "There are a lot of times when I look at her and it just doesn't seem possible that she has leukemia. I mean she looks so happy and healthy and normal. It's not easy having a child and knowing that she may only live a percentage of what should be her normal life span. Every day I face the possibility of the disease coming back, and I feel the anger and the pain surge up inside me. After coming so far, it's pretty hard to accept that it may not yet be behind us."

"The fact that there's not yet a definitive cure for leukemia but only a long stalemate makes it very hard to live with," Davis commented. "You have to live one day at a time, aware that things can turn sour very quickly, but viewing the good times as being all the more precious precisely because they may not last forever. Whatever happens, you should treat your child as if you expect her to live out a normal life span and not spoil her. It may seem cruel to discipline a leukemic child, but it's really in the child's best interests. With young children particularly, it's important to be firm but kind, and set the limits, expecting basically the same good behavior you expected before the illness. Any child whose routine is changed, or whose parents' expectations toward him are clearly altered, becomes frightened and insecure. What a child needs to feel safe and loved is whatever was normal before."

"I often wonder how much my son Danny knows about his illness," Mrs. White began. "We've never actually told him what he has—just that he has a problem with his blood. He came down with leukemia a year ago, when he was six, and he just turned seven. The other day he drew a picture of a cemetery with a headstone that had his name and dates on it. We were totally shocked."

"These kids know a lot more about the disease than we might think," Nelson replied. "We have parents who tell us, 'Please don't say a word to the child.' Some have been coming here for five years and claim that the child doesn't know anything, which is absurd. It's virtually impossible to withhold any diagnosis from a child over eight. Some kids figure out their disease from TV programs or newspapers and magazines, or from their own classmates. Even four-year-olds can really pick up on the tension and anxiety of their parents."

Davis nodded in agreement. "Young children can be amazingly perceptive at piecing together the truth from snatches of overheard conversation and nonverbal communication," she said. "We had a five-year-old here, named Monique, who taught herself to read so that she could have a better sense of what was happening to her. While she was here she got to know another child well, a little boy from Texas, and that child went back home and died there. The little boy's mother wrote Monique's mother a note saying, 'Johnny died in Nov.' Monique got a hold of this letter and not only managed to read it, but she didn't understand what 'Nov.' meant, so she went to the dictionary and looked it up.

"Surprisingly enough, this type of precocious behavior is not uncommon among leukemic children. Since these kids are worked with so intensely and are exposed to all kinds of new stimuli, their reading, writing, and communicating skills are actually accelerated. In this case, the child's need to know was so great, because her life depended on it, that it drove her to this kind of continual monitoring, listening, seeing—a kind of healthy paranoia about her own situation. Negotiating this whole conglomeration of stresses is a maturing experience. As Erik Erikson has said, 'We grow through conflict.' In this situation, the number of stresses and conflicts is enormous. If the leukemic child survives, he has often matured considerably beyond the level of his peers."

Nelson continued along these lines. "When children realize they've been lied to by their parents and doctors, they feel they have been betrayed by the very people they need and trust the most. They also think there must be a reason why we have not told them the truth—that things are worse than they thought, or that the disease is too awful and shameful to talk about. Indeed, most young children experience the illness as a form of

81

punishment for something bad they've done. One young patient told me that he had been sent here because he 'peed too much.' Another said that his mother had gone to the hospital to get a new baby, and that she had brought him back to the hospital in exchange.

"As for older children, they're often in the business of protecting their parents from the very first day, because they know exactly what is going on and are afraid to upset their parents. This leaves the child completely isolated from family and friends, with no one to turn to. When a child, particularly an older child of ten or thirteen, is told the diagnosis, it can defuse a very tense situation. The child can probably live with it a lot better than we can. And discussing the medical facts, although difficult, makes the whole family feel more relaxed and close together and the child less angry and more accepting of treatment. All children respond negatively to dishonesty and lies, so that in the long run, you gain by being honest."

"Some parents are very afraid that we're going to tell the child, 'Tommy, you're going to die,'" Davis went on. "But that isn't it at all. It's presented more factually, stressing what the hopes are. Of course, children of different ages require different degrees of knowledge, but some amount of truth is essential for everyone. A child of four might be told that she has an illness that will last a long time, will get better and worse, and cannot be cured but can be helped by treatment. An eight-year-old can be told that his bone marrow is having trouble making healthy cells. Older children can be told the actual diagnosis.

"Since we see the family of the child with cancer as a unit, the explanation takes place in the presence of the parents and is based on their understanding, ability to convey the information, and willingness to pick up where we left off. It's like sex education: you don't simply list for the child the facts of life. Rather it's a process, a dialogue, that takes place one question at a time. With lots of kids we use less direct techniques such as play therapy or drawing to get their feelings out."

"I think schoolteachers should be given a better understanding of leukemia," Mrs. White said. "Some of Danny's teachers isolated him because they were afraid the disease was catching, or treated him with kid gloves because they were terrified that he was going to keel over and die at any moment."

"People in general are very strange about leukemia," Mrs. Meyers agreed. "They can shy away from your child, or tell their children to do the same. When I first took Chris with me to the shopping center, people stared at him as if he was some kind of freak. I got so angry I wanted to bop them all on the head."

Dr. Nelson nodded. "People just don't know how to react when they see a skinny, bald kid wearing a mask. They may try to say and do the right things, but many times it doesn't come out that way. As far as the fear of contagion is concerned, it's hard to know how much is self-fulfilling: the child expects to be considered contagious and behaves accordingly."

"I think it goes much deeper than that," Mr. Stein objected. "There's a general abhorrence in this society of anything abnormal, crippled, or diseased—anything that doesn't spell Kraft American cheese. School kids taunt the kid who has thick glasses or crutches, and where does it come from? Well, it must come from the parents. Abnormal or different people are not integrated into society; they're cast out as being evil, something to avoid. So you don't help the cripple who falls down on his knees, you just keep on walking. I don't know if it's apathy or rather a fear that the misfortune might touch you in some way."

Mr. Stein paused to catch his breath. He was obviously agitated, extremely intent on what he was saying, and the other parents gave him their undivided attention. "If it were a different society," he went on, "people like Mark would be real heroes. Any patient who has gone through what he has and survived wouldn't be discriminated against but rather admired. It's like the survivors of the Holocaust after the liberation of Poland. Anti-Semitism was worse then than during the German occupation, and they were still killing Jews. So being a survivor doesn't mean anything to some people.

"Of course, if I hadn't been through this experience myself, I'm not sure how sensitized I would be to the problem. If I saw someone on the street with a bald head and purple markings and a mask, how would I react? What would I think? Would I stare? Curiosity is one thing—you can't help being curious. But you have to go beyond that. Because of the public abhorrence of anything abnormal, people are incredibly ignorant about that side of human experience. What about the idea of being old? How sensitive are people to that?"

Everyone around the table seemed moved and saddened by Mr. Stein's outburst. "It's true that children can be terribly cruel," Mrs. White said. "Danny is very afraid of going back to school when his counts come up. He has nightmares and cries when I wake him in the morning. 'They'll laugh at me and make fun of my wig,' he says. He's also afraid that they'll pull off the wig and everyone will see that he's completely bald."

"You should buy him a 'Bald Is Beautiful' T-shirt," Mrs. Jeffries suggested.

"It's not funny," Mr. Meyers objected. "I know what it's like to be teased like that, and it's no fun. I remember when I was a boy, I had my head shaved for a ringworm infection, and there was no end to the abuse."

"Our daughter Robin wore a wig to school," Mr. Jeffries replied, "and she was pleasantly surprised to find that her close friends treated her well and included her in all their games and activities as before. Of course, other children did stare at her, which made her feel uncomfortable and excluded, but she managed to overcome this. For her, the 'Bald Is Beautiful' T-shirt made her feel that everything was out in the open—nothing had to be hidden in shame."

"That's right," Helen Davis said, "it's nothing to be ashamed of. All families have something that makes them different or unique, both in positive and negative ways. One family may have a leukemic child, another may have a child with a handicap or a learning problem, a third may be confronted with a tragic accident. That becomes part of their identity as a family. It's important that you be able to share with the other families here, so that your feeling of separateness from the outside world is coupled with the sense of being alike in this new inside world. The self-isolation felt by families with leukemic children is similar to that experienced by people who have been recently divorced. Their friends treat them differently, and other people may not know what to say or do, for fear of hurting. But you don't have a contagious illness—you don't have to be isolated.

"I think it's particularly important for children to attend school, in spite of the inevitable problems," she went on. "After the prolonged helplessness the child experiences in the hospital, the classroom may be the only area of his life where he feels a sense of achievement and control over his surroundings. Often leukemic children fall behind their peers because they miss so many days of school for checkups, infections, and chicken-pox outbreaks. In such cases it's useful to get home tutoring in conjunction with the school—usually a substitute teacher—who can help the child keep up with his grade and therefore feel less fearful and insecure about returning to school after a long absence."

The discussion continued for several more minutes, covering topics of a more strictly medical nature addressed to Nelson and Fein. Then the meeting ended on a light note. Mrs. White said that she had asked her son Danny if he wanted to be a doctor when he grew up, and he had replied, "No, I don't want to hurt people." Everyone laughed, and as it was after 9:00 P.M., Nelson adjourned the meeting until the following month.

After the doctors had left, several parents remained behind to talk. Mr. Jeffries, a stockbroker, offered Mr. Stein financial advice on how to manage the enormous cost of a planned bone-marrow transplant for his son. Meanwhile, Mrs. Jeffries came up to Sally and introduced herself. "I'm glad you came tonight," she said warmly. "As you could probably tell, all of us here are like members of an exclusive club. We have to support one another, because nobody else can really understand what it's like. When I hear of a kid who's making it, I feel great. It's part of my success, too. We're all in this together."

Sally expressed her admiration for Dr. Nelson, and Mrs. Jeffries agreed. "Our first doctor out on Long Island was extremely patronizing and kept all of the medical information from us," she said. "His attitude was, 'Don't worry about a thing. We're too busy saving your child to talk to you.' We felt we couldn't trust him to tell us the facts, and we had to watch his face to guess what he was really thinking. With Dr. Nelson, though, I feel as if he's giving it to us straight."

After a few minutes, the Murphys excused themselves and took the elevator up to Ellie's room. Although it was comforting to know that there were many other people in the same situation, they still felt very alone with their private agonies. No one could share the fear and vulnerability they felt over the welfare of their own child. And when it came down to it, Ellie was the only one they really cared about.

A few days later, they learned that Billy Gordon had died. They never saw his parents again. Brian was glad he hadn't gotten to know them well.

11 Outpatient

On Thursday, September 28, 1978, twelve days after her admission to the hospital, Ellie was discharged. The intensive chemotherapy had taken its toll: her pale face had broken out in cold sores and her hair was falling out in patches. She was still suffering from diarrhea and stomach cramps, for which Nelson recommended Maalox and Kaopectate. Her platelet count had finally stabilized around 30,000—still very low, but at least above the danger threshold—and her white count was only 1,100, with a marked deficiency of polys. Since polys are the major bacteria-killers among white cells, that meant that Ellie was still highly vulnerable to infection, and Nelson recommended that she avoid crowds and wear a surgical mask whenever she went outside. Once her poly count had reached 1,000, she would be able to play with other children.

Nelson's decision to discharge Ellie did involve a calculated risk of infection, but he felt that the emotional benefits for the child and her family far outweighed it. His philosophy was that leukemic children should be treated on an outpatient basis whenever possible, once they were out of immediate danger. Even if Ellie was not yet in remission, she could be away from the hospital environment much of the time and resume some semblance of a normal life. In addition, having clinic nurses administer Ellie's IV medications would free up a bed on M-5 for an acutely ill patient.

Every Monday, Wednesday, and Friday for the next two months, Ellie would have to come to the Children's Day Hospital on the seventeenth floor of the Memorial Hospital tower for chemotherapy and blood tests; bone-marrow exams would be done once every two weeks during induction, and once every three months thereafter. Sally realized how fortunate it was that they would be able to stay at Barbara's apartment, just a few blocks from the clinic. She didn't know what they would have done otherwise. It would have been impractical and exhausting to commute every day from New Jersey, and they certainly couldn't afford to stay at a New York hotel for two months. She had heard that residential houses for young cancer patients and their families had opened in a few cities with pediatric cancer centers, but no such residence had yet been established in New York.

After the discharge papers had been signed, she and Ellie went directly to Barbara's apartment, where they set up house in the living room. When Barbara came home from work, she and Sally talked and cooked supper together. Although Ellie had always been a finicky eater, the prednisone had the side effect of making her so ravenously hungry that foods she had previously shunned now seemed like delicacies. Barbara and Sally felt free to concoct an exotic supper of mousaka with creamed spinach and rice pilaf. Much to their amusement, Ellie wolfed it down and asked for more.

After dinner, however, she retched repeatedly. In the hospital she had developed the habit of carrying around a plastic mixing bowl in case she felt ill. She would vomit into the bowl, rest, and then continue to play or watch TV. Sally was horrified by this routine, but Ellie merely accepted it. Another constant reminder of the disease was the loss of hair caused by chemotherapy. Ellie had always had beautiful brown hair halfway down her back, and Sally was crushed to see it go. The child would sit on the rug and pull out her hair in clumps, and Sally would get upset and tell her, "Don't do that—don't touch your head. Maybe it will last another day." She had purchased a child's wig, but Ellie hated it and refused to wear it.

The next three days were spent relaxing. Sally put Ellie in the stroller, since the child's legs were still too sore for walking, and took her outside for some fresh air. They stopped on the corner to buy a hot dog from a street vendor, since Ellie was hungry again, and then continued on to Central Park. They passed the model-sailboat pond near Seventy-second Street and Fifth Avenue, and went up to the Alice in Wonderland sculpture. The massive bronze showed Alice standing beside a giant mushroom, surrounded by other famous characters from the book: the Caterpillar, the

Mad Hatter, the White Rabbit, and the Dormouse. As always, the sculpture was aswarm with climbing, jostling, shouting children.

Ignoring the stares of the other mothers, Sally pushed the stroller up to the statue and let Ellie watch for a while. Instead of being entertained, Ellie became whiney and irritable, and Sally suddenly realized that she must feel tremendous frustration at not being able to climb and play like the other children. Feeling guilty and depressed, she wheeled Ellie back to the apartment for her nap.

At ten o'clock Monday morning they were due at the clinic for their first appointment. After breakfast, Sally put Ellie in the stroller and wheeled her down East Sixty-eighth Street to the hospital. Looking down at her child's bloated cheeks and sparse hair, she imagined some little old lady coming up to them and saying, "Oh, what an adorable child! She's really cute. Do you have any more like her at home?" For a moment, Sally didn't know whether to laugh or cry.

Emerging from the elevator on the seventeenth floor, they stopped at the nurses' station and checked in with the receptionist, who gave Sally a slip with a list of the tests that would be done that day. Their first destination was the weigh-in room, where Ellie's height and weight were checked to calculate drug doses, and recorded on a growth grid. Sally appreciated the smiles and cheerfulness of the weigh-in woman.

After weighing, they went to sit in the waiting room, which was already crowded with parents and children of all races: black, white, Hispanic, Oriental. A number of healthy siblings were also present, but the leukemic children could be easily distinguished by their sparse or absent hair and their prednisone-swollen cheeks. Volunteers in pink smocks entertained the young patients, bringing them paints and paper or Play-Doh to work with. To Sally, the sick children seemed remarkably happy and absorbed in their play. One little boy was curled up on a chair beside his mother, dozing, while a bottle of chemotherapy dripped into the IV in his arm. Occasionally a terrible piercing scream would come from the vicinity of the examining rooms, but the children paid no attention; they seemed to know exactly what was going on. The faces of their parents reflected many different emotions: some looked anxious, others depressed, still others resigned or even relaxed.

Sally sat with Ellie and listened to the buzz of conversation. One mother, referring to her little boy in a stroller, said to another, "He's not quite up to par today. He had a lung removed on Friday." Most conversations centered around the clinic: the relative merits of various attendings, residents, and nurses, and how other children were doing. Two mothers were talking about one child who had not shown up for his scheduled appointment, speculating out loud about what could have happened to him. Had he relapsed and gone back to M-5? Had he perhaps died at home?

Sally felt uneasy and alone, surrounded by strangers whose only common bond was their enormous misfortune. The bustle of the clinic was more impersonal than the slow-motion world of the ward, and Sally did not recognize any of the doctors and nurses. She encouraged Ellie to play with some of the other children, but Ellie was not feeling particularly gregarious. Fearful and shy, she clung to her mother's arm with no intention of letting go.

After what felt like an hour's wait, the receptionist called their name and a nurse directed them into one of the small examining rooms along the corridor. A few minutes later a technician came in to do a finger-stick. By this time, Ellie had learned to warm up her fingers by rubbing her hands together, bringing the blood to the surface so that it would flow more easily. "That's right, warm them up," Sally coached her. "Put them under your armpits, Ellie."

The child closed her eyes but did not utter a sound as her finger was jabbed. The technician took up the blood in a thin capillary tube and then placed a square of gauze on Ellie's fingertip to staunch the flow of blood. Ellie lifted up the gauze and stared at her finger in fascination. "Look at all the blood," she said.

"Hold it tight," Sally told her.

When the bleeding had stopped, the technician covered the tiny cut with a Band-Aid and left. A few minutes later Dr. Nelson came in, and Sally was relieved to see him.

"Hello, Ellie," the doctor said. "The weigh-in lady tells me that you've put on four pounds since last week. You must be eating up a storm."

"Oh, she is," Sally said wearily. "I'm beginning to feel like a short-order cook."

Nelson smiled. "It's the prednisone that does it. I'm afraid there's not much we can do, other than keep her on a low-calorie diet. Okay, Ellie, let's have a look at you."

The child was irritable and slightly flushed, although her lips and gums were pale. Old bruises were scattered on her lower arms and legs but there were no new ones. Her abdomen was soft and no longer sensitive and her lymph nodes and spleen had shrunk back to normal size. Her liver, however, was still swollen, extending four centimeters below her right rib-cage.

Nelson checked Ellie's ears, nose, and throat for signs of infection. One eardrum was slightly thickened, but everything else looked normal. Using swabs, he took specimens of her saliva and nasal mucus for culture. The

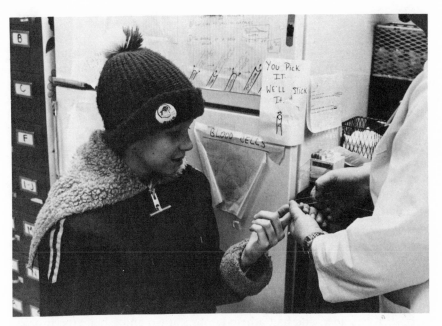

A finger-stick to obtain a drop of blood for cell counts and blood smears is done every time a leukemic child in remission comes to the outpatient clinic for a checkup. *Photo courtesy of the American Cancer Society.*

inside of her mouth showed none of the common side effects of chemotherapy: painful ulcers, bleeding gums, or a white-coated tongue (a fungal infection called "thrush"). With a lighted ophthalmoscope, Nelson peered into Ellie's eyes, telling her to stare straight ahead while he shone the beam at the back of each eyeball. Her optic disks looked sharp, a sign that her central nervous system had still not been invaded by leukemic cells.

Next the doctor took out a key and scratched it lightly across the bottom of Ellie's foot. The child's toes curled downward—a negative Babinski's sign. If they had curled upward, that would have indicated a brain lesion of some kind. He then tested Ellie's deep-tendon reflexes by tapping the tendon just below her knee with a rubber hammer. There was no response in either leg, indicating vincristine toxicity to her peripheral nerves.

Finally Nelson did a couple of coordination tests. He asked Ellie to touch his finger with her finger, then touch her nose, and touch his finger again, repeating this sequence several times with both hands. She became confused and laughed. "You must think I'm crazy, right?" Nelson asked. "Okay, very good."

He picked her up and lowered her down to the floor. "Ellie, let's see if you can walk in a straight line along one of those cracks in the floor. Walk toward Mommy, that's right. Very good. I know some big people who can't do that so well. Now I want to test your balance. I want you to put your hands out in front of you and close your eyes and keep them closed. I won't let you fall, don't worry. Very good, you pass." Nelson turned to Sally. "She's all done now. Can you think of any other problems she's had?"

"She did tell me she's had a few headaches, but I didn't give her anything for it."

"Where did your head hurt, Ellie?" Nelson asked, but the child merely shrugged.

"I don't think it's anything," he said. "I could see by looking at her eyes that her intracranial pressure is fine."

"Thank you, doctor. Should we wait outside for the counts now?"

"Yes. I'll call you when they're ready."

They waited for another ten minutes, until the blood sample had been run through the cell counter and the smears had been stained and examined. Nelson came out with the results and said that Ellie's counts were still very low: she had a hemoglobin of 6.6 and a hematocrit of 20 percent, both less than half normal, and her white count was 1,300 with few polys in the differential.

Sally was upset by the counts. "The fact that her counts are taking so long to come back—is that a bad sign?" she asked Nelson.

"No, some kids just have a more fragile bone marrow that takes a long time to recover after chemotherapy. But I don't think anything else is going on, if that's what you mean. The only problem is that if her counts continue to stay down, we may have to hold her chemotherapy until they come up again."

"That's why I'm worried," Sally said. "I just hope her counts come back."

"I think it's natural to worry," Nelson replied. "There's something to worry about, anyhow. But I think it's just because she has a fragile bone marrow."

Sally looked down at her child with feigned annoyance. "You would!" she said. "But I love you anyway."

"I'll give her the L-asparaginase today and a transfusion of packed red cells for her anemia, and then we'll play it by ear," Nelson said. "You should continue her daily prednisone tablets, and I'll see her again on October third. If her counts don't recover soon, we may have to re-admit her."

"Oh, God, I hope not," Sally said.

By October 3, Ellie's counts had risen modestly, and Nelson felt it was safe for her to receive her vincristine injection, which was given by "IV-push." A clinic nurse administered the drug. By this time Ellie had become quite cooperative during blood tests and chemotherapy, extending her arm when asked to. The nurse inserted a butterfly needle into one of the few good veins left in the child's arm, succeeding on the second attempt. She made sure there was a good backflow of blood into the syringe and then slowly injected the drug over a period of two minutes, talking to Ellie to distract her from the pain. By now Ellie was a veteran and did not cry or even flinch.

A routine was soon established. Barbara would leave the apartment early in the morning, before Sally and Ellie got up. The two of them would awaken by nine, eat breakfast, and then go down to the clinic for Ellie's ten o'clock appointment. On Tuesdays and Thursdays they went for walks in the park or just stayed in the apartment and rested. In the evenings Brian would visit, along with other friends and relatives. Although Ellie was not very responsive to visitors, she did enjoy playing with the toys and dolls they invariably brought with them.

After several visits to the clinic, Ellie began to feel more relaxed in the waiting room and ventured out to meet some of the other children. One little girl named Leslie was Ellie's age but had a high-risk type of ALL that had spread to her spinal cord. She was on a different set of medications and her prognosis was not good. Although she and Ellie were both lethargic and said little to each other, they seemed to share a basic understanding, the bond of a common painful experience. Ellie came to look forward to her clinic visit so that she could play with Leslie. Sally also got to know Leslie's mother, although it was hard for her to talk to a parent whose child was not doing well. She felt fortunate that Ellie's prognosis was so much better, and yet at the same time felt terribly guilty.

By October 8, the twenty-third day of induction, Ellie's appetite was ravenous. Her hair had continued to thin, and she still had diarrhea. The vincristine was causing pain and weakness in her hands and legs, so that she had trouble walking or even lifting a fork. Once Sally accidentally struck Ellie's hand, and the child cried out.

Her drug-induced hunger pangs were also becoming more intense. She had hated the food at the hospital, but now that her mother and aunt were cooking for her she demanded to be fed almost continually. There was no arguing with her: she would shout, "I want food!" and cry if she didn't get it immediately.

Sally could not believe how much Ellie ate. When they were at the apartment, it seemed to Sally that she never left the kitchen. For breakfast every morning Ellie had four eggs with several pieces of buttered toast and two large bowls of cereal. When they went to the hospital, Sally had to pack two bag lunches for Ellie—one for before her appointment, the other for after—and between meals the child was continually nibbling on highly salted junk foods such as DooDads, a mixture of crackers, pretzels, and peanuts that she had become addicted to. When they got back to the apartment, the child could easily consume a family-sized can of ravioli as a snack, and by suppertime she would be ravenous again. Between the fluid retention caused by the prednisone and Ellie's incessant bingeing, she was rapidly getting fat.

The prednisone also caused dramatic swings in her mood, causing her to become even more irritable and demanding than usual. Although Sally often felt guilty about disciplining the child when her bad behavior might be due in part to the drugs, she refused to let Ellie become spoiled and continued to treat her as strictly as she always had. When Ellie was being obnoxious, Sally would tell her so and if necessary shout at her or send her out of the room. It was often very difficult not to give in when Ellie looked so sick and frail, but Sally knew that she was acting in her child's best interests.

From October 9 to October 13, there was a brief interlude between cycles of chemotherapy, and at Ellie's Monday morning checkup Nelson said that she could go home to Menlo Park for the first time since her treatment had begun, nearly a month before. Sally called Brian, and he agreed to drive in and pick them up.

When they got home to New Jersey, Brian carried Ellie from the car into the house and set her down on the living room couch. She sat there lethargically like a diminutive Buddha, only instead of a look of religious bliss her face was twisted in an unhappy grimace. Brian's parents were there, and Sally's sister, Lynn, who had flown in from Chicago for a week. They tried to be cheerful, but Ellie looked awful and Brian and Sally were very anxious about her.

The responsibility of caring for her desperately ill child overwhelmed Sally. As long as they had been at Barbara's apartment, with the hospital just a few blocks away and a registered nurse in residence, Sally had been fairly secure about coping with possible crises. But now she felt totally unprepared, and her mind filled with horrific fantasies of all the things that might go wrong. Once during Ellie's hospitalization her platelets had dropped below 20,000 and she had developed a severe nosebleed in her sleep. By the time a nurse discovered it, her pillow was soaked with blood and an emergency transfusion had to be ordered. What if something like that happened now?

When Beth came home from playing and saw her sister, she was astonished. She stared at Ellie for a moment and then ran outside to round up several of her neighborhood friends. They all trooped into the living room and gathered in a semicircle around Ellie.

"What happened to her hair?" one girl asked.

"The medicine did it," Sally replied. "I'm sorry, kids, I'm afraid you'll have to leave now," she said, shepherding them all out the front door. As they left, Beth explained authoritatively, "You see, they rubbed medicine on her head and it made all her hair fall out."

When Beth came back in, she was whiney and demanding. "Mommy, can I get a haircut like Ellie, too?" she asked, continuing to pester her mother until Sally finally agreed to give her a pixie cut. For Beth it was a matter of principle: she wanted everything that Ellie was getting. She felt neglected by her mother, whom she had not seen in three weeks, and she was intensely jealous of all the attention and presents Ellie was getting. From her perspective, the illness looked like a joyride: you went to New York with Mommy for a long time and came back with lots of toys. "Gee, I wish I could go to the hospital so I could get presents," she kept saying. Sally made a concerted effort to give Beth the attention she demanded; it was almost a repeat of the "new baby syndrome."

That afternoon, Sally sat down with Beth and told her about the disease. "Ellie has a problem with her blood," she explained to the now worried child. "There's a possibility that what Ellie has could get worse. But maybe if we pray real hard and have faith, she'll get better."

"What's the matter with her?" Beth asked, starting to cry.

"She has a problem with her bone marrow, which makes the blood. You know, Beth, swimming around in your blood are millions of tiny cells that do different things for your body. The white cells are like white knights that fight off the bad germs when you catch a cold. The platelets are little tiny cells that stop you from bleeding when you cut yourself; they all rush to the hole in your skin and plug it up, so no more blood runs out, like the little Dutch boy and the dike. The red cells give you energy, so when you're feeling good and your cheeks are red, it's because the red cells are there. The problem is that Ellie's bone marrow isn't making enough of these good cells because she has little bugs in her blood. So she has to get medicines to get rid of the bugs and let her good cells grow. But the medicines will make her feel sick before she gets better. So you should treat her very gently because she isn't as healthy as she should be. You shouldn't jump on her or hug her tight or play rough with her right now, and she can't run because her legs are sore."

"Can I hit her back if she hits me?"

"No, Beth, you can't."

Although Beth was upset that her sister was sick and might die, she remained acutely aware of the fact that Ellie was getting special treatment. She also felt a pang of guilt—had she done something to make Ellie sick? Many times she had wished that something bad would happen to her younger sister, even that Ellie would die so that Beth would have her parents all to herself. Now she was afraid that her wish was coming true, and when her parents found out they would never forgive her.

Cindy Lewis came by later on that afternoon, bearing a tray of cupcakes. She was prepared for Ellie not to look good, but it still came as a shock to see her so bloated and lethargic, with large patches of hair missing. Cindy did not want to intrude on what appeared to be a family gathering, but she did talk to Sally for a few minutes and heard some anecdotes about the hospital.

"My God," she murmured. "I could never handle that."

"Cindy, nobody asks you if you can handle it," Sally replied wearily. "You just handle it."

That evening, Sally asked Ellie what she wanted for supper, and Ellie said that she wanted steak. Since it was a special occasion, Sally decided to humor her and took her along to the supermarket to do the shopping. Ellie had always been able to squeeze into the back seat of the car without pulling the front seat forward, but now she could not fit. "Mommy, you'd better move the seat," she said. "I'm getting too fat and I can't get through."

In spite of the fact that Ellie hated being fat, she could not stop eating and was chewing on crackers all the way to the store. When they arrived, Sally told her, "If you promise to leave your food in the car, we'll buy you some more."

Sally bought a small cut of sirloin that she thought Ellie and Brian could split. As it turned out, Ellie ate the entire piece of meat, along with a large baked potato, two vegetables, a salad, and milk, not to mention the large helping of salad that she ate while Sally was preparing the meal. Just when Sally had finished washing the dishes and putting them away, Ellie came into the kitchen and announced, "I'm hungry."

"You've got to be kidding," Sally said. "You can't be hungry."

"Yes, I am. Can I have a baloney sandwich?"

When Ellie insisted, Sally finally gave in, although she could tell that Beth was upset by all the special meals her sister was getting.

That night, Sally was unable to sleep without Ellie. Finally she asked Brian to sleep on the couch in the living room and put Ellie in the bed beside her. Much to her relief, the night passed uneventfully.

Barbara took advantage of the five days Ellie and Sally were away to let off some emotional steam. The night they left, she spent some time alone in her apartment. She poured herself a drink, put on some sad violin music, and had a good cry, releasing some of her stored-up grief and tension.

Over the next few days, Ellie's continual eating became irritating to her parents because she was becoming so fat. She had developed a moon face and a swollen belly, in grotesque contrast to her matchstick arms and legs, and her face had become so puffy that her eyes were mere slits and all the capillaries in her cheeks were broken. Her body contour had changed so radically that Sally was forced to buy her a new wardrobe, shocked to discover that the child had gone from a 4-Toddlers to 5-Chubbies in the space of a month. With a trace of black humor, Sally thought she looked like Humpty Dumpty.

Things came to a head on Ellie's third day home, October 11, when she devoured an entire large jar of dill pickles that was in the refrigerator. She then began to eat a jar of peanut butter and was halfway through it when Brian discovered her and decided to tape the refrigerator door shut.

Sally worried that the high salt content of the pickles might disrupt Ellie's already fragile bowels, and indeed the child's diarrhea soon worsened. Ellie was growing paler as well, and Sally's nervousness intensified. She called Dr. Nelson and asked if he would see them. He agreed, and Sally and Lynn drove Ellie into the city. When Nelson saw the child at the clinic he shook his head. "My God, Ellie," he said. "You look like you're going to burst."

He examined her. The child's abdomen was protuberant because of her obesity, but her liver had decreased in size and her spleen was no longer palpable. Her gait was still abnormal and her deep-tendon reflexes remained absent. Finding nothing acutely wrong, Nelson prescribed a new medication for her diarrhea.

Over the next two days, Ellie's symptoms improved. On October 13—the twenty-eighth and final day of the induction protocol—they went back to the clinic for a bone-marrow exam. Ellie protested when Sally told her that morning that she would be getting a "bow-and-arrow." Although she was brave about chemotherapy and blood tests, she had never adjusted to the idea of getting stuck in the back. Not being able to see what was going on made the procedure much more painful and frightening than it otherwise would have been. When the finger-stick had been done, Barbara arrived on the floor and accompanied Ellie, squirming and fighting, into the treatment room.

Nelson first did an aspiration and made a set of marrow smears. He then performed a bone-marrow biopsy, inserting a large-bore needle into the marrow space and cutting out a centimeter-long core of bone and tissue, which he removed and placed in a vial of formalin. The biopsy specimen would be sent to Special Pathology for fixation, sectioning, and microscopic examination, and it would take about forty-eight hours to get the results. Whereas the smears provided a quick view of the various types of cells growing in the marrow, the biopsy specimen would reveal the intact architecture of the marrow: the numerous spicules—clusters of blood-cell precursors in various stages of maturation—interspersed with large globules of fat. A biopsy specimen was therefore preferable for determining the marrow's cellularity: the populations of the different blood-cell lines.

After fifteen minutes, Ellie emerged from the treatment room angry and sullen, her cheeks stained with tears. Nelson went off to examine the slides, leaving Sally and Barbara to wait for the results. The minutes dragged by like hours.

Finally Nelson returned, a reassuring smile on his face. "I have good news," he said. "Ellie is in remission. Her marrow is still sparse, but there are no blasts—not even a hint of anything suspicious."

"That's wonderful!" Sally exclaimed, enormously relieved and happy. But Nelson cautioned that the battle had just begun: a remission was not yet a cure, and additional treatments would be necessary for some time yet. First, Ellie would have to receive a special therapy designed to prevent the spread of the disease to her central nervous system.

"Even though no blasts seem to be left in Ellie's bone marrow, they may still be lurking somewhere else in her body," Nelson explained. "Leukemic cells can infiltrate almost every tissue, and a few cells, hidden away in a poorly perfused part of an organ, usually manage to escape being destroyed by antileukemic drugs in the bloodstream. The protected sites are called 'drug sanctuaries,' and include the testes and the central nervous system. These are the places where a relapse of leukemia is most likely to occur."

Nelson went on to explain that the brain and spinal cord provide a particularly favorable breeding ground for leukemic cells. The reason is that the central nervous system is isolated from the circulating blood by a filtration system known as the "blood-brain barrier," which serves to protect the delicate chemical systems of the brain and spinal cord from toxic substances in the blood. Unfortunately, this system also prevents most antileukemic drugs from entering the CNS. As a result, the meninges—the three protective membranes sheathing the brain and spinal cord within which the cerebrospinal fluid circulates—provide a protected environment where leukemic cells that have migrated out of the cerebral blood vessels can proliferate, unimpeded by drugs.

"In order to eliminate such leukemic infiltrates even before they can be detected," Nelson continued, "the cooperative groups have developed a therapeutic regimen known as 'CNS prophylaxis,' which involves injecting the drug methotrexate intrathecally—into the cerebrospinal fluid—and giving radiation to the brain. This approach has been very successful in reducing the incidence of CNS leukemia, which until recently was the major cause of relapse in children with ALL. In the past few months, though, there has been some controversy about the long-term effects of this therapy."

Nelson explained that a few recent studies had indicated that almost every child who received cranial irradiation and intrathecal methotrexate developed some permanent intellectual impairment as a result. The manifestations were usually subtle and revealed only by psychological testing, but indications of lowered IQ were more evident in young children. One study had found that 45 percent of children who received treatment before the age of eight showed significant intellectual impairments years later: short-term memory loss, reduced ability to concentrate, and a decrease in fine motor skills. About 10 percent had developed serious disorders, such as uncoordination or seizures.

Although Nelson was disturbed by the evidence that CNS prophylaxis produced marked intellectual impairment in some younger children, he felt that there should not be any hesitation in using aggressive treatment when it was essential for cure. If by doing CNS prophylaxis they had gained an increasing number of children who would survive the disease, then they were balancing the evil of long-term toxicity against a much greater one. Still, the cooperative groups should not just rest on their laurels and put up with the adverse effects of their protocols; they had to keep searching for ways to control the disease with less extreme remedies. In a few years, one out of every thousand people aged twenty would be a cured cancer patient, so there was an urgent need to make sure that the treatment these children received today would have as few harmful effects as possible on their future lives. That was why CCSG and the other groups were developing protocols that reserved intensive therapy, with its associated risks, to children with poor prognostic forms of leukemia. For example, CCSG Protocol 161, designed for children with relatively low white counts at diagnosis, used intrathecal methotrexate alone—without cranial irradiation—to prevent CNS leukemia. Since Ellie had the average-risk type of ALL, however, Nelson was convinced that both methotrexate and radiation would be necessary to prevent the complication. "Until we come up with a safer way of doing things," he concluded, "this treatment is the best we have."

Sally dreaded the possibility of more side effects, but she had also grown inured to the constant trade-offs involved in cancer therapy. As long as the treatment would prolong Ellie's life and prevent the leukemia cells from invading her brain, they would live with it and take their chances. She and Brian were gamblers at heart, anyway, and the whole thing had been like one big gamble.

Sally went to call Brian at his office to give him the news of Ellie's remission and the next phase of treatment. Meanwhile, Barbara stayed with Ellie while Nelson did the spinal tap. After he had drawn off a sample of spinal fluid for analysis and culture, the doctor filled a syringe with bright yellow methotrexate solution and attached it to the open needle. He first drew some more cerebrospinal fluid into the syringe in order to dilute the drug and then injected it slowly into Ellie's back.

When the procedure was over, Nelson met with Sally and told her that Ellie would be getting three more intrathecal injections of methotrexate over the next four weeks, concurrent with her radiation treatments. Before Ellie could begin her radiotherapy, however, she would have to be taken off prednisone. Since prolonged administration of prednisone induced a state of physical dependence, the dose of the drug would have to be reduced gradually over the next eight days to allow the body to adapt to its absence, a process called "tapering."

Every other day, Nelson instructed, Ellie's dose of prednisone should be divided in half. Since the full dose was 40 milligrams, that meant she should only take 20 milligrams on each of the first two days of tapering, 10 milligrams on the second two days, 5 milligrams on the third two days, and 2.5 milligrams on the last two days. The doctor recommended that Sally use a wall calendar to keep track, since it was easy to get confused. He also set up an appointment for Ellie on October 24 with Dr. Beatrice Gerson, a radiation therapist at Memorial who specialized in the treatment of leukemic children.

12 Radiation

The week of tapering passed uneventfully, except for a few episodes of nausea and vomiting, and on October 24 Sally took Ellie to the Radiation Therapy Department on the second floor of the hospital. Signs directed them to a large waiting room with blue vinyl chairs and bland landscape paintings on the walls. Sally put their appointment slip and red hospital charge card in the box near the reception desk and sat down to wait, holding Ellie in her lap. It seemed they were always waiting these days. What a waste of time, when every minute was so precious!

Sally looked around her. Nearly all of the waiting patients were middle-aged or elderly and accompanied by their spouses; many had a look of puzzled resignation that Sally found depressing. When the man on her right was called for therapy, she struck up a conversation with his wife, who seemed preoccupied but was eager to talk. After they had exchanged a few pleasantries, the woman suddenly announced that her husband had incurable lung cancer and had been given only a few more weeks to live. He had not been informed of his prognosis, and she was agonizing over whether to tell him. This revelation stunned Sally but she tried not to react. When the couple finally left, she resolved not to get involved in any more "casual" conversations.

Meanwhile, Ellie napped peacefully in Sally's arms. Farther down the row of seats, a little boy had arrived with his mother. He looked unusually healthy and energetic, although it was clear from his sparse hair that he was undergoing treatment for some form of cancer. His mother gave him a rubber ball and he began playing catch with himself, tossing the ball up and down on the floor in front of his mother's chair. Sally watched him for a while, enjoying his happy smile, in such contrast to the glum faces of the adults around him. Suddenly the boy missed a catch and the ball rolled across the carpet and bounced off the foot of an elderly patient. "Stop that!" the man snapped, and the little boy ran weeping to his mother. Sally was furious at the old man. Although she realized that he was probably in pain and irritable, the sight of a child acting healthy and normal should have brought him some joy instead of annoying him.

As the long minutes passed, Sally's anxiety grew. She had been told that the radiation treatments were important, but she was still terrified of those invisible, deadly rays that could wreak such havoc on the human body. It seemed starkly ironic that they were using radiation to treat leukemia when the aftermath of Hiroshima had shown so clearly that radiation could induce the disease. Indeed, the whole idea of radiation was inextricably caught up in Sally's mind with the terror of the atom bomb, the undercurrent of fear that had been the backdrop of her Sixties adolescence. Sally also worried that the radiation would do Ellie some permanent damage, such as preventing her from having children. It was perhaps silly to worry about that now, when Ellie was still a child herself, but the prospect of her growing up without even the option of children haunted Sally.

Finally Ellie's name was called. Sally, carrying the child in her arms, followed the orderly into the therapy area. In an open space, three patients on stretchers awaited their treatments. The rest of the room was taken up by the receptionist's desk and several small cubicles, marked off by low partitions, containing the control panels for the radiation machines. Along the far wall were the massive lead-shielded doors of the radiotherapy rooms. Yellow-and-red warning signs shouted CAUTION HIGH RADIATION AREA.

Sally's anguish was building as Dr. Gerson walked up and introduced herself. She was a pleasant woman in her late forties with graying hair pulled back into a bun and a warm, toothy smile. Very few cancer hospitals treated enough leukemic children to justify employing a specialist like Gerson, but Memorial did; Nelson had told Sally that Gerson usually had between fifteen and twenty leukemic children in her care at any one time. She had begun her career as a radiotherapist working primarily with adults, but her interest shifted to the radiotherapy of childhood leukemia in the early 1960s when, largely because of the conquest of the major infectious diseases of childhood, acute leukemia became the leading cause of nonaccidental death in the industrialized West for children between the ages of two and fifteen.

Detecting Sally's anxiety, Gerson gave her an explanatory tour of Treatment Room 242, which had just been vacated. The room was dominated by the massive radiation machine, a Theratron 80 with a cobalt-60 source. Large plastic representations of Dumbo, Donald Duck, and Mickey Mouse had been hung on the back wall in a well-intentioned effort to make the room slightly less intimidating; another wall was lined with shelves displaying dozens of plastic molds of patients' heads. Gerson explained that the molds were used to hold the patient perfectly still during focal radiotherapy of tumors of the head and neck.

Gerson then showed Sally and Ellie the console that controlled the machine. Calibrated dials indicated treatment time, dose rate (in rads per minute), and the orientation of the machine along two axes. Gerson also demonstrated the closed-circuit TV monitor and intercom that Sally would use to watch and talk to Ellie during the session.

"Ellie will be getting treatments every weekday afternoon at this time for the next two weeks," Gerson said. "During each session she will receive an exposure to each side of her head for a total of 200 rads. Each exposure takes only a few minutes."

"What's a rad?" Sally asked, while Ellie stared at the TV monitors.

"It's a unit of radiation exposure. One rad is approximately equal to the amount of radiation you're exposed to by a dental X-ray."

"Will Ellie be sedated during the procedure?" Sally asked. "I doubt she'll be too cooperative."

"I can sedate her, but only if you insist," Gerson replied. "I generally prefer not to. It's not too good for a child to be groggy for two weeks, not eating well and not being active. You'll be happier taking her home awake rather than asleep."

"But what if she moves when she shouldn't?"

"I'll explain to her the importance of staying still, and you should talk to her continuously over the intercom while she's in there, so she won't panic. In any case, the technician will watch closely on the monitor, and if she moves at all he'll turn off the beam immediately."

"All right," Sally said. "It's worth a try." She felt relieved; the radiation was not as frightening as she had expected.

They went back into the treatment room, where a nurse and a technician were setting up. There was a high-pitched whirring sound as the machine rotated into position over the table. The nurse picked Ellie up and placed her down on the table on her left side, with her head resting on a cushioned lead block. Although Sally held her hand, Ellie was terrified and began to cry. The machine loomed above her with its black gaping mouth, looking like a sea monster about to swallow her up.

The room lights were dimmed and a set of cross hairs was projected from the machine onto the side of Ellie's head. While the nurse tied the child's head down to the table with a wide band of elastic material, the technician arranged some lead blocks on a clear plastic shelf beneath the radiation source. The blocks cast sharp shadows, indicating the shielding pattern that would protect Ellie's eyes and face from the beam. If her eyes were exposed to too much radiation, the lenses could eventually turn opaque, causing cataracts.

"You're a good girl, Ellie," the nurse was saying, trying to comfort the screaming child. "It's not necessary to cry. Mommy's going to talk to you on the intercom. Remember, you've got to hold nice and still. Then when it's all done we'll give you a lollipop."

The nurse wound up a carousel music-box, which she set down on the table so that the child could see it. "Okay, Ellie, watch the carousel," she said. "We have to go bye-bye now, but only for a little while." The music-box tinkled sweetly, almost drowned out by Ellie's howls.

Everyone quickly left the room. The massive shielded door with its tiny window slid shut, and the warning light above it changed from green to red. Standing at the console, Sally anxiously watched her daughter on the TV monitor. Ellie looked very tiny and frail under the giant machine. She was still crying, but at least she did not move.

"You be a good girl and behave yourself, Ellie," Sally said into the intercom. "Mommy's in the next room, watching you on TV. What would your friends think if they knew you were on television? Stay nice and still, okay? It will be over in a few minutes." Sally was grateful that she could

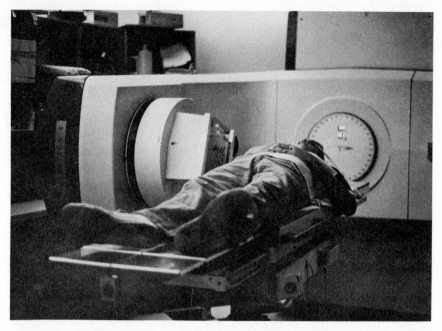

Radiation to the brain in order to prevent the multiplication of leukemic cells in the central nervous system, which is largely inaccessible to antileukemic drugs, has long been an essential component of therapy for ALL. The radiation, from a cobalt-60 source, is usually done in conjunction with injections of methotrexate into the spinal fluid. *Photo by Jonathan B. Tucker.*

talk to Ellie during the session. Her active participation served to lessen somewhat her lingering feelings of powerlessness and guilt.

After about five minutes, the machine was switched off and Ellie was turned over on her right side. The nurse rewound the carousel and the process was repeated. When the second exposure was over and the huge door slid back, Sally rushed in and held her daughter close until the child's sobbing subsided. Then the nurse offered Ellie her choice of a bunch of lollipops. "Which one do you want? Cherry? Okay. Bye now, Ellie. See you tomorrow."

"Say, 'bye,'" Sally coached. "Blow the nice nurse a kiss."

The child stuck out her tongue and grimaced. Everyone laughed, except Ellie.

Over the next two weeks, Sally took Ellie to the Day Hospital each morning for her medication and blood work and then to Radiation Therapy after lunch. Although Ellie was scheduled for a 1:00 P.M. appointment, the radiation session usually consumed most of the afternoon. Some problem would always arise: the machine would break down, another patient would be late, or Ellie would not cooperate. The tension of waiting was sometimes unbearable, and Sally began to count down the days.

By the end of the first week, Ellie's terror of the procedure had diminished, although she still complained about it. As predicted, the radiation caused the rest of her hair to fall out. The apartment was soon littered with clumps of light-brown hair like those of a shedding cat, and Barbara would find strands of hair clinging to food in the refrigerator or mixed up in the mayonnaise.

When the grandparents heard about the details of the radiotherapy, they were appalled. They felt the disease was hopeless and that putting a child through this torture was a crime. "Why do all this?" Brian's mother kept asking. But Sally saw it all differently. For her, anything that might work was worth trying, and nothing was too much if it gave some hope that Ellie would be with them for a few more days. She got very angry at parents who refused to give their child the best therapies modern medicine could offer, resorting instead to faith healing and quack cures. As long as any hope remained, she felt that she and Brian were morally obligated to keep Ellie in treatment.

On Monday, November 6, Ellie received her last dose of radiation. Beyond a few episodes of nausea, she had not suffered any skin burns or other immediate side effects from the radiation treatments. Nonetheless, Nelson prescribed a two-week rest period to make sure she did not develop any delayed symptoms. During this period, Ellie was allowed to return home to Menlo Park.

The child was now entirely bald, with only a few fine strands of baby hair clinging to her blue-veined scalp. The complete loss of hair disturbed her: that afternoon she appeared in the living room of Barbara's apartment with a towel draped around her head and said to her mother, "See my beautiful hair. See my long hair." She was also preoccupied with fears of injury, insisting on a Band-Aid for the tiniest scratch.

Although Sally had hoped that life would return to near normal soon after their arrival home, Ellie continued to have behavior problems. She followed her mother around the house wherever she went, demanding Sally's constant attention and becoming enraged when anyone infringed on it, including Beth. Ellie was impatient and demanding, and her feelings could be hurt very easily: if Sally said something to her in the wrong tone of voice she would start to cry. She had also become very selfish about her possessions. Whereas before the illness she had been a generous child, she now screamed, "Mine!" if Beth touched one of her toys.

The day-to-day strain culminated in a full-blown tantrum over a beautiful doll that Barbara had given Ellie before she went home. After much deliberation, Ellie had decided to leave it at Barbara's apartment so that she would have something to play with on future visits. But a few days later she regretted her decision and insisted that her mother drive back into the city and pick it up. "Mommy, I want my doll!" she whined.

"Honey, you have to accept the fact that the doll's there," Sally replied patiently. "Aunt Barbara said she'd take good care of it for you."

Ellie stamped her foot and frowned. "Well, I want it now!"

"I think you should go to your room."

"NO!" Ellie howled, and began to cry.

"Okay, that's enough of that. The next fresh word out of you is going to require a spanking."

"I want my doll!"

"I guess Aunt Barbara should never buy anything for you anymore, so we don't have to go through this. You're the one who made the decision to leave it there."

"No! I left it 'cause you said to."

"I did not say that."

"Yes, you did!" Ellie insisted tearfully. "You said, 'Put it back.'" Sobbing, she threw herself on the floor.

Sally let her lie there. "No, you never asked me," she said. "Come on, honey, be a good girl."

"Mommy, come here!" Ellie sobbed, wanting to be comforted.

"What do you want me to do?" Sally asked, exasperated.

"Nothing!" Ellie shouted. She got up and ran off to her room, slamming the door behind her.

Sally hoped that Ellie's bad behavior was her way of reasserting control over her environment after feeling helpless and victimized for so long in the hospital, and that it was a passing phase. Although Sally was sometimes tempted to give in just so that Ellie would stop her tantrum, she knew that children, sick or well, require limits to feel secure and loved, and that she would not be doing Ellie any favors by satisfying her every whim. "It isn't fair to Ellie," she told herself. "Whatever happens, she has to live like a normal child." When visitors came over, Sally asked them not to make a special fuss over her.

It came as a shock when Sally discovered that Brian was working at cross-purposes. Doubtless guilty about his infrequent visits to the hospital while Ellie was an inpatient, he overloaded the child with toys and gifts and caved in to her every demand—however outrageous—even a late-night request for an ice-cream sundae. From his perspective, Ellie could be dead in a few weeks for all they knew, and he certainly wasn't going to deprive her of anything she wanted. He hoped to make up for all of her suffering by making her as happy as possible.

But Ellie wanted the impossible—for her sickness and pain to go away—and as a result, no gift or indulgence was enough to satisfy her. Sally could see that Brian's special treatment and coddling were just making Ellie more selfish and demanding, and Beth more jealous and resentful. Increasingly, the Murphys argued over how best to handle Ellie.

Beth, for her part, remained confused and frightened about this strange illness that continued to cast a shadow over their lives, even now that Ellie had returned from the hospital. Beth was angry at her mother for deserting her and at her sister for stealing away her parents' love and affection; yet at the same time she feared that her anger might have precipitated the illness in the first place. Fearing retribution in the form of getting sick herself, she was troubled by doubts about her own health. There was also the guilt she felt about being active and playing outside while her sister was weak, nauseated, and confined to the house, unable to play with other children.

For the first few days, Beth treated Ellie with distanced respect, unsure if her sister was really sick or well. Then they had their first quarrel—over whether Beth had the right to play with Ellie's new toys—and the ice was broken. Although Beth knew that she was not allowed to hit her sister, they had frequent verbal battles. But in spite of their intense rivalry, Beth clearly cared for Ellie, since she always came to her sister's defense when other children made fun of her.

It was already the week before Thanksgiving. Every Thanksgiving Day since the Murphys had moved to New Jersey, Sally had prepared a turkey dinner for a large gathering of relatives and friends. This year everyone assumed that someone else would be giving the party, but Sally insisted on planning for the banquet as she always had. It was therapeutic in the sense that it forced her back into some semblance of her normal routine.

A few days after their return home, Sally went shopping for a turkey at the A & P. She was pushing her cart down the aisle when she caught sight of her neighbor Lois Clark, who had sent over a little stuffed animal for Ellie. Sally started to thank her for the gift, but Lois suddenly put her hands up in front of her face. "I can't even look at you," she said. "I feel so awful, I don't know what to say. Is everything okay?"

"So-so," Sally replied. She knew that Lois wanted to hear that things were fine, but who was she to go around consoling other people? She was aware that several of their friends had been reluctant to call or confront them, either out of fear of invading their privacy or due to anxieties of their own. The people who provided the greatest support, like Cindy Lewis and her husband, Dan, were those who treated them spontaneously and naturally, providing tangible help and understanding rather than useless words of sympathy or advice. A cooked supper in the refrigerator or an offer to baby-sit was worth a hundred condolence letters.

In spite of the daily tensions in the family, Thanksgiving dinner turned out to be a joyous occasion. There was much celebration of Ellie, who looked plump but healthy and wore a pretty cotton scarf over her bald head. Sally's oven disgorged one aromatic dish after another, supplemented by potluck specialties contributed by various relatives. When they were all seated at the long table, Brian uncorked some bottles of champagne and offered a toast. "Let's all thank God we're here together, and Ellie's with us. We have a lot to be grateful for."

13 Maintenance

Ellie returned to the Children's Day Hospital on November 29, three weeks after the end of her radiotherapy, for a complete examination. Nelson found that she had tolerated the radiation well, without fever, skin rash, or markedly lowered blood counts, and a bone-marrow aspiration confirmed that she was still in remission. Since Ellie appeared to be in good shape, Nelson decided to start the maintenance phase of her chemotherapy, which was the experimental part of Protocol 162.

The protocol had six different "arms," or maintenance regimens, to which Ellie could be assigned: the regimen currently considered best and five modifications of it believed to be less toxic, more effective in preventing relapse, or both. Since the optimal therapy was not known in advance but could be determined only through statistical analysis of the outcomes of a large number of patients, random assignment of patients to the various arms was considered ethical. Nelson hoped to randomize as many children as possible in order to distribute equal numbers of patients to the different regimens, but first he had to inform the parents of the six options and obtain consent. If parents had a strong preference for one arm over the others, they had the right to select it without going through the randomization process. The Murphys did not feel strongly about any of the regimens, however, and agreed for Ellie to be randomized. As a result, it was left to the computer at the Children's Cancer Study Group operations center in Los Angeles to assign Ellie to the arm designated I-A.

This regimen included four drugs, administered according to a schedule that repeated itself every three months for a total of twelve cycles over three years. Ellie would receive oral 6-mercaptopurine (6-MP) every day, oral methotrexate once a week, an intravenous injection of vincristine once a month, and seven days of oral prednisone per month. She would be seen in the clinic every two weeks for a physical and blood tests, and a bone-marrow aspiration would be done every three months. Nelson also prescribed Bactrim, an antibiotic, to prevent a variety of bacterial infections.

Nelson told Sally that since it was highly unlikely that Ellie's treatment to date had eliminated all her leukemic cells, two or three years of maintenance chemotherapy would be necessary before she could come off medication. The doctor stressed the importance of giving Ellie her drugs on schedule and making sure that she took every one of them, since that was the only way to keep the disease under control.

Nelson was particularly concerned because recent studies had shown that a phenomenal number of outpatients on chemotherapy simply did not take their medications as directed: about 60 percent of adolescent patients and between 18 and 30 percent of children. Even when the mother was responsible for administering the drugs there were often problems with compliance. While the illness was acute and life-threatening, patients tended to get their pills, but after the child had been in remission for several months and the symptoms went away, compliance went down. Compliance also declined with highly complex drug regimens and when there were a large number of side effects.

The discovery of the magnitude of the noncompliance problem had raised disturbing questions about the validity of research protocols, on which current treatments for leukemia were based. When the protocols were designed, the planners had assumed that all patients would take their maintenance chemotherapy as directed. The fact that many did not put the results of the studies in doubt. Was it primarily the noncompliant patients who relapsed and succumbed to the disease? No one knew, and more research was clearly needed to identify the at-risk population and find ways of encouraging better compliance. Until then, Nelson did his best to frighten or cajole parents into giving their children the medications faithfully.

Nelson wrote up the drug schedule for Sally in chart form, giving her a wall calendar to keep track of which drugs and dosages to give on each day. Then he went over the possible side effects associated with each medication, including liver toxicity and bone-marrow depression. Since 6-MP was capable of sensitizing the skin of some individuals, causing it to react with a rash or exaggerated burn on exposure to ultraviolet light, Nelson cautioned that Ellie might have to stay out of the sun while she was on maintenance. "You really have to play it by ear," he suggested. "Let her try a little sun, and if she doesn't seem to be breaking out, try a little more, and so forth." Nelson added that he had kept Dr. Warner in Plainfield informed of Ellie's progress and that they should go to him for treatment of any routine problems or side effects.

On their way back to New Jersey, Sally explained to Ellie that her blood problem was not completely cured but had merely gone away for now. At first the pills and shots had been to make her better; now they were keeping her well. Sally never used the word "leukemia" with Ellie, fearing that the child would eventually learn it was a form of cancer and think she was going to die.

"Will I have to keep going to the doctor forever?" Ellie asked.

"No, Ellie, not forever. Just for another year and a half, if you stay well." As Sally said this, she realized that for Ellie a year and a half was tantamount to forever.

Over the next few weeks, the Murphys returned to a near-normal routine and achieved a fragile emotional equilibrium, although they knew they would never be quite the same again. Brian and Sally continued to argue about how best to treat Ellie. Brian reminded his wife what Nelson had told them: that the first year of remission was the riskiest in terms of complications and the chance of relapse, and that there were still no guarantees of how long Ellie would live. Why not have as much fun with her as possible now, when she was still with them? Sally, on the other hand, believed that Ellie would continue to do well and that if they did not treat her like a normal child, she would turn into a real monster. Brian's special treatment was making her increasingly selfish and demanding: Ellie was always upping the ante without ever really enjoying what she had. Sally was annoyed by her husband's fatalistic attitude and did her best to counteract his influence, refusing to give in to Ellie's demands and letting the child know she would be punished for her obnoxious behavior.

Soon after Ellie came home, Beth began doing poorly in school. She had always been an excellent student, but now she was reversing the letters in words and getting fifteen out of twenty problems wrong on math tests. At first the Murphys suspected a learning problem such as dyslexia, and sent her to a psychologist for testing. In sessions with the psychologist it soon became clear that Beth was merely acting out. She had felt angry and abandoned when her mother and sister were away at the hospital, and when they came home she had assumed that everything would return to normal. But Ellie had continued to receive special treatment, making Beth even more jealous and resentful. By this time she was so insecure about her position in the family that she was afraid to express her feelings directly, and instead they were reflected in her poor work at school.

When the Murphys confronted the issue at home, it came out that Beth objected to hundreds of little things, such as the fact that she had only a bottom sheet whereas Ellie had both a top sheet and a bottom sheet. The litany of complaints continued: "Why can't Ellie eat the same thing as everyone else in the family?" "Why can she hit me and I can't hit her back?" "Why doesn't she have to clean up her things like I do?" After this crisis, Brian became less blatant in his favoritism of Ellie, and both he and Sally made a concerted effort to give Beth the attention she required. Not long afterward, her schoolwork improved.

Another stressful aspect of home care was the inevitable series of medical—and hence emotional—ups and downs. Because the maintenance chemotherapy had the side effect of lowering Ellie's poly count, she was highly susceptible to bacterial infections. One day she could be perfectly healthy, and the next she could have a raging fever or a bad case of bronchitis, necessitating a trip to Dr. Warner. If Ellie fell down and cut herself, there was always the possibility that her platelet count was low and she would bleed profusely. Just when Sally felt she could begin to breathe easily again after one scare, everything would blow up again.

One afternoon in mid-December, Cindy Lewis caught a glimpse of what life was like for the Murphys. She had come to visit during the day to be with Sally, since the two of them were becoming increasingly close. When Ellie awoke from her nap, Sally felt her forehead and discovered that it was red hot. She took Ellie's temperature with a child's thermometer, and Cindy was shocked to see how fast the mercury rose, shooting past the maximum on the little thermometer—over 104 degrees! Sally did not seem surprised, but she was clearly scared. "I'm going to call Dr. Warner," she said urgently. "Get Ellie in the tub and bathe her with lukewarm water."

Stunned, Cindy did as she was told.

When Ellie got sick, Brian became distant and Sally found it harder to fight off her negative thoughts. She had learned it was essential to maintain a positive attitude, since otherwise she became very depressed and it was a major struggle to get up again. She never let herself cry in front of the children, knowing that it would only confuse and frighten them. Whenever she felt the tears coming unbidden, she immediately complained that her allergies were making her eyes water.

Her primary source of support when times were bad was Cindy, who of all of her friends had been the most loyal and giving. Their friendship had deepened to the point where they no longer bothered with formalities and pretenses and got right down to honest feelings. Every Saturday afternoon the two of them went grocery shopping, and a few times they sat for a while together in the parking lot of the A & P and cried, letting out their anguish and rage over the things they could do nothing about.

Cindy was impressed that Sally, in spite of the real dangers, refused to overprotect Ellie, letting her rejoin the play group and participate in most of the children's activities in the basement and the backyard, providing they were not too rough. Although Jennifer Lewis and Chrissie Bradley were fascinated at first with Ellie's lack of hair, they soon took it for granted, along with the fact that Ellie went to see the doctor in New York twice a month. Had Sally begun treating Ellie as if she were different or special, the other children and adults probably would have followed her lead.

Cindy often worried that her children might give Ellie a cold or an infection that could be serious or even fatal because of her lowered resistance. If one of her daughters awoke with cold symptoms on a morning the play group was scheduled to meet, she would call Sally up and give her the option. "Becky's nose is running. It's fine with me if Ellie comes over, but it's up to you."

Sally would always reply, "Don't be silly. Their noses are all running constantly."

When the play group did not meet and Ellie's counts were high enough, she would try to tag along with Beth and some of her neighborhood friends. The chemotherapy impaired her coordination, and Brian found it heart-wrenching to watch his little misshapen child limping around after the older, taller girls, who often wanted nothing to do with her.

Beth was acutely aware that, because of her sister, their family was now "different" from other families. At times she felt isolated in the house because her friends would not come over to play. Part of the reason was that when Ellie's counts were low, Sally did not want Beth's friends bringing in germs that could make Ellie very sick. But the other reason was that several parents believed in that old, false notion that leukemia is contagious and did not want their children exposed to Ellie. Beth also felt the impact of the disease at school. One day she came home from school in tears; a classmate had told her that, according to his parents, Ellie had cancer of the blood and was going to die. Sally was distraught but kept her emotions concealed while she explained to Beth that yes, Ellie was still sick, but she was going to be with them for a very long time to come.

Sally found the frequent trips into the city for Ellie's checkups to be a major strain. She could go from day to day without thinking constantly about the disease, but every time she went into the clinic and saw other leukemic children, she faced its harsh realities. On the days they went in, Beth would stay with Cindy after school.

By now Ellie knew all about her blood counts. After the finger-stick, she would wait with her mother until the technician came back with the print-out, and Sally would let her read it. Ellie knew that if her white count was a four (4,000), that was good, and if it was a two (2,000), that meant she would have to stay in the house and could not go out and play with other children.

On those clinic visits during which Ellie had just a physical, a blood test, and an injection of vincristine, she would return home in great spirits, causing the other children to believe that she had had a wonderful time in New York. Sally would have taken her out to her favorite fast-food restaurant, and Ellie would return home clutching a couple of plastic syringes, which made excellent squirt-guns. The times Ellie had a bone marrow or a spinal tap, however, she would return home sad and cranky. She never got used to them and let it be generally known each time that she hated what was going on. Even so, she insisted on knowing two or three days in advance when it was going to happen, so she could prepare herself.

If Ellie dreaded the bone marrows, she looked forward to playing with the other children she had gotten to know at the clinic who had regular appointments on the same day. During one visit she realized she had not seen her old playmate Leslie in a long time. "Where's Leslie?" she asked her mother. Sally questioned one of the nurses and was told that Leslie had died. The reality of the child's death came as a brutal shock, and Sally felt she had to protect Ellie. "Leslie isn't coming to the Day Hospital anymore," she said. "She got all better and doesn't need any more shots or blood tests." Ellie was clearly disappointed, but she seemed to accept Sally's explanation.

Although Sally kept her anxiety about Ellie's well-being under control, there were two fears that never went away: that the leukemia would return, and that Ellie would get chicken pox, a potentially life-threatening infection in leukemic children. The illness was of no concern for the majority of children who had chicken pox before they got leukemia and hence were immune to it; unfortunately Ellie had never been exposed. Dr. Nelson told Sally that although most leukemic children who got chicken pox experienced mild symptoms and recovered normally, in about one third of cases the usually benign virus ran rampant in the body, invading the liver, lungs, or brain as well as the skin and causing serious complications. In about one fourth of these serious cases, the complications proved fatal.

Since such a catastrophe was rare even among the small minority of leukemic children who did develop chicken pox, Nelson urged Sally not to worry excessively or to overprotect Ellie. Careful precautions did have to be taken, however, to avoid the disease as much as possible and to make sure that all significant exposures were reported immediately. If Ellie ever did become exposed, there was a special antiserum she could get, called ZIG, that contained large numbers of antibodies to the chicken pox virus. When administered within ninety-six hours of exposure, this antiserum could prevent or attenuate the severity of the infection and reduce the risk of major complications.

Sally alerted all her neighbors to the seriousness of the threat, and urged them to inform her immediately if any of their children were exposed to the virus. For Cindy Lewis and Pat Bradley, the fear of the disease became a real phobia. If Cindy heard that a child at school had come down with chicken pox, she would be terrified that one of her own children would be exposed and transmit the infection to Ellie. They were all more relaxed now that it was winter, since chicken pox outbreaks usually occurred in the spring and fall.

By Christmastime, Ellie's appearance was improving. Her face was no longer round and puffy and her hair was growing back—it looked like a short crew cut. Sally lifted Ellie up every morning so that she could look at herself in the mirror of the medicine cabinet and admire the night's added growth. Ellie's obese belly was also shrinking slowly, leaving behind stretch marks and lumpy fat-tissue that would take months to disappear.

Ellie was still getting a week of prednisone per month, and she continued to overeat during those periods. She also developed strange cravings like those of a pregnant woman, particularly for salty foods. In addition to pickles, bacon and eggs became an obsession. Whenever the family went out to a restaurant, all Ellie ever ordered was bacon and eggs. It was such a pleasure for her that she would prolong the meal as much as possible, cutting the bacon into tiny bits with her fork and eating them one by one. Her mood during the week of prednisone was also erratic, vacillating from euphoria to extreme irritability.

Since Ellie's remission was holding, Brian decided to take a week off from work after Christmas so that the whole family could vacation in Florida. Although the trip meant borrowing $1,000 from the bank at a time when they could not really afford it, Brian wanted Ellie to start having fun and forget as much as possible the horrible two months she had spent in treatment. Still, although he did not admit it to Sally, he was concerned about finances. Blue Cross/Blue Shield continued to send them rejection slips, asserting that outpatient chemotherapy was not covered under their basic plan. Although Major Medical picked up 80 percent of the medical costs, they were still left with a substantial bill—one that could really add up if Ellie ever had to be hospitalized again for a long time. But what did money matter when Ellie might not be with them much longer?

They took the train down from Newark and spent three days with Brian's parents at their winter apartment in West Palm Beach. Then they rented a car and drove north to Orlando, checked into the Contemporary Hotel at Disney World, and spent three active days. Brian took Ellie on all the best rides, including the Octopus, the bumper cars, the Haunted House, and the roller coaster, although Sally had cringed at the idea. As Brian had predicted, Ellie returned from the rides beaming and excited; she was also thrilled at having shaken hands with Mickey Mouse.

Although Ellie enjoyed the rides and the various exhibits, she was as spoiled and recalcitrant as ever. One evening she was looking drawn and pale, and Sally refused to let her go watch the fireworks display at the Enchanted Castle. Ellie threw a terrible tantrum and Sally made her stay in the room. The child carried on for nearly an hour, screaming and crying. Sally was amazed at her endurance, the way she would go to such lengths to get her own way. It was as if the illness had made her tough—had got her defenses up. She had always been an assertive child, and the hospitalization had exaggerated it.

During the last night of their stay, Brian and Sally went for cocktails at the bar. As usual, Sally ordered a gin and tonic. The drink gave her heartburn, and the thought passed through her mind that the only time drinking upset her stomach was when she was pregnant. The possibility terrified her, and she quickly reassured herself that it could not be true.

Although the trip had been mostly fun, Brian was disappointed that Ellie had not been quite as happy as he would have hoped. He had taken several rolls of film and had them processed immediately. When they looked at the pictures, the effects of the chemotherapy were still evident in Ellie's round face and very short hair. One picture was so ugly that Brian tore it up, afraid that Beth would get hold of it and tease Ellie.

Shortly after their return home, there was a parents' group meeting at the hospital. They had not been to the group for two months, due to conflicting social engagements and the Florida trip. Brian talked about the vacation and was surprised to learn that half of the parents present had taken their leukemic child to Disney World soon after he or she was in remission.

Sally looked around at all the new faces and wondered what had become of the parents she knew from before. Perhaps they had simply lost interest and dropped out, or their children had died. She thought of asking Dr. Nelson, but then decided that she really didn't want to know.

14 Complications

Toward the end of January 1979, when Sally's menstrual period was three weeks late, she went to her gynecologist for a pregnancy test. The positive result indicating that she was five weeks pregnant came as a real shock, and she returned home upset and confused. During the first few weeks after Ellie's return from the hospital, she and Brian had made love with an intense, almost desperate passion that they had not experienced since the first months of their marriage. Preoccupied and swept away, Sally had neglected to use birth control because she thought she was in a "safe" part of her cycle. In retrospect, she could guess when the conception had probably taken place. Ironically, their initial passion had soon been replaced by resentment and had become by now a near-total absence of desire.

Before the illness, Sally had considered having a third child, but after Ellie's diagnosis she had decided against it. "I just couldn't go through this again," she had told Barbara. "I'd be a terrible mother, constantly checking to make sure that the baby was healthy." Now that the pregnancy was a fait accompli, however, Sally decided that she wanted the baby. The fact that Ellie was doing well diminished her anxiety somewhat.

Perhaps subconsciously Sally had wanted a third child, and the conception had not really been "careless." Now if anything happened to Ellie, they would still have the two children they wanted initially. And by producing an additional normal child, she could prove to herself that the fault for Ellie's leukemia did not lie within her own body.

Brian was stunned when Sally told him she was pregnant. He refused to believe it had been accidental, convinced that Sally had decided on her own to have a third child without consulting him. He felt angry and excluded, as he had while Ellie was in the hospital. If Sally had asked him, he probably would have said no—not because he was afraid of having another sick child, but because of the financial burden. Since the Murphys were Irish Catholics, although non-churchgoers, they never seriously considered an abortion.

Once the initial shock had passed, the pregnancy provided Sally with a new focus for her attentions and anxieties. She often brooded that there would be something wrong with the baby and, if so, that she would be unable to cope with it. "I've endured all I can," she told Cindy. "I just can't handle any more problems." With Cindy's encouragement, she resolved to stop smoking during her pregnancy, something she had not done with either Beth or Ellie.

On February 19, Ellie celebrated her fifth birthday. Sally gave her a party to which several neighborhood children were invited. They wore party hats, blew balloons, and got icing all over their faces. Except for Jennifer Lewis, who spilled grape juice all over her new dress and cried bitterly, everyone had a good time.

Ellie's next checkup revealed fewer than 5 percent blasts in the marrow aspirate; the remission was holding. Other than a case of bronchitis and an ear infection there were no major complications in February, and Nelson continued Ellie on standard doses of all four of her drugs. During the first months of maintenance, Brian and Sally had been very anxious about the results of the blood tests and bone marrows, and Sally would call her husband at the office as soon as she heard the news. Now that Ellie's checkups continued to be uniformly good, they began to relax. Sally once again became active in the Junior Women's Club, Brian worked hard at expanding his list of clients, and Beth was caught up in the social intrigues and academic challenges of the first grade. The hospital, which for months had been the major focus of Sally's life, now occupied progressively less of her time and energy, particularly after Nelson cut back Ellie's clinic visits to once a month.

March and April passed uneventfully. The high point was Easter Sunday, when the Murphys went to Mass at St. Patrick's Cathedral in New York and joined the elegantly dressed throngs on Fifth Avenue for the Easter Parade. Brian bought Ellie a live Easter bunny, which she adored. She never tired of holding the warm furry animal in her hands, and named him Fluffy. With some prodding from Sally, Brian bought Beth one as well.

On May 15, Ellie had her monthly checkup in the city. Dr. Nelson did a bone-marrow exam and found that her marrow contained 5 percent blasts—the maximum acceptable number for a complete remission. This percentage was ominous, perhaps suggestive of an imminent recurrence, but it was also possible that the high count might be due to an error in diluting the aspirate. To make sure, Nelson decided to repeat the bone marrow on Ellie's next visit. He did not tell Sally about the worrisome result, wanting to avoid unnecessary alarm should the whole thing turn out to be a mistake. When Ellie's marrow was sampled a month later, she was back in complete remission. Either there *had* been a dilution error, or the maintenance chemotherapy had done the trick.

During June, Ellie was healthy and vigorous: an active, growing child with a dimpled smile and close-cropped brown hair that, once straight and thick, was growing in fine and curly. Her young beauty was enhanced at times by Sally's realization of her vulnerability, which brought with it a mixture of sadness and the positive feeling that life was precious. Increasingly, though, the basic truth that Ellie was merely in remission and not yet cured was submerged beneath the flow of daily living.

Toward the end of June, the Murphys were confronted with a dilemma: there was an upcoming movie on television called *Something for Joey*, about a little boy with ALL. Beth's teacher had told her class about the show, and Beth brought it up at supper the day before it was scheduled to appear. Brian wanted Ellie to watch it, since he thought it would help her understand what she had gone through, but Sally felt she was still too young to know that she had a potentially fatal illness. Sally had read a summary of the movie in *TV Guide* and knew that the child died in the end, and she did not think it was a good idea at all. But the whole debate was really moot. Once the children knew about the show and asked to watch it, it was really too late to refuse.

Sally did not watch the movie at all the next evening, but Brian caught snatches of it with the children. After the little boy relapsed, he could not bear to watch any longer and stayed out of the room. The movie had shown most of the procedures Ellie had been through many times—bone marrows, spinal taps, and chemotherapy—and he wondered to what extent she identified with the little boy.

When the movie was over, Beth ran out into the living room, crying, "Daddy, he died! The little boy died!"

Ellie seemed upset by what she had seen. "Mommy, I don't want to die," she moaned.

"I don't blame you," Sally said. She explained to Ellie that she did have leukemia, which could be very serious, but that she was fortunate to be in remission. "That's why," she added, "when you complain about going to the doctor every month, he's just checking to make sure that everything's okay."

Ellie accepted her mother's answers and did not want to discuss the subject any more, but Beth was fascinated and kept asking questions. She wanted to know if Ellie had gotten all those shots, and the needle in her back. When Sally said yes, Beth looked at her sister with new pity and respect. "Oh, poor Ellie," she murmured, which displeased Sally. The last thing Ellie needed was to feel any sorrier for herself.

Later on that evening, when Sally mentioned something about Ellie's leukemia, the child interrupted, "You mean I *had* leukemia. I don't have it anymore." Sally hesitated, but she didn't have the heart to disagree. She doubted that Ellie could understand the concept of a chronic illness, and she did not want her to think she was going to die.

On the last Saturday in June, the Murphys gave a party for all the friends and relatives who had helped out while Ellie was in the hospital. Sally had been meaning to for months, but first the trip to Florida and then the pregnancy had come in the way. She was now six months pregnant and wore a maternity dress as she wove among her guests in the backyard, where Brian was cooking a barbecue of hot dogs and hamburgers. Many of Brian's cousins were there, including the ones who had organized the raffle on

Ellie's behalf, and all the members of the Junior Women's Club who had participated in the blood drive. It was a festive occasion, and everyone commented on how well Ellie looked. The Murphys found themselves agreeing when people told them that she must be cured.

More than eight months had now passed since Ellie's remission, and Cindy began to notice that Sally no longer mentioned the disease to outsiders when it might have been appropriate to do so—for example, when people were discussing leukemia. The illness had never been a taboo subject before, and Sally had always talked openly about her feelings at meetings of the Junior Women's Club. Cindy wondered why she had suddenly decided not to discuss it. Perhaps she had experienced people turning off to the subject or treating Ellie differently after they knew she had a serious disease.

This impression was strengthened by an episode that took place at the end of June. Both Cindy and Sally had become friendly with Martha Harris, a new member of the Junior Women's Club who had a daughter the same age as Ellie. Martha's daughter had joined the play group, and they had begun shuttling their children among their respective houses. They had been doing this for nearly six months when Cindy mentioned to Martha one day, in Sally's absence, that Ellie would not be joining the play group the next morning because she had an appointment with her doctor in New York.

Martha was clearly puzzled by this. "Why does Sally take her all the way into the city to see a doctor?" she asked. "It's an awfully long trip. Can't she find somebody local?"

"Because of Ellie's leukemia, she has to go to a specialist at Memorial Sloan-Kettering," Cindy explained.

Martha looked blank. "Leukemia? What are you talking about?"

"Surely you know that Ellie has leukemia," Cindy replied.

Martha was totally shocked. "What? No, I didn't have the faintest idea."

"Oh, I thought Sally told you," Cindy said, feeling her heart sink. Oh, my God, she thought to herself. Maybe Sally didn't want her to know.

"She's never mentioned a thing about it to me," Martha replied, slightly annoyed. "You know, I've always wondered why she keeps Ellie's hair so short. Now it suddenly makes sense."

They all laughed about it afterward, and Sally made some excuse, but Cindy realized that she clearly did not want any more people to know about Ellie's leukemia because of their possible negative reactions. As long as the child was well, there was no reason why she should not be treated exactly like any normal five-year-old.

Sally and Cindy spent the month of July together, sharing a rented cottage on the Jersey shore. Their children were with them, and their husbands came down on weekends. Ellie was active and healthy-looking except for her short, frizzy hair and a facial rash; the 6-MP and methotrexate made her skin more sensitive to sunlight, but Sally found it all but impossible to keep her inside. Sally had brought along all of Ellie's pills and would lay them out on the kitchen table every morning, watching to make sure that she swallowed them with her orange juice.

On weekends they lived in very close quarters, and tensions often flared up. Cindy and Dan had the misfortune to be present several times when Brian and Sally argued. Although Cindy knew she was not an objective observer, she had the strong impression that Brian was mainly angry at himself, and that he was lashing out at Sally because he envied her strength. Cindy often got annoyed at him because he definitely played favorites with Ellie, which was unfair to the other children. He could never seem to say no to her, and it made her even more demanding. When they had just finished exploring the boardwalk, Ellie immediately wanted to know if they could go to the amusement park tomorrow, and somewhere else the next day. She was never satisfied with the present and always had to be looking forward to something bigger and better.

It was in August, after the Murphys returned home, that things began to go wrong again, and all their familiar fears resurfaced with their original intensity. First Ellie developed an eruption of red acne on her cheeks and forehead. Her face also became slightly bloated, and hairs surfaced on her cheeks. When Dr. Nelson saw the rash and facial hair at Ellie's August checkup, he suspected that she was having an adverse reaction to the prednisone reinforcement therapy she was still receiving for a week each month. Either Ellie had become unusually sensitive to the drug, or her liver was breaking it down in an atypical way to yield toxic byproducts. In any case, Nelson decided to discontinue Ellie's prednisone.

Although Ellie's acne soon healed, the other drugs began to cause even more serious problems. All along, Ellie had been given liver-function tests at regular intervals to monitor the harmful side effects of her maintenance chemotherapy, since both 6-MP and methotrexate were known to cause cirrhosis or scarring of the liver in some patients. Because liver cells, when injured or killed, release their store of specialized enzymes into the blood, a rise in blood levels of one or more of these enzymes would indicate liver damage.

Ellie's liver-function tests had vacillated up and down for several months now, and Nelson had modified her dose of 6-MP and methotrexate accordingly. In August, the blood level of one of her liver enzymes rose precipitously. Although this enzyme subsequently fell again, Nelson felt it would be prudent for Ellie to undergo a liver-scan and a liver biopsy. Since the liver-function tests merely reflected the destruction of tissue occurring at any one time, a biopsy was the only accurate way to determine the extent of permanent damage to the organ caused by the drugs.

On August 16, Ellie was admitted to M-5 for the tests. The question to be answered was whether her liver damage was extensive enough to require lowering her dose of chemotherapy significantly. Judging from what Nelson told them, the Murphys found the alternatives frightening. If the drugs were indeed causing damage, they could jeopardize this vital organ and seriously impair Ellie's functioning in later life. On the other hand, if Nelson cut back on the drugs now after less than a year of maintenance, they would be risking a recurrence of Ellie's leukemia. Moreover, they would be throwing away their last psychological crutch, since the daily routine of chemotherapy provided the security—probably more emotional than real—that the disease would not return. The choice before them was between the terrors of the known and those of the unknown, and either way Ellie might lose out.

The Murphys were also concerned about the biopsy itself, since Nelson told them that there was a small but significant risk of complications. Nevertheless, he conveyed to them the importance of the test, and they signed the consent form. At this point, Sally realized painfully, they just had to have faith in Nelson's judgment.

At least Ellie was not as frightened by the hospital as she had been the first time. She chatted happily with her roommate—a little black girl undergoing an umbilical hernia repair operation—and watched TV. For lunch, she asked Barbara to bring her up a hamburger from outside, since she hated the hospital food.

In the early afternoon, Ellie was taken down on a stretcher to Special Procedures for the liver/spleen scan. Then she was brought back up to M-5 and wheeled into the treatment room. While Sally held her hand, an anesthesiologist injected a few cc's of ketamine into the tubing of her IV, and a few seconds later Ellie was unconscious. Sally left the room as the scrub nurse began prepping the child's abdomen for the biopsy. When it was ready, a specialist passed a large-bore needle through Ellie's abdominal wall into her liver and removed a small core of tissue that would be fixed and sectioned for microscopic examination. Since she was already under anesthesia, he also did a bone-marrow aspiration and biopsy.

The procedures went smoothly, and Ellie awoke quickly from the anesthesia. She was frightened—the drug had given her a nightmare—but Sally was there to console her. Nelson came in the next day with good news: the amount of liver damage caused by the chemotherapy was not excessive, and Ellie could continue her maintenance at the standard doses. Moreover, her bone marrow was still "M-1": in remission, with fewer than 5 percent blasts and normal numbers of precursor cells for red cells, white cells, and platelets. The Murphys were very relieved, and Ellie was discharged the following morning.

The last week in August, just a few days before Ellie was to begin kindergarten at Menlo Park's elementary school, she had a recurrence of moderate hair loss, and Nelson cut her vincristine to half the standard dose. It was hard for Sally to send Ellie to school with her hair still short and sparse, but Ellie seemed resilient enough by now to accept some teasing without its leaving any lasting scars. Nelson cautioned that, although Ellie's poly count was now high enough to protect her against common bacterial infections, if there were any major outbreaks of chicken pox in the school she would have to be tutored at home. An occasional case of chicken pox did not warrant keeping her away, however. Nelson had known some parents to get overprotective, isolating their children completely, which could be harmful.

On the first day of school, the schoolyard swarmed with noisy, active children and nervous parents. Ellie clung tightly to her mother's hand. Some of the other mothers stared at her curiously, no doubt wondering why her hair was so short, but Sally had resolved not to say a word about the illness. She did tell Ellie's teacher, in confidence, so that if there were any cases of chicken pox in the school Sally would be notified immediately and Ellie could be tutored at home.

After the initial pangs of separation from her mother, Ellie decided that she liked school. The kindergarten was a large, unstructured class of twenty-eight students and one teacher in a room cluttered with toys and materials. Ellie gave most of her attention to paints, crayons, scissors, and paste, materials she was quite adept at using. She drew several pictures based on her hospital experiences, one depicting the pain of a bone-marrow exam in a scribble of yellow and green, with the puncture site on her hip marked with a big red X. Dr. Nelson loomed over her tiny form on the treatment table like a giant monster with huge, grinning teeth. Ellie's other favorite activities were singing, making rhythmic music, and playing in the doll corner with the other girls, shrieking and being silly.

Ellie wore a cap to cover her short hair, and some of the other children would pull it off and tease her. When they asked her why her hair was so funny, she explained, "I have a sickness, but I can go to school most of the time." She often felt compelled to prove her normality by doing risky things, such as swinging very high or hanging upside down from the jungle gym.

Ellie missed school fairly often due to clinic appointments or ear and bronchial infections, and this impaired her participation in class activities. Nonetheless, her regular visits to New York were having a positive effect on her intellectual development. Few children in her class had spent so much time in the city, and she had an understanding of her body, illness, and death far beyond her years. Since such knowledge was critical to her survival, she had a strong motivation to learn and make better sense of her environment. At school, she enjoyed playing doctor-and-nurse games with other children.

In late September, Ellie's pet rabbit, Fluffy, caught pneumonia and died after she left his cage in front of a drafty window. She cried a great deal and helped her father bury it in a corner of the backyard, placing a large stone over the site. When Sally went into Ellie's room to try to comfort her, the child said, "Fluffy was sick and he died. Am I going to die, too?"

Sally was stunned. "No, Ellie, you're going to be fine," she said quickly. "Fluffy never went to a doctor or a hospital, and he never got any medicines or IV's or blood tests like you did. It's different for you because we know you're sick and we're taking care of it."

"Is Fluffy ever coming back?"

"No, he won't ever come back, Ellie. He won't eat or breathe or feel anything anymore, but his body is very peaceful now. It will go into the earth and become other things, such as grass and flowers."

Ellie thought for a moment. "So after you die you turn into a flower?" she asked.

Sally nodded, biting her lip.

On October 3, Sally gave birth to a six-pound baby girl at Muhlenberg Hospital. They decided to call her Amy. Although Ellie must have resented all the attention focused on the newest Murphy, she was excited about having a younger sister. She was not the baby of the family anymore.

15 Crisis

On October 21, Jennifer Lewis came down with a fever that turned out to be the chicken pox. Cindy Lewis, overwhelmed by guilt, called Sally with the news. Although Ellie had not been near Jennifer for some time, Beth had played in the Lewises' house the day before.

Terrified, Sally immediately called Dr. Nelson. He was concerned by the news and instructed her to call him as soon as Beth developed any clinical symptoms of infection. If Beth did come down with the chicken pox, Ellie could still be protected with the injection of a special antiserum containing high levels of antibodies to the chicken pox virus. It was ZIG, short for zoster immune globulin.

After hanging up, Sally knelt down in the privacy of her bedroom and prayed that one of her greatest fears would not be realized. Recently she had been praying more than she ever had before; it seemed to help her through the most trying times. She decided to move Beth into the guest room to reduce the risk of exposure to Ellie.

On October 23, Sally noticed a single red pock on Beth's cheek. It was early evening, and she could not reach Nelson in his office. Finally his answering service located him at his home in Riverdale. Nelson called Sally back and said that since it now seemed almost certain that Ellie had been exposed to the virus, he would arrange for her to get an injection of ZIG. Because the supply of ZIG was limited, a child was eligible for it only if he or she had never had chicken pox before, had been exposed to the virus within ninety-six hours but had not yet developed clinical symptoms, and had an impaired immune response due to leukemia, lymphoma (a solid tumor of the lymphatic system), immunity-suppressing drugs, or a congenital or acquired immune deficiency.

Nelson was particularly concerned in Ellie's case because blood tests done at her last checkup had revealed a shortage of antibodies in her blood. The reason appeared to be her lack of healthy lymphocytes. Although her white count was 3,800 she had 87 percent polys and only 4 percent lymphocytes, instead of the usual 20 percent. Ellie's high poly count was useless against the varicella (chicken pox) virus because polys kill mainly bacteria; only the more sophisticated, antibody-secreting lymphocytes could neutralize the viral invaders. Without sufficient numbers of antibodies, the virus would be able to enter Ellie's lungs, causing viral pneumonia, or gain access to her central nervous system, resulting in a serious case of encephalitis, an inflammation of the brain. Nelson could only hope that ZIG would be able to keep the virus at bay.

When Nelson had ended his conversation with Sally, he immediately placed a call to the Clinical Microbiology Division of the Sidney Farber Cancer Institute in Boston, which was the central releasing authority for the distribution of ZIG. The administrator there took down Ellie's basic medical information. Once the request for the antiserum had been cleared by her superior, she called the quarantine station closest to Memorial Sloan-Kettering—the one at John F. Kennedy Airport—and gave them the authority to release the required number of vials of ZIG for this patient. The drug was administered according to body weight: since Ellie weighed 50 pounds, she would be given three vials.

The administrator then called Dr. Nelson back, and he in turn called Sally and told her that the ZIG had been approved and could be picked up at the airport that night. After considerable prodding by Sally, Brian agreed to go, even though he did not believe that Ellie had the chicken pox, let alone that it could be life threatening. The whole thing seemed to be a wild-goose chase.

Ellie was clearly excited to be going off on an expedition with her father, so it was with mixed feelings that Brian climbed into his station wagon about 8:00 P.M. As they turned onto the highway, however, he fancied himself on an important mission. Surely they deserved a police escort, with sirens blaring and lights flashing!

It took them nearly an hour and a half to get to the airport in Queens. Brian parked in front of the International Arrivals Building and they found their way to room 23–39, the quarantine station where certain vaccinations for foreign travel were done. At the desk, a public-health officer took Ellie's name and returned with the vials of antiserum, still cold from the refrigerator. They were packed in a small cardboard box and looked very unimpressive.

With the box in his lap, Brian drove back into Manhattan, arriving on the pediatrics floor of Memorial just after midnight. The resident expected them, having been briefed over the phone by Dr. Nelson. He read over the material enclosed in the box along with the vials: a consent form and a response sheet for the physician to fill out, noting any reactions and the date and time of administration. Brian glanced at the consent form, which asserted that the drug was associated occasionally with mild side effects such as local pain and tenderness at the injection site, malaise, headache, fever, rash, and hives. It added in neutral legal prose: "While no severe or life-threatening reactions have been reported, their occurrence is possible."

Brian shrugged and signed the form. He was pleased to note that because the drug was still experimental, it would be provided at no cost. The resident then took them into an examining room, where he drew a blood sample from Ellie for baseline antibody levels and then gave her two injections of ZIG, one into the muscle of each buttock. He wished them good luck, and they drove back home to New Jersey, arriving at 2:00 A.M. with Ellie sound asleep in the back seat.

For almost three weeks the serum seemed to be working. Beth broke out in pocks all over her body, yet Ellie remained symptom free. Then, on November 9, twenty days after her exposure, Ellie awoke with five pocks on her face. Although she had no fever, Sally was very scared, much more so than she had been when she first learned that Ellie had leukemia. That time she had been in shock and had little inkling of what the disease was all about. Now she knew precisely what the consequences of chicken pox might be.

She called Dr. Nelson, who noted that Ellie had not developed symptoms until the tail end of the varicella incubation period, so perhaps the ZIG was providing some protection. He told Sally to discontinue Ellie's chemotherapy immediately so that her lymphocyte population would be able to recover from the suppressive effect of the drugs and fight off the virus.

Nelson realized that he had made a mistake: it would have been wiser to stop Ellie's chemotherapy before she came down with the infection. He had planned to do so initially, but then when Ellie had appeared to respond to the ZIG he had changed his mind. Now that clinical symptoms of chicken pox had developed, administration of more ZIG would be useless; they would just have to hope that the infection would be mild. If it was not, Nelson privately doubted that Ellie's immune system could recover in time. All he could say to Sally was, "I just don't know."

The doctor's guarded remarks alarmed Sally. When Ellie's leukemia had first been diagnosed, Nelson had been confident and reassuring, and had given them a good idea of what to expect. Now even he could not predict what was going to happen. By abdicating the traditional godlike authority of the physician, Nelson had revealed to them the imprecision of the medical art: how little doctors really know. Although that realization made Nelson more human and accessible, it was also very frightening. In spite of everything, Sally still had hope that the infection would be mild and that Ellie was going to be all right. "If you don't have hope," she told herself, "you don't have anything."

The illness stayed moderate that weekend. Although Beth had sores all over her body, Ellie's pocks remained sparsely scattered and her fever was only slightly elevated.

Everything seemed under control until the night of November 12. Sometime after midnight Ellie began crying loudly, and Sally awoke and rushed into her room. At first she thought the child was having a nightmare, but then she realized that Ellie's eyes were open: she was hallucinating. "Don't step in—there's a hole!" Ellie screamed.

Sally turned on the light and saw to her horror that Ellie's face was covered with innumerable red, oozing sores. She folded back the covers and saw that the pocks were everywhere: covering the child's arms, legs, and trunk, under her arms and on her genitals, eyelids, scalp, and lips. It was a gruesome sight. How bad it would have been without the antiserum, Sally could not begin to imagine.

Ellie's forehead was blazing hot, and she had a profusely runny nose and a bad cough. Sally ran for a thermometer and took the child's temperature, which was 103°. She gave Ellie some Tylenol for her fever and bathed her in a tub of cool water. Brian never volunteered to help, but carried out Sally's instructions in silence. Afterward, Sally was afraid to return to her own room, so she climbed into bed with Ellie instead.

She got little sleep that night. Ellie would doze off for a while and then wake delirious, in the grips of that terrible fever, and Sally would have to cool her body with damp washcloths. Once, in her crazed state, Ellie fought back and bit hard on her mother's hand, drawing blood. Sally cried out in pain, waking Beth and the baby, who began to howl. At Sally's request, Brian crawled out of bed to feed Amy, swearing under his breath.

It was a terrible night. First thing in the morning, Sally called Dr. Nelson and told him what had happened, her voice cracking with emotion and exhaustion. At first the doctor did not seem unduly concerned, merely telling her to keep watching the child and giving her more fluids and Tylenol. There was a trace of annoyance in his voice, as if he thought Sally was just being a hysterical mother—a species with whom he was no doubt familiar. But Sally knew she was not exaggerating when she insisted that there was something seriously wrong. "This is no mild case anymore," she said. "It's really gotten bad. She bit me last night in her delirium. I'm very scared."

"All right," Nelson said finally. "Bring her in."

Sally called Cindy and asked whether she would be willing to look after Beth and Amy if Ellie had to stay at the hospital, and Cindy graciously agreed. Then Sally called Barbara to tell her that Ellie still had a high fever and that they would be driving to Memorial later that morning. Barbara said that she was on jury duty and would be unable to be with them in the morning, but that she would join them at the clinic as soon as she got off in the afternoon.

The entire Murphy family, including Amy, arrived at the clinic around 10:00 A.M. After a short wait, Ellie was taken into a small examining room and looked at by Dr. Nelson. Dr. Ann Falk, a fellow in infectious diseases, was also present to consult on the case.

Ellie was alert and in no distress, with a temperature of 102°. When Nelson listened to her chest with his stethoscope, he heard abnormal respiratory sounds: dry, coarse rales in her bronchial tubes, due to partial obstruction. He sent her down to Radiology for a chest X-ray, which revealed patchy infiltrates in the lungs suggestive of pneumonia.

Blood also had to be drawn for blood gases—an index of lung function. To determine the concentrations of oxygen and carbon dioxide in Ellie's blood, it was necessary to obtain a sample of oxygenated blood from one of her arteries before its content of oxygen was distributed to her tissues. A resident probed with a hypodermic deep into Ellie's wrist in search of the artery, which he would recognize from the bright color of the blood sucked into the syringe. Although the test was done under local anesthesia, it was still excruciating and Ellie howled. Failing to find an artery on the first try, the resident decided to put off another attempt until the next day. He did, however, manage to draw blood from a superficial vein for blood counts and chemistries.

The results came back an hour later. Although Ellie had a white count of 4,300, her differential showed only 3 percent lymphocytes—still ominously low. Nelson sent a blood sample to the Immunology Lab at the hospital for functional assays of her lymphocytes. He then did a spinal tap: Ellie's cerebrospinal fluid was normal and clear, revealing no signs of encephalitis, but a sample was taken for viral culture.

After some discussion with Dr. Falk, Nelson decided to admit Ellie. Since she was still highly contagious, he had her placed in a private room on an adult floor so that none of the other susceptible children on M-5 would be exposed to her. It took a few hours to arrange for the room and fill out the admitting forms, and it was early afternoon by the time the Murphys went up to the floor.

Barbara arrived back at her apartment at 4:00 P.M., having spent a long, frustrating day at the courthouse. She called the nurses' station at the Children's Day Hospital and asked if the Murphys were still there. The duty nurse told her that Ellie had been admitted and was now in isolation, with viral pneumonia in both lungs.

Fearing the worst, Barbara hurried to the hospital and went up to Ellie's room. When she arrived, Brian was preparing to leave with Beth and Amy. Although Sally wanted very much for him to stay and help her through this ordeal, Brian's refusal to accept the seriousness of the situation made it impossible for him to comprehend her anxiety. Sally was very relieved to see Barbara, and after Brian and the children left, they talked in low tones while Ellie slept.

Looking over at her desperately ill child, Sally was reminded of all the times during the past months when she had felt bored with her life: the long days of cleaning house and picking up after the children, with only soap operas for stimulation. But now she thought: "Please, God, give me back my boring days, and I'll never complain again." She was ready to bargain, to make sacrifices, just so long as Ellie did not have to die.

When Ellie had been doing well, Sally had quickly come to take it for granted. That was the way things were: you didn't appreciate something until you were about to lose it. A month ago, when everything was fine, why hadn't she realized how good it was? It seemed that it was only when life itself hung in the balance that she could realize the preciousness, the gift of being alive.

About 5:00 P.M., Dr. Nelson came in to examine Ellie. She was awake by this time and watching television while an IV dripped in antibiotics to treat a secondary bacterial infection of her oozing pocks. Nelson looked at her throat, which was still very inflamed, and listened to her chest with his stethoscope, asking Ellie to take deep breaths. Her lung sounds indicated that the pneumonia was worsening, so he decided to order another X-ray, to be done on a portable machine.

Ellie's deteriorating condition, combined with lab findings that she had a deficiency of all classes of antibodies as well as decreased lymphocyte function, meant that her prognosis was guarded. Antibiotics could do nothing against the virus, and it was questionable whether her lymphocyte population could recover from the suppressing effects of the chemotherapy in time. Nelson decided to put Ellie on an antiviral drug, ara-A (adenine arabinoside), although he doubted that the drug could be of benefit to a patient who already had internal-organ involvement. They would just have to wait and see.

Sally left the room for a few minutes to smoke a cigarette, leaving Barbara alone with Nelson. The doctor went into the bathroom to wash his hands, and when he emerged Barbara asked him how Ellie was doing. Since Nelson knew that Barbara was a nurse, he felt he could confide in her and admitted that the outlook was grim. "There's a forty-eight-hour critical period," he said. "If she can survive that long, she'll pull through. But frankly I don't think she'll make it."

Barbara was stunned by this news; she could not maintain her customary clinical distance when the patient was her own niece. It had been lonely and stressful all along, knowing so much about the disease but having to package the truth into small, digestible bits that the Murphys could accept. Now, once again, she was aware of a terrible piece of information that should not be fully revealed.

Just then Sally returned, having seen Nelson on his way out. She asked Barbara to come out into the hall for a moment and then whispered, "I think there's something Dr. Nelson isn't telling me. Did he mention anything to you about Ellie's condition?"

Barbara hedged for a while. Finally she admitted that he had.

"Did he say there's a chance she might not make it?"

"Yes, there is a chance."

"Why wasn't he honest with me?" Sally said angrily. "I could tell from his eyes that things are bad."

"He was just trying to protect you, Sally. But he also said that if Ellie makes it through tomorrow, she'll be okay."

Sally felt her tears welling up, the ones she had been holding back for so long. She and Barbara embraced tightly. It was so good to cry, to get everything out, to face it! Through her pain Sally felt a kind of relief, as if a deep abscess had been lanced.

Ellie continued to be very sick that night and into the morning of November 14. She was still developing new pocks and her high fever persisted. Sally hardly ate or slept at all, continuing to care nonstop for Ellie: taking her temperature with the electronic thermometer, applying cool compresses to her forehead, trying to feed her. Because Ellie remained in critical condition, a nurse by the name of Michelle was assigned to her bedside full-time. Every fifteen minutes she took Ellie's vital signs and wrote them down on the nursing flow-sheet. Graphed, Ellie's temperatures looked like a jagged mountain range, with the peaks representing her spiking fever.

In medical dramas, the family is often depicted hoping fervently that the patient will survive the night; if he can just live to see the dawn, the crisis will be over and his survival assured. Sally, however, prayed that Ellie would survive the day, convinced that the night would bring some relief from her suffering. Occasionally she thought guiltily about her two other children, who were staying at Cindy's house. Amy was less than two months old, and what kind of a mother had Sally been to her? All of her energies were being directed toward Ellie, and she had almost forgotten that the others existed.

By late afternoon, Ellie was still spiking fevers up to 104° and her breathing was labored. Brian drove to the hospital after work and spent a few hours at his daughter's bedside. He tried to cheer her up, but Ellie was miserable and angry at her parents. She turned away from her father and absorbed herself in TV. Brian found it hard to accept her rejection and unresponsiveness; finally the strain became unbearable and he got up to go. The amateur basketball team he belonged to was playing a rival club at the Menlo Park Sport and Social Club that evening and he was eager to get home in time for it. What was the point of worrying about things over which he had no control?

When he told Sally that he was leaving to play basketball, she was too shocked to protest. It was only later, when Barbara came up to relieve her for supper, that her anger came out. Barbara was equally outraged. She felt that she was constantly taking over Brian's responsibilities in addition to her own, and the stress was beginning to overwhelm her. If Brian cared so much about his daughter, why wasn't he doing something?

In a fury, Barbara went down to the lobby to call her brother from a pay phone. A part of her had long resented being a nurse, always ending up with the rotten side of life: blood and excrement and pain. People were constantly coming to her with problems and at times she got fed up with all of them. Why didn't they go pester somebody else for a change? She picked up the receiver of the pay phone and punched out the Murphys' New Jersey number. Brian answered.

"Hello, Brian?" she said bitterly. "Look, this is getting ridiculous! I think you should drive back here tonight and take over for Sally. That poor woman has been going for forty hours straight, and she's about to drop. How you could even think of playing basketball when your child is on the brink of . . . Brian, do you realize how serious this is? Ellie could die!"

"I didn't know that," he said in a muted voice. "I thought she was doing fine."

"Well, she isn't at all fine, and I'm getting tired of relieving Sally all the time. You're at home and going to work and doing your own thing, and here I am taking care of your child! Why does it always have to be Sally and me? Christ, Brian, you're the father!"

Brian repeated that he had no idea it was so serious, but there was nothing he could do about it now. "I love Ellie just as much as you or Sally," he added. "It's just that my way is different." Saying that he would be at the hospital first thing the next morning, he hung up.

Meanwhile at the hospital, Sally decided she was going to stay at Ellie's bedside the entire night, determined to break this fever. By now she had lapsed into a blank state in which she existed physically but not mentally, functioning by instinct rather than by thought or feeling. Ellie's temperature was still around 104°, and an oxygen mist tent had been set up over her bed to facilitate breathing and control her temperature. Michelle would give her some Tylenol, which would start her sweating, and her temperature would drop to 103° or 102° before rising again. Watching the sweat flow like water from her child's face, Sally reached into the plastic tent every few minutes to swab her brow with a cool washcloth. Ellie lifted up her head and murmured, "Gee, it's wet on my pillow."

On the Celsius scale, in which normal body temperature is 37°, Ellie's fevers ranged between 39° and 40°. Each time Michelle read off the child's temperature, Sally would say, "Think thirty-seven, Ellie. Think thirty-seven." Soon it became a kind of game and they were all chanting it, until the words became as hypnotic as the spell of an African witch-doctor.

Perhaps it was an effect of the incantation, but at 2:30 A.M. Ellie's temperature fell to 37.5°, almost normal. By this time Michelle was on overtime and the night nurse was on duty as well. "It looks as if things are finally getting better," Michelle said with a sigh of relief. When Sally realized that the fever was going down and the crisis was over, she was too drained even to smile. She collapsed on her cot in utter exhaustion and fell asleep almost immediately.

The next morning, Ellie's fevers continued to be less high and spiking and there were no new skin lesions or evidence of progressive lung disease on her X-rays. She was still very sick but no longer in grave danger, and Dr. Nelson now felt confident she was going to make it. If her disease had continued to progress, with the pneumonia spreading to additional parts of her lungs, he would not have been as optimistic. Even so, Ellie's breathing was still labored and it would be a couple of days before she could be weaned from the oxygen tent. An additional week or two of hospitalization would be needed to allow her lungs time to repair themselves; there was still the danger that she might be a pulmonary cripple afterward from permanent lung damage.

Brian came in that morning, but Sally could not forgive him. He seemed nonchalant and uncontrite, as if there had not been a chance in the world that things might turn out badly. Brian's inability to face reality disappointed and vexed Sally, and she realized that she had many needs and wants that he would never fulfill. She wondered if he might have been stronger in this situation had he been married to a weaker partner. If she had fallen apart emotionally under the strain, perhaps he would have taken over and been the strong one. But the fact that she had remained intact and able to mobilize herself on Ellie's behalf had perhaps made him feel unneeded and superfluous. Maybe his own fallibilities had seemed all the more disastrous to him.

For a few hours, Sally seriously considered leaving him in the near future, but because of the children and her fear of having to cope alone she decided to stick it out for at least a few more years. She was also unsure whether she was reacting merely to Brian's inability to handle the illness or whether there were more fundamental and ultimately unreconcilable problems with the marriage.

Over the next two days, Ellie showed a marked improvement. Her temperature gradually returned to normal, her blood gases stabilized sufficiently for her to be taken off oxygen, and significant numbers of new lymphocytes appeared in her differential count. On examination, Nelson heard scattered dry, coarse rales throughout Ellie's lung fields, but her pneumonia was resolving well.

A week later, Ellie was discharged and allowed to go home. Although she still had a cough and a runny nose, her pocks were drying and she had no fever. Her white count was close to normal, with a differential of 67 percent polys and 15 percent lymphocytes. Nelson decided to keep her off maintenance chemotherapy until November 30, at which time the drugs would be resumed at the standard doses. It was truly remarkable: for a week Ellie had been on the brink of death, and now she was doing fine. Sally felt an enormous relief. If they could get through this, they could get through anything.

By Ellie's December checkup, she had recovered completely from the chicken pox: all of her skin lesions had healed and her antibody levels were in the normal range. A bone-marrow aspiration revealed a normal marrow with no increase in blasts. Ellie's remission was holding, and her family felt confident that the worst was over. At least they would not have the chicken pox to worry about anymore.

Later that month, Dr. Nelson gave a party for his young leukemic patients in remission in order to give them a better understanding of their disease. Only children were allowed to attend; their mothers dropped them off at the clinic and picked them up two hours later. Ice cream and cookies were served in the playroom, and Nelson showed slides of blood cells and marrow cells and explained in simple terms why bone-marrow exams and spinal taps were necessary. Then he opened up the floor to questions. Ellie was particularly interested in the chicken pox, since she had recently had it; she believed that was what her disease was, not leukemia.

When Sally picked Ellie up after the party, the children were all talking excitedly and Dr. Nelson looked totally worn out; handling a roomful of children had apparently been too much for him. Watching the children leave with their parents, Sally found it hard to believe that they all had leukemia, even though many were bald or had very short hair. Far from the depressing scene one would have expected, the room seemed to be overflowing with life.

16 On Shifting Sands

In January 1980, there was a scare with Beth. She had been getting increasingly pale, and Sally panicked and took her to Dr. Warner for blood tests. "If this is going to be something serious," Sally thought, "I just won't be able to handle it." It turned out to be very minor—a mild case of iron-deficiency anemia—and Dr. Warner prescribed iron supplements that worked in a short time. Sally discussed this incident with Cindy and they agreed that they were both becoming more paranoid the more children they had. With the first child they had simply assumed that everything was going to be perfect, but by now they had heard and lived through too much not to be aware of all the things that could go wrong.

By March, Ellie was six years old and doing well in kindergarten. The months since her recovery from chicken pox had passed smoothly and with few complications other than bronchitis and colds. Now that she was off prednisone her swelling and excess weight had gone down and she had become an attractive child, with bright blue eyes, dimpled cheeks, and light-brown hair that she usually wore in short pigtails. Having lost her hair twice she now treasured it and refused to have it cut, even though it was becoming scraggly. She was an imaginative child who often conducted elaborate conversations with her dolls. Although she was still extremely demanding, her all-out temper tantrums had become infrequent.

Whenever the family looked at slides or pictures taken when Ellie was an outpatient, she would point and say, "Look at me, that's when I was a baldie!" She did not like the pictures much, but Beth was fascinated by them and insisted on seeing them over and over again. Otherwise, the only reminders that Ellie was different from other children were her daily pills and monthly visits to New York. The Murphys did not consciously avoid discussing the disease, but the subject rarely came up. Ellie often asked her mother, "Why do I have to keep going to the doctor? I feel fine, and Beth doesn't have to go except once in a while." Sally would always explain that with Ellie, they had to be extra sure that everything was fine.

Sally had relaxed after the chicken pox crisis, but she was still very aware of Ellie's vulnerability. This awareness was not with her at every moment but it did lurk in some dark corner of her mind, poised to leap into consciousness at the slightest indication of something amiss: undue fatigue, a sore leg, a swollen gland, a slight pallor, a cut that was slow to clot. . . .

Barbara, too, had occasional flashes of awareness. She brought each of her nieces into the city to spend occasional weekends with her. One day when Ellie was visiting, Barbara watched unnoticed while the child played with her favorite doll. Suddenly Barbara remembered that Ellie still had leukemia and that a remission could never be taken for granted. Ellie was too young to comprehend that even years from now her disease could return. Perhaps only when she was a teenager would she fully come to grips with the long shadow that the disease cast across her future.

For Brian, Ellie remained more fragile and hence more precious than his other daughters. He did not want to think about the long-range expectations and resented it when people, even close friends, asked him about Ellie's prognosis. It was idle speculation anyway, and what difference did it make? He himself could get run over by a car tomorrow, but he did not spend his time pondering the odds of that happening. Whenever the question came up in conversation, Brian simply avoided it.

Privately, however, he longed for the ordeal to be over and for Ellie to be finally considered cured. He had a recurring fantasy that Dr. Nelson would call him in the middle of the night to bring Ellie to the hospital for the injection of a revolutionary new drug that would destroy every last leukemic cell in her body without harming any healthy tissues. One shot of this "magic bullet" and the specter of the disease would no longer haunt them. Such a miracle drug was not yet visible on the horizon, but they had to keep hoping. Meanwhile, they had much to be thankful for.

Dr. Nelson, for his part, was cautiously optimistic about Ellie. But he had seen success turn sour many times and had even known patients to relapse eight or ten years after diagnosis, although that was extremely rare. Between 10 and 20 percent of children who came off treatment entirely after years of maintenance chemotherapy subsequently relapsed. So there were no guarantees.

On the afternoon of Thursday, April 3, 1980, Sally answered her ringing phone. It was the nurse at the elementary school calling to say that Ellie had suddenly developed a fever. Feeling a chill of fear run down her spine, Sally said she would be right over. She picked up Amy and ran out to the car.

It took her only minutes to reach the school, a modern one-story building. Carrying Amy, she walked down the corridor to the principal's office, hearing voices of children and teachers in the classrooms on either side. Passing a display of student paintings, she searched automatically for Ellie's or Beth's work but nothing really registered in her mind. She hurried on to the office and walked up to the desk to speak to the school secretary. When Sally mentioned Ellie's name, the woman directed her to the teachers' lounge.

Ellie was lying on the couch, looking very feverish and pale, her eyes closed. The school nurse was sitting beside her and began to explain, but Sally merely nodded distractedly, leaned over her child, and spoke her name. There were several tiny red dots scattered on Ellie's face, as if her skin had been pricked with needles from the inside. Petechiae, Sally thought, her fears mounting.

The child blinked her eyes open painfully in the harsh fluorescent light. "Hi, Mommy," she said. "Are you taking me to the doctor?"

"Do you feel sick?"

Ellie nodded.

"Okay, don't move. I'm going to call Dr. Nelson."

Sally went to use the phone in the front office. As she dialed, she kept telling herself that the skin hemorrhages were due to the fact that the chemotherapy had suppressed Ellie's platelet count. The child was too healthy, too full of life, for it to be anything more serious.

Nelson was not in his office, but his secretary offered to have him paged. When he finally got on the line, Sally described Ellie's petechiae, pallor, and fever. Nelson tried to be reassuring, but she could detect the concern in his voice. "Bring her to the hospital this evening," he said. "I'll arrange for a bed, and one of the residents will admit her and treat her fever. I'll be in tomorrow morning to examine her and do a bone marrow."

When Sally had hung up, she asked the secretary if she could have Beth called from her second-grade classroom for a few minutes, since she had something important to tell her. A short while later the office monitor returned with Beth, who looked scared and mystified. As soon as she saw her mother and the baby, she smiled happily. "Hi, Mom. What are you and Amy doing at school?"

"Ellie's sick and Daddy and I have to take her to the doctor in New York," Sally replied. "After school today you should go to the Lewises' and stay there, the way you do when Ellie has her checkup. Daddy will pick you up later on tonight."

Beth was about to protest, but she was muted by the tension and sadness in her mother's face and voice. She nodded solemnly, allowed herself to be kissed, and returned alone to her classroom.

Sally tried to get in touch with Brian at his Newark office but he was out on a sales call. She left a message with the company receptionist. Then she drove home with Amy and Ellie. As soon as they arrived, Sally gave Ellie some Tylenol and put her to bed.

Lying on her bottom bunk, Ellie felt her old fears of mutilation and abandonment begin to surface once more. Like many children, she was able to read the smoke signals of nonverbal communication to which the adults around her were less consciously attuned. Her mother's nervous excitation, the frequent taking of her temperature, the secretive talking on the phone, all suggested that something was seriously wrong. She was even more frightened when, half-closing her eyes and pretending to sleep, she saw her mother look in on her and quickly wipe away a tear.

Sally got Amy changed and fed and put her in the crib to nap. Then, feeling as if a lead weight were pressing on her chest and making it difficult for her to breathe, she poured herself a stiff gin and tonic and sat down in the empty living room. She felt very alone and confused. What if the leukemia had returned? What then? She forced the thought out of her mind. She would just have to relax and not let herself jump to conclusions. . . .

Two hours and two drinks later, Sally was feeling groggy but still quite anxious. When the phone rang, it took her to the sixth ring to answer it. Brian was returning her call. When he heard about Ellie's petechiae and fever, he said he would drive home immediately and take them to the hospital. He was convinced that Ellie's symptoms were due merely to a complication of chemotherapy, requiring nothing more than an adjustment of dosage. Sally also called Barbara, who agreed to meet them at Memorial.

By the time Brian arrived at the house, Sally had her bag packed and Ellie and Amy were dressed and ready to go. They got into the car and, after a few unsuccessful attempts by Brian to ease the tension with some forced jokes and wisecracks, drove most of the way to the city in gloomy silence.

It was after 7:00 P.M. when they arrived on M-5; Barbara was waiting for them, looking drawn and anxious. The resident on duty that night, Susan Drake, was expecting them. Ellie was put in a private room so that Sally would be able to stay with her overnight. Then Drake did an admitting interview and a physical exam. Ellie had a fever of 103° and increased heart and respiration rates. She looked very anemic and had bruises and numerous petechiae on her arms and legs. The lymph nodes in her neck were swollen and her spleen was enlarged and palpable. Drake did a finger-stick and made some smears, which she sent off immediately to the Hematology Lab for a CBC (complete blood counts). When the results came back fifteen minutes later, they were ominous: Ellie's white count was 8,900 with few polys and a large number of atypical lymphocytes, her hematocrit was 25, and her platelet count was 8,000.

Drake asked the Murphys to join her out in the hall. She cleared her throat, looking very uncomfortable. "On the basis of the physical exam and the counts, I presume it's a relapse," she said. "But I can't be sure until the bone-marrow aspiration is done in the morning."

Sally felt as if she stood on shifting sands, utterly lost and adrift. Any control she had ever felt over her life, any security and order, was now an empty illusion, shattered by this cruel, unpredictable growth. Just when she had begun to believe that Ellie was really cured—when she was able to mouth the word *leukemia* without intolerable anguish—it had returned.

Brian refused to believe the diagnosis, just as he had initially two years ago. For him, Drake's hesitation—"I presume it's a relapse"—left the door slightly ajar; there was still time for a miracle. "Did you say that until you have the results of the bone marrow, you can't be sure what it is?" he asked.

Drake nodded. "The atypical lymphocytes in the smear and the enlarged nodes and spleen are suggestive of leukemia, but her white count is not sufficiently high. What we may be seeing is what's called a 'subleukemic leukemia.' In the early stages of a leukemic relapse, blasts can proliferate and accumulate in the blood-forming tissues, disrupting the formation of normal blood cells without being released in large numbers into the peripheral blood. That would explain Ellie's anemia and low levels of platelets and polys. There's a chance that it may be something else, like a viral infection, but the odds of that are small. In any case, with her polys so low, we'll have to start her on antibiotics immediately."

When the Murphys went back into the room, Ellie asked her mother if they could go home now. When she finally realized that she would be spending the night in the hospital, and getting an IV and a bone marrow as well, she felt terribly betrayed by her parents. "Why do I always get sick?" she screamed, and began thrashing around on the bed. Suddenly she picked up the telephone from the table beside the bed and threw it on the floor. The plastic housing cracked, sending a fragment skittering across the linoleum. Drake was finally forced to sedate her with Valium.

Because Ellie had an FUO—fever of unknown origin—Drake did a complete bacteriological work-up, taking bacterial, fungal, and viral surveillance cultures of her nose, throat, urine, blood, and stool. A systemic bacterial infection in a child with low poly counts could be fatal in two or three days—before the culture results were known—so broad-spectrum antibiotics had to be started immediately. Drake ordered intravenous antibiotic therapy with a combination of three drugs: Keflin, gentamicin, and carbenicillin. This combination would cover the most common fever-causing microbes seen in leukemic children—staph, E. coli, and *Pseudomonas*—until the particular organism involved could be identified.

When Sally learned that an IV would have to be started to administer the antibiotics, she was extremely concerned that Ellie not suffer any more pain than was absolutely necessary. She knew that chemo nurses could usually start an IV with one stick, whereas it took the average resident four or five tries. It would not be easy to tell Ellie that she would have to endure multiple sticks because there were no IV nurses around at night. So Sally insisted, "I don't want a doctor trying to start her IV. I'd rather wait until morning, when the IV team will be here."

Dr. Drake was taken aback. "If we don't start an IV on her now, it's going to delay her antibiotics and transfusions. That could be serious."

Sally shook her head. "Ellie's been through enough. It has to be a chemo nurse or nobody."

Frustrated, Drake sought out Marianne, one of the night nurses, and asked her to try to convince Sally to let the IV be started immediately. After much discussion, Sally finally agreed, but only under the condition that Drake try only once; if it did not go in the first time, they were going to wait until morning.

While Sally held Ellie, Marianne rubbed the underside of the child's thin forearm, trying to raise one of her delicate veins. Detecting a fine bluish streak, Drake opened a butterfly pack and slid the small-gauge needle into Ellie's pale skin, while the child squirmed and cried. There was a long moment of tension; then came a good backflow of red blood into the IV tubing and everyone breathed her own sigh of relief.

At 9:00 P.M., Brian left to drive Amy back to Menlo Park, and Barbara

136

went home shortly afterward, promising to return early the next morning. Sally set up the cot in Ellie's room. She slept little that night, fearing what the bone-marrow aspiration would reveal and hoping against hope that Dr. Drake might have made a mistaken diagnosis. "Dear God," she prayed, looking over at her sleeping child. "Please let her live."

It seemed to Sally that whenever she dozed off, she would be awakened by one of the night nurses coming in to check on Ellie or to change the transfusion bags of packed red cells and platelets that she was getting. As a result, Sally was bleary eyed and stiff the next morning when Dr. Nelson came in with a stretcher to take Ellie to the treatment room. Barbara had come up to be with Ellie during the procedure, since Sally felt too queasy to watch. Instead, she sat outside and listened to her daughter's screams, while tears ran silently down her cheeks.

After rinsing her face in the bathroom, she followed Ellie's stretcher back to the room and waited anxiously for the results of the bone marrow. Meanwhile Brian arrived, having left Amy at home with his parents. He looked haggard, with dark bags under his eyes and deep lines in his forehead. While they waited he and Sally held Ellie's hands.

After what seemed like hours, Nelson appeared in the doorway and beckoned the Murphys to follow him. Leaving Ellie with Barbara, they went into a small, unused examining room off the corridor and sat down reluctantly. Sally's heart was beating furiously, as if she were about to hear a sentence of life or death. The doctor looked grim and she felt her hope seeping away. Even so, it came as a shock when Nelson told them that Ellie's bone marrow had contained 20 percent blasts; 5 percent or less was normal.

Sally started shaking. "Oh, my God, this is the end. . . ." she thought. She wondered how much Ellie would have to suffer and how much warning they would have. She didn't want to be alone with her when it happened; she definitely couldn't handle that. . . .

Brian was stunned, his mouth open in astonishment. "What the hell happened?" he demanded. "She looked so well, and we were so sure she was cured. What caused the relapse?"

Nelson shook his head. "Leukemia is an insidious and deceptive disease. When chemotherapy reduced the population of leukemic blasts in Ellie's blood below a billion, she went into a remission in which all visible traces of the disease were gone. But she was not cured yet. In the fortunate patients—about half of all kids with ALL—the cycles of maintenance chemotherapy wipe out the remaining leukemic blasts and do achieve a cure. But in the less-fortunate fifty percent, some of the leukemic cells become resistant to the drugs or hide out in some poorly perfused tissue where the drugs can't reach them, and these cells can multiply later on and cause a relapse. That, I'm afraid, is what happened to Ellie."

"Will you be able to get her back into remission?" Sally asked desperately.

To her surprise, Nelson's voice was reassuring. "Yes, our chances of getting her back into remission are excellent. We can achieve a second remission in sixty percent of children with ALL who relapse. Since Ellie relapsed so early, after only a year and a half of treatment, I'll try to reinduce her remission with a more intensive drug regimen. Another course of radiotherapy shouldn't be necessary."

Sally felt a surge of hope. "Does that mean she might still be cured?"

Nelson shook his head. "The outlook for a cure at this point is not good. Since she has already failed fairly aggressive therapy, it's doubtful that a second round of chemotherapy could produce a cure."

"Why not?" Brian asked. "Why can't you just give her higher doses of the drugs to kill off the resistant cells?"

"Unfortunately, the toxic side effects of the drugs on normal tissues limit the dose of chemotherapy we can give to a level that will induce remission but probably not kill every last leukemic cell. There are some specialists who believe that it may not be necessary to destroy every last cell to cure leukemia; if we can just get rid of most of them, the patient's immune system will be able to search out and eliminate the few remaining ones. Ironically, chemotherapy has the serious side effect of suppressing the immune system, thereby compromising its antileukemic effect. So although we may be able to achieve additional remissions by trying different drug combinations, the chance for cure with chemotherapy is now only about ten percent."

Sally felt as if she were riding a roller coaster, from despair to hope and back to despair again. "How long do you expect the remissions will last?" she asked faintly.

"Several months at first," Nelson replied. "But they will get increasingly shorter, and eventually the treatments will probably fail."

All the anguish and tension of Ellie's first hospitalization and the chicken pox crisis flashed through Sally's mind with the clarity of a nightmare. Now the whole ordeal was starting over, only this time they would have lost the hope of a cure. She would have to take Ellie into the city three times a week for chemotherapy injections and then, later on, for the weekly finger-sticks and monthly bone marrows, terrified each time that the blasts might have returned, unable to control the pounding of her heart and the cold sweat while she awaited the results. Once again, the hospital would become the focal point of their lives. Sally dreaded the idea of a series of remissions, each one shorter than the last, until there were no more drugs left to try and the leukemia finally won out. She was angry, full of rage at this doctor before her. "What's the use of more drugs that will make her sick and miserable, when it will only postpone the inevitable?" she blurted out. "Are you telling us that there's no hope that Ellie will ever be cured?"

Nelson licked his lips nervously. "As I said before, the outlook for a cure with chemotherapy is not good. There is one other possibility, however." He took a deep breath.

"What's that?" Sally asked impatiently, sounding strained and exhausted.

"A bone-marrow transplant," Nelson replied, "providing that Ellie has a compatible donor, which may or may not be the case. The purpose of the transplant would be to provide Ellie with replacement marrow from a healthy donor so that we could administer massive, potentially curative doses of chemotherapy without having to worry about protecting her healthy marrow cells. Without the transplant, such extreme therapy would be fatal. Bone-marrow transplantation is not just a means of prolonging life for a few months; it offers real hope of a long-term remission and perhaps even a cure. But you should realize from the outset that if the graft does not take, or if complications develop, the treatment will probably kill her."

"So it's a choice between a few more remissions with chemotherapy and a possible cure with the transplant?" Brian asked.

"Yes, but with a few big ifs. We don't know yet whether Ellie has a compatible donor. And before she can be considered for a transplant, we'll have to get her back into remission. I'd like to start her on the reinduction protocol immediately."

Sally looked over at Brian. Getting no hint of a reaction, she turned back to Nelson. "What would you do in our situation, doctor?"

"I definitely think you should have your family tissue-typed to see if Ellie does have a compatible donor. Then, if and when the transplant is a real possibility and Ellie achieves a good second remission, you should think long and hard about the transplant before coming to a decision. It's a question of gambling the time Ellie has left for a potentially curative treatment that is very unpleasant and has about a fifty-percent chance of working. What I'm saying is that the transplant is not necessarily right for you. It's a terribly difficult thing."

Brian nodded, his brow furrowing with tension. "Would I be able to donate marrow to Ellie?" he asked.

"I'm afraid not," Nelson replied. "Parents often find this very difficult to accept, but it's purely a question of genetics." The doctor explained that each individual has a unique set of identifying markers on the surface of his or her tissue cells, white blood cells, and platelets that enables the body's immune system to distinguish between them and "foreign" cells, such as tumor cells or bacteria. For this reason, a graft of tissue carrying the wrong molecular code will be rejected from the body as if it were a colony of invading bacteria. If the graft is to survive in its new host, it must carry a code identical to—or, at the very least, extremely similar to—that of the host's own cells. The match can only be perfect between identical twins, who share all the same genes, but close matches such as those that exist between some nonidentical siblings can also be accepted.

Because of the nature of genetic inheritance, Nelson added, children hardly ever have the same set of genetic markers as either parent. The siblings do, however, have a one-in-four chance of matching up with one another. Clearly, the more siblings there are, the better the chance of a match. So before the transplant option could be discussed further, Ellie's sisters would have to be tissue-typed to determine if one was a suitable donor. Only a simple blood test was required.

Brian hoped desperately that the drugs would work so well that Nelson would decide that a transplant was not necessary. Still, he agreed to have Beth and Amy tissue-typed. The family could not afford to burn any bridges. "When do you want me to bring my other daughters in?" he asked.

"Monday, to the Children's Day Hospital," Nelson replied. "A nurse will draw the blood samples, and we should have the results within a week. I must tell you that even if Ellie does have a match and you decide to go ahead with the transplant, there may be a delay of weeks or even months before we can find her a bed. There are only a few cancer centers in the country that do bone-marrow transplants on a routine basis, and most of them have long waiting lists. But we'll confront that problem when we come to it."

Brian thought about that. What a feeling it would be: to know there was something that could save your child's life, and then to have to endure a waiting list. . . . It would drive him crazy to sit patiently while time passed by.

Sally could imagine such a predicament a little better. She was used to waiting. It seemed she had spent the past year and a half waiting for something to happen. Now yet another month of agonizing uncertainty lay before her. Would Ellie get back into remission? Would she have a match? And if so, could a bed be found in a transplant center?

Nelson accompanied the Murphys to the door and said good-bye. Privately he hoped that one of Ellie's sisters would prove to be tissue-compatible. Since Ellie had relapsed so soon it was very unlikely that additional chemotherapy-induced remissions would be of long duration—probably six months at the most. A marrow transplant, although risky, seemed to offer the only hope of long-term survival.

The next day, Ellie was started on the reinduction protocol, which included vincristine, prednisone, L-asparaginase, and an additional drug, daunomycin. She cried when she heard that she would be getting more needles and that her hair would fall out again. "Why me?" she protested. "Why do I always have to get sick?" She felt sad, as she had after her pet rabbit died, and she was scared because her parents were obviously very upset and preoccupied.

The most dangerous side effect of the new drug, daunomycin, was known to be cardiac toxicity. Before this effect had been realized, a number of young patients who had been apparently cured of their leukemia had later succumbed to heart failure. Since then it had been found that the drug's cardiotoxicity was related to the total dose administered over several months, so lower total doses were now being used. As an additional precaution, Ellie received a baseline evaluation of her heart function, including an electrocardiogram. Her heart function would be monitored after each dose of the drug and compared with this original observation. After Nelson had informed the Murphys of all the possible side effects of daunomycin, he asked them to sign yet another informed-consent waiver.

Brian and Sally went through several phases in trying to deal with Ellie's relapse. After the initial reluctance to accept the truth, there came great anger, both at the injustice of it and the fact that the disease would again disrupt their lives. They had waged a great battle and won, only to have final victory slip through their fingers. Sally was tormented by the thought that something she had done had allowed the leukemia to return: letting Ellie out in the rain, allowing her to stay up two nights in a row, not keeping a closer watch on her. . . . Whenever Sally passed normal families in the street, she resented their happiness and how they seemed to take their good fortune for granted. Moments later, she would feel guilty for being so selfish.

This phase was followed by a rather bitter resignation and a search for some tangible meaning, a reason why. Increasingly, Sally found solace in religion. Although she had attended parochial school as a child in Chicago, she had largely neglected her faith until now, when it seemed to offer some shelter against the terrifying unpredictability of the disease. She began going to a small church across from Memorial. Two or three times a day she retraced her steps to the church, seeking out a few moments of relief from the starkness of the ward.

During the day, the church was nearly empty, with only a few older women in black scattered among the pews. The colored light from the stained glass windows filtered gently onto the altar, with its suspended, agonizing Christ. Sally went into one of the back pews and knelt down on the prayer stool, folding her hands and closing her eyes. She stayed there for long minutes, murmuring half-remembered prayers and picturing Ellie well again. These daily meditations gave her the strength to return to her daughter's bedside. Every night before Sally went to sleep, she would listen to Ellie's regular breathing in the room and pray to God not to take her that night. In the morning, her first thought was, "Thank you, God, for this night. We have another day."

On Monday, Brian drove Beth and Amy to the Day Hospital for the blood tests. Beth was old enough to understand that Ellie's bone marrow was not producing enough blood cells, and Brian explained that if one of them could give Ellie some new bone marrow, it would start to grow inside her body and make healthy blood cells again. The test was to find out whether Beth or Amy had the right kind of marrow. Beth was anxious about the test, but she wanted to help her sister. She also relished missing a day of school and spending time with her father. Amy, only six months old, just enjoyed the ride.

One of the clinic nurses drew the blood; Brian held his daughters' hands but could not bear to watch. Both children cried but it was over quickly. Then the specimens were sent down to the Histocompatibility Testing Laboratory, where the specific molecular markers on the surface of Beth's and Amy's white cells would be determined by means of reactions with standard solutions of different antibodies. Three of the four major cell markers, known as HLA antigens, could be detected in this way. For a marrow transplant to be possible without undue risk of rejection, the donor and recipient had to have identical (or nearly identical) HLA antigens. In addition to these major cell markers, there were several minor ones, not detectable with antibody reactions, that could provoke a more subtle but no less dangerous rejection reaction. In order to predict the ability of Ellie's body to reject a graft of her sister's marrow (or conversely, the ability of Beth's or Amy's white cells, once transplanted, to attack Ellie's tissues), a second test was required: a "mixed-lymphocyte culture," or MLC.

The principle behind the MLC was simple. Lymphocytes obtained from the blood of Beth and Amy would be mixed in separate culture dishes with lymphocytes from Ellie's blood to determine if the white cells recognized one another and attacked. The activated lymphocytes would take up a radioactive substance present in the incubation mixture, enabling them to be detected. If there was a strong reaction (a large amount of radioactivity in the cells), that meant that Ellie would most likely reject the transplanted marrow or that the grafted cells would attack their new host. If the reaction was weak, the transplant stood a good chance of working. Recent research had shown that even if two siblings were not HLA identical, transplantation could still be successful if their mutual reactivity on the MLC test was low. The nurse told Brian it would take a week before the results of the tests were known.

17 Psychosocial Conference

On the morning of April 10, Dr. Nelson walked down the corridor toward Ellie's room, hearing the child crying through the closed door. She had now been on the reinduction protocol for a week. Although she was responding well to the drugs, the daunomycin had made her nauseated and lowered her blood counts to a dangerous degree, requiring multiple transfusions of concentrated platelets and red cells. A small cut on her left third finger had recently become red and swollen (her white count was too low for there to be pus), but bacterial and fungal cultures had been negative so far. Nelson knocked twice on the door of the room and entered.

Ellie was lying in bed, her cheeks wet with tears; her mother was sitting in a chair beside her. The child's hair had already begun to fall out and her skin was pale, with a yellowish cast. Two IV's, one delivering antibiotics, the other a bright red solution of daunomycin, dripped into her thin arms. The life in her seemed concentrated in her bright, angry eyes, glaring out of her gaunt face. She frowned when she saw the doctor, fearing some new pain.

"Good morning, Ellie," Nelson said cheerfully. "What seems to be the problem? I could hear you making noise all the way down the hall. What's the complaint this morning?"

Ellie turned her head away from the doctor in disgust. When Nelson tried to examine the sore on her finger, she pulled it away, shouting, "Don't touch it! I don't want that medicine on it, either! It stings!"

"I can give it to you as a pill," he offered.

"I want it by mouth, by liquid!" she demanded.

"Ellie, please don't talk to Dr. Nelson like that," Sally scolded.

"All right, we'll give it to you by liquid," Nelson said. The child was spirited, but a brat. Still, he admired her determination. It was hard not to want to appease her.

143

"The same kind of liquid I get up on seventeen, right?" Ellie asked.

"The very same bottle," Nelson reassured her.

"Am I going to have blood taken today?" she asked fearfully.

"Probably."

Sally sighed. "Will they take enough blood this time so that they don't have to come back? Apparently to do the cross-match, they didn't take enough blood."

"No, that wasn't the reason," Nelson replied. "Ellie has developed an unusual problem. She's made some antibodies to her transfused blood cells, which can happen after multiple transfusions. It's not dangerous; it will just make it more difficult for us to get blood for her."

The disease often seemed purposefully malicious, Nelson thought. Here was a child whose immune system was unable to defend her against common infections, yet it had produced an antibody that was complicating their efforts to treat her! Fighting leukemia was akin to battling the Hydra, the multiheaded monster of Greek myth: when one head was cut off, two more immediately grew back in its place.

"We have to do further tests to see what the antibodies are, so we can decide what blood we can give her," he went on. "But that's the blood bank's headache, not yours. They say they need eight cc's of blood today for the tests."

Sally shook her head wearily. "All right."

"Another thing is yesterday's chest X-ray," Nelson continued. "We found some haziness on her right side, but we're not sure if it's significant. So we want to repeat it today to see if anything's developing."

"Repeat what?" Ellie asked, suspicious.

"Your chest X-ray," Nelson replied gently. Turning to Sally, he said, "Sometime today or whenever we can squeeze it in. Perhaps tomorrow morning."

"I just don't like her getting all that radiation," Sally said.

"I know, but this is important," Nelson stressed. "She may be brewing something in there."

"Oh, all right." Sally's weariness was evident. "You know, yesterday they called for her while she was getting a transfusion."

"I realize that. Unfortunately we don't have much control over when they call for a chest X-ray. We send a slip down and when they're ready they call for her. It's not by appointment."

Sally just shrugged.

"By the way," Nelson added, "we should have the results of the mixed-lymphocyte culture in a few days. As soon as they're in, I'll let you know."

"Oh, good," Sally said apathetically, her eyes focused beyond Nelson at some secret configuration in the air.

Troubled, Nelson thanked her for her cooperation and left the room. Both mother and child seemed to him very depressed and anxious.

Not long after, Susan Drake came in to draw the blood specimen for the antibody studies. Sally was furious when she realized that the resident would be sticking Ellie instead of one of the chemo nurses, who were much more skilled at finding veins. She held tightly onto Ellie's hand while Drake removed the needle from its sterile pack and began to probe the child's forearm with it.

Ellie cried and squirmed, and Sally bit her lip until it bled. No sooner had Drake gotten the needle into the vein than it collapsed. The resident swore under her breath, sweat glistening on her brow as she withdrew the needle and started again on another fragile vein. Ellie was crying harder now, and flinched as the needle went in.

"Stop moving!" Drake snapped at her.

"I can't help it!" Ellie screamed. "You're hurting me! Mommy, she's hurting me!"

Ellie's pathetic cry tore Sally from her paralysis, and she suddenly exploded in a rage. "Goddammit! Can't you find someone to practice on who isn't getting stuck twenty times a day?" she demanded, trembling with anger. "This poor child has had so many needles she must feel like a pincushion. Get out of here and find an IV therapist who knows what she's doing!"

Shaken and intimidated, Drake backed off and left the room. When she had gone, Sally calmed down a little, feeling a pang of regret for having allowed herself to get so angry. But she realized that she would have to be Ellie's advocate and defender—the child was just too small and weak to protect herself.

At 2:00 P.M. was the Psychosocial Conference, a weekly meeting sponsored by the Department of Psychiatry for the discussion of staff problems in their interactions with patients and families. Dr. Nelson went into the small lounge in one corner of the nurses' station and sat down, already exhausted although the day was only half over. The room was rapidly filling up with residents and nurses. Soon all of the seats and benches along the four walls had been taken and a few more chairs were brought in. Finally someone closed the door and the session began.

Leading the discussion were Dr. Saul Eisenberg, the child psychiatrist on the floor, and Helen Davis, the pediatric social worker. Eisenberg asked if anyone had a specific problem to discuss, and Susan Drake raised her hand. "I'd like to talk about Mrs. Murphy," she said, and Eisenberg nodded for her to go ahead.

"Mrs. Murphy told the resident who was on over the weekend that she felt we were ignoring Ellie this time around," Drake began, an angry edge to her voice. "In fact, the only reason Ellie's care hasn't been optimal is because her mother makes things difficult for us. She has refused to have anyone but an IV nurse take blood from Ellie or start an IV, she's objected to chest X-rays, and it's just been one thing after another. She says she's tired of taking everything from the doctors and being told what to do. Ellie herself is sick, feels lousy, and has been through enough so that she is objecting to anything that causes her more discomfort. So between the two of them . . . I've had to ask Dr. Nelson, Ellie's private attending, to intervene several times."

"Has it been effective?" Eisenberg asked.

"Temporarily," Drake replied sharply.

Nelson shook his head. "A relapse is an emotionally devastating thing, and I don't blame the Murphys for being upset. It's been a tremendous letdown for us as well as them, and for a six-year-old kid who had been doing well to have to start over from scratch is really difficult. She's very clear about it: 'I'm tired and I'm fed up.' "

"Ellie has always been a difficult child," Sue Kramer said. "It's really a problem to take blood from her or start an IV. She starts screaming, and you can't blame her. Doctors have started IV's on her and it's taken three or four sticks. That's why her Mom refuses. But I think she's reality-oriented enough to know that if Ellie's IV stops flowing in the middle of the night, a doctor is going to have to restart it."

"No, she's not," Drake insisted. "When she came in that first night, when Ellie had a fever and we didn't know why and she needed antibiotics, Mrs. Murphy told me point-blank that she was not going to let me start an IV on her. That was at nine P.M., and she knew it was going to delay Ellie's antibiotics and transfusions, but she wanted to wait until morning and would not let me touch her. The night nurse finally persuaded her to give me one chance. Luckily, it was all I needed."

"Have you seen a change in Mrs. Murphy since Ellie came back to the hospital this time?" Davis asked.

Several nurses nodded. "Especially in the last few days," Margaret O'Connor, the head nurse, replied. "She's very anxious, she's not really focused, and she's not willing to sit down and talk about what's going on. She wants to know why this or that can't be done, and although she gets the same answers from everyone, she keeps going from one nurse to another. She doesn't come out of the room to talk to you, and Ellie's in the background screaming her head off. You feel sorry for her because the kid's yelling, but at the same time . . ."

Karen Lagano, another nurse, agreed. "We're trying to take care of Ellie, but at the same time Mrs. Murphy is trying to take over. It's getting to the point where she'll come into the nurses' station and pick up the electronic thermometer and take Ellie's temp every half hour. I've tried to explain to her that there are a limited number of things we can do to control a child's temp anyway, so that taking it every half hour is only going to make her daughter very anxious. But she keeps coming back for the thermometer and the poor child is just freaking out. We've been asking Mrs. Murphy to let us do more of the routine care to relieve her, but she just won't sit down and let us talk to her about it."

"She's driven, and she seems totally exhausted," Pat said.

Nurse O'Connor nodded. "You'd be tired, too, if you were taking temps every half hour all night long."

There was a brief silence, and then Nelson spoke up. "I've noticed that Mrs. Murphy has also become very religious since the relapse. She goes to the church across the street a couple of times a day. She may get some strength from this, but on the other hand, it may prevent her from seeing some of the reality."

Nurse O'Connor nodded. "When I came back from my trip, I told Mrs. Murphy where I went. She said, 'If only I had known you were going to Jerusalem, I would have asked you to say a prayer for Ellie, and maybe she wouldn't be in this hospital today.' I said, 'Well, saying a prayer in Jerusalem wouldn't necessarily mean that Ellie could leave here.' And she said, 'God would hear you better, because that's where Jesus walked.'"

Dr. Eisenberg cleared his throat. "I think that beyond her religious faith, she believes in miracles. She's not facing reality very well."

"That's one of her defense mechanisms," Nelson replied. "To believe in the supernatural."

"Yes, the Lazarus syndrome," the psychiatrist agreed. "Last year, Ellie survived a bad case of chicken pox complicated by pneumonia that brought her to the brink of death. Since she made an almost miraculous recovery against all odds, perhaps Mrs. Murphy now refuses to believe that God would let her die. I think there's the danger that she's going to become more and more involved in her faith while Ellie gets sicker and sicker, and pretty soon she's going to be overwhelmed."

"We're considering Ellie now for a bone-marrow transplant," Nelson said, "which is all the more reason to make her more realistic. It was very difficult for her to accept the fact that Ellie relapsed. If her faith depends on Ellie being cured, then I'm afraid she's going to be destroyed. Our job is to try and preserve her faith in the face of this, and I'm not sure how one goes about that."

"Have you spoken with the father, Dr. Nelson?" Eisenberg asked.

"Very little. He comes in on weekends and an occasional evening."

"He doesn't call?"

"Rarely."

"I'm not sure how much support she gets from her husband," Sue Kramer interjected. "He was supposed to come in on Friday and stay with Ellie so that Mrs. Murphy could go home and do the laundry and get some rest. I was in the room when she asked him if she could stay home for two days and spend some time with her other daughters. He sounded angry and not at all supportive. He said, 'If you get the hell out of here already, you'll have more time to spend at home.' He really didn't sound sympathetic. So I don't know what's happening between them. There must be quite a bit of strain."

"Are there any suggestions about how to handle Ellie emotionally?" Eisenberg asked.

"I definitely think we should try to get the father more involved," Nelson said. "I'll speak to him the next time he comes in. In the meantime, you should all try to be as supportive as you possibly can."

Eisenberg nodded, and the conference moved on to the next case.

Helen Davis called Brian at work that afternoon, and he reluctantly agreed to meet with her the following Monday. He wanted to come in alone, but Helen insisted that Sally be with him. She felt that it was destructive to see a husband individually if he was isolating himself from his wife and child; not treating them as a couple would merely worsen the situation. When the Murphys had sat down in her office, looking noticeably strained and uncomfortable, she asked Brian point-blank how he was feeling.

He shrugged. "Oh, all right, I suppose, under the circumstances. I'm working hard to pay those damn medical bills, but otherwise . . ."

"Have things changed for you since Ellie's relapse?"

"Well, it was quite a blow, but the doctors are obviously doing everything they can to get her back into remission. I'm quite optimistic."

Helen shook her head. "Somehow I'm getting a very different picture of how things are going from your wife. She tells me that ever since the relapse you've been withdrawing progressively from her and from Ellie."

"Well, I do have to work extra hard to get new accounts if we're going to pay for all those medical bills, not to mention keeping up with the mortgage payments and putting food on the table for the rest of the family. I just don't have that much time to spend at the hospital."

"You should make time!" Sally snapped. "Your child's happiness should come first. I'm tired of carrying the load for both of us."

Helen turned to look at Brian; he avoided eye contact. "It sounds as if things are really worse than you've been letting yourself believe," she said. "Perhaps you feel that not admitting the seriousness of the relapse makes it less of a reality, as if there's a power in the denial that prevents the feared event from happening. In fact, that's not true. But if you deny yourself the opportunity to spend time with Ellie because you're refusing to confront your negative thoughts and feelings, then you're going to feel terribly guilty later on if she doesn't do well."

Brian sighed. "I guess it's just very hard for me to be with her. She's suffering so much, and I can't prevent her pain. It makes me so mad."

"That's a perfectly normal feeling," Helen said. "Parents—fathers especially—have a need to be the protector and strength of the family. After all, the major charge to a parent is to protect your children, to guide them and help them grow. So parents in this situation often feel weaker and less in control than at any other time in their lives. But you have to realize that you haven't failed as a parent. Medicine has failed, science has failed, but you as a parent could not have prevented your child from having a relapse—that's truly something beyond your control.

"Men often think," she went on, "that it's necessary to be strong and not to show emotion—that they have to be a pillar of strength all the time. You probably assume that since Sally is obviously upset already, the last thing she needs is to hear how bad you feel. But in fact one of the best ways to get through the rough times in life is to share feelings together. You don't have to fall apart—just let yourself feel. It's not weak to show emotion, and it doesn't take away from your manliness. Of course, your emotions don't have to be worn on your sleeve; they can be expressed in privacy without the world becoming involved."

Brian nodded. "It's just been hard for me to talk to Sally lately, since she's been so totally involved with Ellie and the hospital. Nothing else has any importance for her."

Sally glared at him. "Brian, if I didn't take care of Ellie, who would? You certainly haven't been doing your share."

"Wait a minute," Helen interjected, trying to forestall an argument. "Sally, it's important for you not to neglect Brian, either. While Ellie was in remission you both went back to having two focuses in your lives—your children and yourselves—so it must be very hard for both of you to have all of the attention suddenly going to Ellie again. In fact, it's not at all uncommon for a husband or wife in this situation to be a little jealous of the child, and that in turn can lead to feelings of guilt. But there are ways to get back to being a loving, devoted couple again, and the most important is communication. Nobody else in the world knows better what you two people are feeling than you do yourselves, since you share the same basic feelings of love and concern for Ellie. So there's really no need to protect each other from those feelings, and you're not likely to do the other person harm by sharing. On the contrary, you can help each other get through this hard time.

"I would also encourage you to take an evening out alone, having a friend or a grandparent stay with Ellie for a while. Go out to a quiet restaurant and don't talk about the illness but rather about yourselves, putting everything else aside for the evening, if you can. Talk about what each of you is doing and feeling, and what your plans for the future are, so that you're back focusing on your relationship instead of solely on Ellie."

That evening, Brian and Sally went out to dinner together not far from the hospital. Later, in the car, they wept quietly in each other's arms.

Two days later, the tissue-typing report from the Histocompatibility Testing Laboratory arrived on Nelson's desk. The tests had revealed that while Amy and Ellie had incompatible bone marrow, Beth and Ellie were as well matched as could be expected for nonidentical siblings: they shared all four major tissue markers (HLA antigens) and were mutually non-stimulatory in the mixed-lymphocyte-culture test. The only major hurdle in the match was the existence of different blood types: Ellie was type O and Beth was type A. Such a mismatch could occur even in the presence of perfect tissue compatibility, since the ABO markers on red cells are coded for by a different chromosome from the one that specifies the histocompatibility markers on white cells, platelets, and tissue cells. This finding meant that if Beth's marrow, containing large quantities of red cells, were given to Ellie without further processing, a massive and probably fatal transfusion reaction would result.

Nevertheless, the director of the Histocompatibility Testing Lab had attached a memo to the results in which he concluded, "Beth Murphy should not be excluded from further consideration, because techniques exist for crossing major blood-type barriers." A reference was given, but Nelson was already familiar with these developments. There were now a few methods available for getting around a blood-type incompatibility, once an insurmountable obstacle; the simplest method involved removing the mismatched red cells from the donor's bone marrow by spinning the marrow in a continuous-flow centrifuge.

The fact that Beth was the compatible sibling was fortunate, since she was now eight years old and sufficiently mature to donate substantial amounts of marrow without significant risk to herself. Working with Amy, now six months old, would have made the procedure much more difficult, although it would still have been possible. The youngest transplant donor to date had been a five-month-old infant who had donated marrow to her five-year-old sister in January 1980, at the Children's Hospital Medical Center in Boston.

Encouraged by the news of the tissue match, Nelson went to Ellie's room to tell Sally that the transplant was now a real possibility, providing they got Ellie back into remission. When that time came, the decision to do a transplant would no longer be a medical one but a parental one. "Why don't you call your husband?" he suggested.

Over the next week, Ellie responded well to the antibiotics and her fever went down. Two days later she was discharged from the hospital and her treatment continued on an outpatient basis, with Sally planning to commute in from New Jersey for the weekly injections of chemotherapy at the Day Hospital.

On Thursday, May 1, day twenty-eight of the reinduction protocol, Ellie was scheduled for a bone-marrow aspiration to determine if she was back in remission. She had continued to be very pale and weak, and Sally worried that the leukemia might still be there. Since Beth had wanted for some time to visit the clinic, Sally took her along. Beth waited outside the treatment room during the bone-marrow exam, cringing at Ellie's screams. When her mother emerged from the room, she was clearly upset. "Oh, it's so icky, it's so icky!" she kept saying.

The slides were sent off to the lab for immediate analysis, and Sally waited for the results as she had so many times before. She chatted with some of the other mothers in the waiting room, talking about everything but her real concerns. After about forty minutes, Nelson returned with the results. When Sally saw the smile on his face, she let out a great sigh of relief.

"Good news!" Nelson said. "Ellie's marrow looks fine. Everything is there that should be, and there are no blasts, no sign of the leukemia. She's back in remission, but it will take a few weeks before her poly count returns to normal, so she should stay away from crowds."

Sally fought back her tears, barely managing a whispered "Thank you, doctor."

A week later, at Ellie's next checkup, Nelson again brought up the subject of a bone-marrow transplant. Now that Ellie was feeling better and regaining her strength, Sally felt ambivalent about the procedure. She was torn between believing what Nelson said—that Ellie would probably relapse within six months—and her heart, which told her that Ellie was now a healthy child and that to give her a transplant would be putting her through something that might end her life.

Nelson understood her doubts, but he encouraged her to have Ellie evaluated by one or more of the transplant centers. If the child proved to be a suitable candidate for transplantation, she could then be put on the waiting list. At least then the option would be kept open. Sally appreciated the chance to defer a decision, so she asked Nelson to go ahead and refer Ellie for evaluation.

Nelson first inquired at the seven-bed transplant unit on the nineteenth floor of Memorial Hospital. He was informed by the director that there were no immediate openings, and that the waiting list was long and moving slowly. Since Nelson was reluctant to postpone the transplant evaluation too long, he decided to explore other possibilities. He did not know how long Ellie's remission would last, and if she developed a drug-resistant relapse she might no longer be a suitable candidate for transplantation.

Nelson knew that the Murphys felt strongly about staying in the East. They were anxious to be close to grandparents and friends and to avoid uprooting their other children. While Nelson understood their concerns, he felt uncomfortably constrained at the same time. Transplant centers in Los Angeles, Seattle, and Minnesota became out of the question. Since the units in Philadelphia and Boston were very small—only a few beds each—the fourteen-bed unit at Baltimore's Johns Hopkins Oncology Center seemed the next best bet. Although the transplant unit there treated mostly adolescents and young adults, they did accept a few young children.

Nelson called Baltimore and spoke to Dr. Paul Wood, one of the attending physicians affiliated with the transplant unit, who was responsible for accepting patient referrals that month. Nelson stressed that Ellie was currently in second remission, was in good clinical condition, and had an HLA-matched sibling, aged eight. Wood took down this information and said that because their waiting list was running between eight and ten patients, it would probably be a few weeks before Ellie could come down to Baltimore for an evaluation. He promised that her case would be brought up at their Wednesday census meeting, and that he would get back to Nelson as soon as a decision had been made.

Part **II**
A SEA OF TROUBLES

18 Census Meeting

Shortly before 4:00 P.M. on Wednesday, May 14, 1980, a group of white-coated personnel associated with the Johns Hopkins Bone Marrow Transplant Unit began to gather in the boardroom on the ground floor of the Oncology Center, at the end of a corridor lined with doctors' offices. The boardroom, starkly lit by fluorescent bulbs, was dominated by a large oak conference table, around which were modern armchairs made of steel and bright-yellow upholstering. Other than a blackboard, the walls were bare.

Dr. Charles Saunders, director of the Transplant Unit, sat down at the head of the table. Flanking him were the eight attending physicians affiliated with the Unit, the oncology fellow, a technician from the Immunogenetics Lab, two transplant coordinators, two senior nurses, two physician's assistants, a social worker, and a statistician.

Each of the eight attendings was on active duty for only six weeks a year because the work was so emotionally and physically draining. When the attendings were not treating patients they did clinical or basic research in some area relevant to bone-marrow transplantation, since Hopkins was an academic institution with a "publish-or-perish" mentality. One of the attendings specialized in the exotic bacterial, fungal, and viral infections that occur at high frequency in bone-marrow recipients; a second was studying the formation of the blood, which could be investigated to great advantage in the regenerating blood-forming tissues of marrow recipients; a third was interested in the mechanisms and management of graft-versus-host disease, a complication of marrow transplantation. As staff physicians

155

on salary, they made about half what they could have in private practice, but had the satisfaction of working on the frontiers of medical research.

Even when the attendings were not on active duty on the ward, they all came to the weekly census meeting in order to learn about the medical status of all of the inpatients and outpatients, so that they would be up to date when it was their turn to go on service. Because of this diffusion of knowledge among the various members of the transplant team, there were few abrupt transitions in the plan of patient care in spite of the frequent changes in personnel.

Another key member of the team was the oncology fellow: a young physician who, having completed his residency in internal medicine, was doing a two-year fellowship to receive specialized training in medical oncology, including a three-month rotation through the Transplant Unit. In addition to working on a research project, the fellow's role was to supervise the house staff, mostly first-year residents, who were responsible for the hour-to-hour management of the patients. There were three residents on duty at a time, each rotating through the Unit for a month, although they were not present at the census meeting.

When everyone had arrived, Diane Marks, one of the transplant coordinators, distributed photocopies of the computer print-out patient list, which was divided into five sections: Prospective Candidates, Waiting for Beds, Inpatients, Outpatients, and Six-Month Checkup. Saunders opened the meeting by reviewing the new referrals they had received over the past week. "What we have here is a list of patients, but we just don't have enough beds," he said, shaking his head. "I'll try to streamline the list over the next week, but it's more than we can handle at the moment. We now have seven patients waiting for beds, so the new referrals will have to wait at least a few weeks to get one. Okay, let's see what we have. . . ."

Every week, the referrals came in much faster than beds became available; the demand for bone-marrow transplants was still much greater than the supply. With a total of only eighty-five beds, the eight active transplant centers in the United States could do at most 510 transplants annually (assuming an average of six transplants per bed per year); the need was for several times that number.

The intensive nursing care and in-depth lab studies required for bone-marrow transplants elevated costs to about $1,000 a day for inpatient care, and, if complications developed, the hospital stay could be a long one. On average, the cost of a single transplant ranged from $60,000 to more than $100,000 in 1980, with inflation causing expenses to spiral upward. Even so, a study had shown that, in the long run, bone-marrow transplantation might be cheaper than conventional drug regimens for the poor prognostic types of leukemia, since maintenance chemotherapy often required repeated hospitalizations for complications and was ultimately less effective.

Since Hopkins was a private hospital, most of its funding came from third-party insurance coverage, such as Blue Cross/Blue Shield, Medicaid, and Major Medical. These agencies had agreed to pay for bone-marrow transplants, but only for those patients who had adequate coverage. The Transplant Unit also received funding from the National Cancer Institute to cover the research aspects of its activities. Dr. Saunders did allocate some of the grant money to help out the poorer families, so they would not have to sell their homes and possessions to pay for a transplant. But his entire research grant would have been sufficient to pay the complete hospital expenses of only five patients.

Given the limited number of beds and the center's finite economic resources, the transplant team had no choice but to pick the patients with the best possible chances of survival. Although the team had originally attempted to transplant leukemic patients in the end stages of their disease, the success rate with these patients had been extremely low. Now they almost always required that transplants be reserved for leukemics who were in their first or second remission. Moreover, all transplant recipients were required to have an identical-twin or HLA-identical donor; patients with identical twins were given priority because of the relative lack of complications. Factors that ruled out acceptance or lowered priority on the waiting list included a serious infection within six weeks prior to referral, life expectancy seriously limited by diseases other than leukemia, a severe personality disorder or mental illness, or damage to a vital organ. A patient without a history of central-nervous-system leukemia had preference over someone who had had CNS disease. Finally, a young person generally had priority over an older person, because transplants had so far been more successful in younger patients.

If a newly referred patient was very likely to do well—say, a preadolescent with AML in first remission and an identical-twin donor—he or she might move immediately to the top of the waiting list. The selection process was therefore akin to the triage system practiced on the battlefield, in which seriously wounded soldiers with a good chance of recovery were treated first, and those with hopeless injuries were simply passed over. There were some patients on the waiting list who would probably never get a transplant, since their chances of benefiting from the procedure were slim and other patients would be accepted in preference over them. For example, it made little sense to transplant a patient with ALL in drug-resistant relapse, since only about 10 or 15 percent of such patients would survive more than a year. Even so, when several beds on the unit opened up and the waiting list was short, patients who might otherwise not be accepted could get in. When the unit had 100 percent occupancy (which was increasingly the case), Saunders usually referred prospective patients to other transplant centers as well. Patients were encouraged to be on the waiting list at two or three centers, standing by for the first available bed.

There was also a "political" aspect to the selection process. Hopkins had to compete with the other transplant centers for good patients and federal grant money from the NCI. The better their results, the easier it would be to attract more patient referrals and government funds. That would mean acquiring additional treatment facilities, additional staff, and theoretically better results, which would bring still more referrals and money. It was an ever-enlarging circle of cause and effect. Most of the time the choice of patients for transplantation was a fairly straightforward matter. Since Saunders had the most experience and seniority, he was the one who made the final decisions.

Saunders now quickly went over the list of patients waiting for beds. "There's a Bruce Solomon, age thirty-four, with T-cell ALL in first remission. Apparently everything is cleared, so as soon as we have a bed we'll admit him. Then there's Tracy Stevens, with aplastic anemia, some data pending but everything looks okay except maybe the finances. Jackie Higgins went home. She arrived here when John was attending and he saw that she obviously had an aberration in her liver enzymes, a flare-up of her hepatitis, so we'll have to wait until that's straightened out. Jerry Kovak will be here with his family tomorrow for us to tell them what the transplant is all about, and then they'll have to decide whether they want us to go ahead. On the next page, Marsha O'Mally is still uncertain. I've talked to her parents and they haven't answered, so I presume they don't want to do it now, unless they call."

"Is that a first-remission AML?" Wood asked.

"Yes, it is. I went through everything with them, and they were supposed to give me a decision some time ago. Moving on, Ray Lewis, a twelve-year-old aplastic, will be ready to go as soon as we get a bed."

"What about Susan Lenox?" asked James Krueger, the attending physician currently on service. "That's page two, number six."

"She recently developed a few fractures of her lumbar vertebrae," Wood replied.

"Due to steroids?" Krueger asked.

"That, and perhaps not moving. There were also leukemic infiltrates in there. She's still in quite a lot of pain. The question is, should it discourage us from doing the transplant?"

"Did she have radiation to that area?" Saunders asked.

"I don't think so," Wood replied. "Just chemotherapy."

Saunders shook his head. "I'll put a question mark down on that one."

The fellow, Wade Peters, looked concerned. "Does that immediately exclude her?" he asked.

"No," Saunders said. "I'll get back to her next week. Then I'll get the complete story and have a chance to digest the data."

It was an extremely painful task for Saunders to have to inform patients that they were no longer eligible for a transplant, particularly if they were already on the waiting list. A few weeks before, a young man with ALL in remission, who had been a good candidate for a transplant, had developed a bone-marrow relapse after he had arrived in Baltimore. Saunders had had to tell him the bad news, something he much preferred to do over the phone rather than face to face. He dreaded such confrontations. "Look," he had said, "we wouldn't be doing you any favors by going through with the procedure now. Your chances of survival would be less than 10 percent."

"But I don't have any alternatives!" the young man had protested.

"I know, but at least you can be at home. . . ." Saunders had replied. He hated to play God in that way, and such conversations lingered in his mind for weeks afterward. That was why he was constantly pushing for more grant money and clinical research to improve the transplant procedure, making it more successful, less expensive, and hence available to more of the patients who needed it.

Saunders finished up his discussion of the waiting list and moved on to the latest referrals. "The next patient is Ellen Murphy, a six-year-old with ALL in second remission, referred to us by Dr. Nelson at Memorial Sloan-Kettering. Apparently their transplant unit is filled up for the foreseeable future. Nelson said she is a good candidate, although she is very young for us."

They all looked at the data on the print-out:

```
MURPHY, ELLEN        LEUKEMIA, ACUTE LYM

INITIAL CONTACT: 050980
TYPING: SLOAN-KETTERING
RESULTS: 1 HLA ID SIB (BETH, AGE 8)
MLC: SAME PLACE
RESULTS: NEG
FINANCES: BEING CHKD
DATA REC'D: TYPING
STATUS: 2ND REM
MEDICAL FACTORS: DX 9/16/78, INDUCED ON CCSG-162, 1ST REM
10/13/78, BM RELAPSE 4/3/80, 2ND REM 5/1/80
```

159

COMMENTS: NO CNS DISEASE, IN GOOD CLINICAL CONDITION
REF SOURCE: DR. ROGER T. NELSON
PEDIATRIC HEMATOLOGY/ONCOLOGY
MEMORIAL SLOAN-KETTERING

"According to Dr. Nelson's office, she has adequate coverage," Saunders went on. "Major Medical, I think. There's some data pending on this patient, but everything looks basically okay. Since her prognosis appears excellent, it would put her near the top of the waiting list. I think we should bring her down here soon for an evaluation." Saunders paused, awaiting a reaction from the group. The other attendings all nodded, a few somewhat hesitantly, but no one challenged his decision. Saunders moved on to a brief summary of the medical status of the inpatients, outpatients, and long-term survivors due in for their annual checkup, which brought the meeting to a close. Afterward, the doctors and other personnel quickly dispersed and Saunders retired to his office, thinking about the new referral from Memorial Sloan-Kettering.

He was aware that some of the attendings had been ambivalent about the possibility of transplanting a six-year-old, since they found it more of a strain. Why they should feel worse about a six-year-old going through the procedure than a functional man of forty-five, he did not know, but so they did. If transplants were in fact a reasonable approach to treating leukemia, however, Saunders felt they should not be denied to children, particularly since children tended to respond better to the treatment than adults. He remembered a confrontation he had had with a pediatrician on the hospital's Clinical Investigation Committee while their latest protocol was being evaluated for its ethics. "Is it ethical to do this on kids?" she had demanded. Saunders had replied by turning the question around. "You know we're doing everything we can to improve a terrible situation," he had said. "Now, is it ethical not to offer this treatment to kids?" The pediatrician had acknowledged his point.

Nevertheless, it was still a very tough business, not unlike the Burn Unit. The incidence of complications with marrow transplants was high, and the mortality rate was hovering near 50 percent. At times, when there was a run of bad luck on the service, Saunders found himself questioning what they were trying to do. "I want to get out of this business," he would tell himself. All the other marrow-transplant specialists he knew went through similar crises, during which they agonized over whether they were doing the right thing. The religious ones among them prayed, asking God to give them a sign if they were doing wrong; the others, like Saunders, just hoped that when the results were added up, the good would outweigh the bad.

When Saunders felt most troubled by doubts about transplantation, he would look back and realize how far they had come. He remembered what it had been like to say, "Here's a person with leukemia in third or fourth remission, and there's nothing we can do." With young patients, he had felt even worse. Looking back over the past three decades, he could see how the long years of research and frustration were only now beginning to bear fruit.

The concept of bone-marrow transplantation had arisen initially out of an intense interest among medical scientists in the effects of ionizing radiation on living systems following the use of the atomic bomb in World War II. Many A-bomb victims in Hiroshima and Nagasaki, although not killed instantly by the explosion, died hours or days later due to bone-marrow failure. Accordingly, much U.S. government–sponsored research was directed toward understanding the mechanism of radiation-induced marrow failure and developing ways to protect against it.

In 1949, working at the Institute of Radiobiology and Biophysics of the University of Chicago, L. O. Jacobson and his colleagues discovered that mice could be protected from otherwise lethal irradiation by shielding their spleens with lead. Even if the spleen was removed an hour after the irradiation, the mice still survived, whereas unprotected mice died within twenty-four hours. The following year, Egon Lorenz and his coworkers at the Laboratory of Biophysics of the National Cancer Institute took this experiment one step further. Having exposed a population of mice to a lethal dose of radiation, they gave half of the mice an injection of bone marrow which had been extracted previously from other mice of the same genetic type. Within twenty-four hours the control mice had died, but the mice that had received the injections of marrow were scampering about as if nothing had happened. Still, the mechanism by which the transplanted bone marrow had protected the mice was as yet unclear.

Lorenz came up with two opposing hypotheses: (1) the donor marrow was releasing a chemical factor that caused the host's own marrow to regenerate, thereby rescuing the irradiated mice from death, or (2) the donor's marrow cells were actually multiplying within the marrow spaces of the host, which had been emptied by the radiation, and were resulting in the production of new blood cells.

After much discussion, an experiment designed to distinguish between these two possibilities was conducted in 1956 by C. E. Ford and his coworkers at the Medical Research Council Radiobiological Research Unit in England. These researchers injected bone marrow from Wistar *rats* into laboratory *mice* that had received a lethal dose of radiation. Again, the mice that received the marrow were protected against the radiation, whereas all

161

of the control animals died. Ford then examined the marrow cells that had multiplied in the marrow spaces of the surviving mice. Since the cells of rats and mice differ in the number and shape of their chromosomes, the British investigators were able to determine the source of the regenerated marrow. Microscopic examination revealed that all of the cells in the mice's new marrow contained rat chromosomes.

Ford's experiment clearly indicated that the injected rat marrow cells had migrated from the blood to the marrow spaces inside the pelvis, ribs, and long bones of the host mice and had begun to multiply, turning out life-saving blood cells of all types. Since these mice were now composites of more than one genetic type, he termed them "radiation chimeras," after the mythical Greek Chimera: a freakish blend of lion, goat, and serpent. In a paper published in the March 10, 1956, issue of the British journal *Nature*, Ford concluded, "Although the very term *chimera* points to the antiquity of the idea, it is believed that the experiment reported here provides the first decisive evidence in animals that normal cells of one species may, in special circumstances, not merely survive and multiply in another, but even replace the corresponding cells of the host and take over their functions."

Such genetic mixtures do not normally occur in nature because of the remarkable ability of the body's immune system to reject any cells of a different genetic lineage from its own, whether they be bacteria or transplanted tissue cells that are not genetically matched. Indeed, Ford's belief that he had created a chimera of rat and mouse turned out to be incorrect (although true chimeras have since been produced by "gene-splicing" techniques). After three or four weeks, Ford noted that his "chimeric" mice were beginning to die off, victims of a delayed immunological reaction of the grafted marrow cells against their new host. This ominous development foreshadowed the serious immunological complications that would hinder the development of successful therapeutic bone-marrow transplantation in human beings.

In 1957, Peter C. Nowell and his colleagues at the U.S. Naval Radiological Defense Laboratory in San Francisco studied the most effective way to administer bone marrow to irradiated animals. Transplantation was attempted by four different injection routes: directly into the bones, into the abdominal cavity, under the skin, and intravenously. Both the abdominal and the intravenous routes worked, although in monkeys an abdominal injection required three times as much marrow as an intravenous injection to yield the same protective effect. Remarkably enough, it seemed that marrow injected into the bloodstream managed to find its way into the cavities of the bones, which are extensively supplied with tiny blood vessels.

Further research in other laboratories revealed that intravenously injected marrow cells do not "home" directly to the marrow spaces but first circulate throughout the body. When mice were sacrificed and autopsied immediately after an injection of marrow, small foci of marrow cells were found in the lungs. This finding indicated that injected marrow cells can lodge outside the bone marrow, but soon die off; they can survive and multiply only in the marrow spaces, which evolution has shaped in such a way as to be optimal for the survival and growth of the blood-forming tissues.

The first attempt to extend the promising results of lab-animal studies to therapeutic use of marrow transplantation in human beings was made in 1957 by E. Donnall Thomas, then an associate professor of medicine at Columbia University and a staff physician at the Mary Imogene Bassett Hospital in Cooperstown, New York. In a pioneering clinical research study, Thomas and his colleagues collected human bone marrow from three sources: cadavers, ribs removed during surgery, and living donors. They then transfused the marrow into several terminal cancer patients, all of whom had failed to respond to conventional treatments. Although in one patient the graft took temporarily and began to produce blood cells for a few days, none of the graft recipients survived more than a few weeks. Thomas concluded that human marrow could be collected, stored, and administered without harmful effects, but he suspected that prolonged "takes" would be possible only if the preexisting diseased marrow was first eliminated with intensive radiation treatments, making room for the grafted cells to grow and also suppressing the immune response of the host.

The following year, Thomas and his coworkers attempted transplants in two young children with ALL, both of whom had healthy identical twins as donors and hence would not be expected to reject the graft. Both patients were prepared for transplantation with 1,000 rads of total-body irradiation. The grafts were successful, as evidenced by the return of marrow function in both patients after less than two weeks, but the leukemia recurred after remissions of seven weeks in one patient and twelve weeks in the other. Although this study indicated that bone-marrow transplantation would not be an easy cure for leukemia, it provided hope that marrow grafts could be achieved between identical twins.

Human identical twins are exceedingly rare, however, and few leukemic children are fortunate enough to have one. In an effort to better define the immunological barriers between nontwin siblings that were known to cause graft rejection, tissue typing and matching were developed. In addition, several other medical advances in the 1960s improved the outlook for bone-marrow transplantation: powerful new antibiotics, techniques for separating blood into its various components for transfusion, intravenous nutrition, and the use of immunosuppressive drugs to reduce the frequency and severity of immunological rejection reactions.

In 1962, Georges Mathé of the Institut Gustave-Roussy in Paris transplanted marrow grafts that functioned for as long as eight months, but it was not until 1968 that the first permanent bone-marrow transplant between HLA-matched siblings was achieved by Robert A. Good of the University of Minnesota Medical Center in a child with severe combined immune-deficiency disease (a congenital lack of body defenses against infection). Four years later, in 1972, the first successful matched-sibling transplant was achieved for another blood disease, aplastic anemia (the total failure of the bone marrow to produce blood cells). In each case, engraftment occurred over a period of about three weeks, and blood counts returned to normal within two or three months.

Attempts to apply marrow transplantation to the treatment of leukemia, however, continued to be met by repeated frustration and disappointment. In order to eliminate the leukemic cells from the body, high doses of chemotherapy and radiation were needed prior to transplantation, resulting in damage to vital organs and prolonged aplasia (low blood counts). This drastic therapy often led to fatal bleeding and infection. As an experimental procedure with a very small chance of working, marrow transplantation was considered an option of last resort, ethically justifiable only for patients in the end stages of leukemia whose disease had proved resistant to all conventional therapies. All of these patients were seriously ill, however, and as a result most died of complications before the graft could even be evaluated. In 1973, two out of every three transplant patients died within a month of the procedure, usually of overwhelming infection, and the odds of long-term survival were less than 10 percent. Bone-marrow transplantation had thus become trapped in a vicious circle.

Gradually, however, the pioneering transplant teams at the Fred Hutchinson Cancer Research Center in Seattle (where E. Donnall Thomas had since moved), Johns Hopkins, UCLA, Memorial Sloan-Kettering, Minnesota, and City of Hope Medical Center in California improved their ability to support patients through the hazardous period of aplasia immediately following the transplant. With the use of protective, germ-free environments, powerful antibiotics, and multiple transfusions of concentrated platelets, red cells, and white cells, the statistics began to improve. By the spring of 1975, the Seattle team, now headed by Thomas, had carried out more than one hundred transplants on leukemic patients in the end stages of their disease. Of these, fifteen patients had survived between two and nine years after the transplant, and were tentatively considered cured of their otherwise untreatable leukemia. The Seattle group concluded their report in *The New England Journal of Medicine* on a cautiously optimistic note: "Although [the] overall surviving fraction is small, it is encouraging to find that it is possible to cure some of these end-stage patients, and this has inspired renewed efforts to overcome some of the problems."

The Seattle group now felt ethically justified in attempting transplantation earlier in the course of the illness. In January 1976, they began to transplant leukemic patients in remission who were known to have a prognostically poor form of the disease. Since these patients had a lower tumor load and were in better clinical condition than patients in relapse, they were more likely to withstand the rigors of chemotherapy and radiation and also less likely to develop a recurrence of their leukemia after the transplant.

Indeed, the results of the Seattle study showed this to be the case. Of twenty-two patients with ALL who were transplanted during their second or subsequent remissions, all survived the hazardous first fifty days after the transplant and were successfully engrafted. Moreover, because their bone marrow was healthy at the time of the transplant, they had much less need for transfusions of white cells and platelets than did patients transplanted in relapse, and they spent considerably fewer days in the hospital. Of the original twenty-two patients, three died from nonleukemic complications, eight died of recurrent leukemia, and eleven (50 percent) survived, including two in whom the leukemia returned but was controlled with chemotherapy. The results were even better in patients with AML who were transplanted in first remission: after three to six years, 60 percent were alive and in complete remission.

This watershed study (and others conducted at City of Hope and the University of Minnesota) did much to alter oncologists' perceptions of bone-marrow transplantation. No longer was it considered a desperate therapeutic maneuver for hopelessly ill patients but rather a promising approach for those patients whose leukemia failed to be eradicated by chemotherapy protocols. The risks and complications of marrow transplantation, although major, were now seen to be offset by the possibility of obtaining a long-term remission or cure where none had been previously imaginable. As a result, the number of referrals to transplant centers of leukemic patients in remission increased dramatically. By 1980, the Seattle group was doing more than two hundred transplants a year, all of them on patients in remission, and other centers were beginning to follow suit.

The transplant centers were also getting a clearer idea of the optimal candidates and conditions for bone-marrow transplantation. Patients with

AML in first remission virtually always relapsed without a transplant, and were therefore given preference. For high-risk types of ALL, such as T-cell leukemia in adolescents and adults, first-remission transplants also appeared to be justified. A major exception was the outlook for children with the good-prognostic types of ALL, since the majority of them could be apparently cured with chemotherapy alone. Once such a child relapsed, however, the prognosis became poor and transplantation was then a realistic option.

The Hopkins transplant team had been one of the last groups in the country to start transplanting leukemics in remission, but they had been convinced by the Seattle data. Although they had felt ethically good about transplanting patients in relapse, they had had very little success in getting them through the procedure alive. Now almost every leukemic they transplanted was in remission, and they were doing about fifty transplants per year and receiving more than two hundred referrals annually.

In addition, for patients who had no available donor, they had begun doing "autologous" transplants in increasing numbers. When the patient was in first remission, he donated a sample of his own presumably healthy marrow, which was then frozen for future use. In the event of a relapse, he was induced into a second remission and then given a transplant of his own thawed marrow. The advantage of this approach was that there was no risk of graft rejection, but there was always the danger that the frozen marrow contained leukemic cells. If a patient did not relapse within three months after his bone marrow had been stored, however, chances were good that his marrow was "clean."

In spite of these innovations, there were still many problems to be overcome before marrow transplantation could be considered a safe and reliable treatment for recurrent leukemia. The success rate in 1980 was still between 50 and 65 percent, and the remaining 35 to 50 percent were claimed by rejection reactions, infection, graft-versus-host disease, and recurrent leukemia. Nevertheless, the risks of conventional chemotherapy were also high, and drugs alone showed little promise of curing the disease after the first relapse.

Saunders was often asked if the country could afford to pay vast sums for highly complex procedures such as bone-marrow transplantation. He did not believe there was any dilemma, from either a financial or an ethical standpoint. Actually only about 3 percent of the national health-care budget went for such "heroic" procedures. The bottom line was always: What is one life worth? Leukemia was a rare disease, but if you had it, it was not rare at all. Saunders often presented the problem to critics who questioned spending so much on marrow transplants by reducing it to its starkest fundamentals. "If you have a limited amount of money to treat leukemia," he would say, "then do as follows: Treat patients with drugs, and if they go into remission, beautiful. Then when they relapse, if they can die peacefully, let them. Otherwise, shoot them. It sounds terrible, but that's the implication of not doing marrow transplants."

In fact, Saunders was a visionary about the future of marrow transplantation. He believed that it was a good research investment with a number of exciting therapeutic applications beyond the treatment of rare blood diseases. Already solid tumors such as neuroblastoma (a cancer of nerve cells in children that often spreads to the bone marrow) were being treated with bone-marrow transplantation on an experimental basis at the Children's Hospital of Philadelphia. If the technique could be made safer and more reliable, it might prove suitable for the treatment of more common solid tumors in adults, permitting the use of potentially curative levels of radiation and chemotherapy without concern about their toxicity to the healthy bone marrow.

Other potential applications included treating victims of radiation accidents and curing genetic blood disorders such as thalassemia and sickle-cell anemia. Saunders even speculated that organ transplants in the future might be achieved by first doing a bone-marrow transplant. Since the graft of new bone marrow would change the recipient's immune system to that of the donor, it would then be possible to transplant any organ or tissue—skin, kidney, or heart—without fear of a rejection reaction. Clearly, investigations into the possible benefits of marrow transplantation were just beginning.

19 Three-South

Two weeks passed without word from Hopkins. Then on Wednesday, May 28, Diane Marks, one of the two transplant coordinators who handled all the logistics of setting up evaluations and transplants, called Dr. Nelson in New York and informed him that Ellie had been selected as a candidate. She asked him to notify the Murphys that she would be calling them later on that afternoon.

After speaking with Nelson, Sally Murphy stayed home all afternoon so as not to miss the call from Hopkins. She cleaned the house and tried not to think too much about the transplant, but she jumped every time the phone rang. There were two false alarms: a call from Brian, followed by one from

Cindy. Sally kept the conversations short, promising to call back as soon as she heard any news.

Finally the phone rang again. This time it was Diane Marks, telling her that Ellie had been selected for evaluation, and were they still interested in a transplant? Sally hesitated, but Diane assured her that the evaluation process would not commit them to anything. It would involve three days of tests to make sure that Ellie's systems were functioning well enough to give her a good chance of surviving the rigors of the transplant procedure. If Ellie turned out to be suitable for a transplant, the Murphys would be extensively informed by the doctors about the risks and benefits involved. Only then would they have to come to a decision, and they would have as long as they needed to make up their minds.

Sally thanked her and agreed to call back as soon as she had talked it over with her husband. She hung up, at once thrilled and frightened by the news. What had seemed for so long merely a hazy possibility had now become an undeniable reality. She called Brian and they agreed to go through with the evaluation, since Nelson had said that the transplant offered Ellie the best chance. Sally then called Diane back and made an appointment to bring Ellie to Hopkins on Sunday, June 1.

Since Beth was the potential donor, she had to go along to the hospital for a separate battery of tests, but the Murphys left Amy behind with Brian's parents. During the three-hour drive to Baltimore the family was tense, but Sally tried to be cheerful and optimistic for the children's sake. She joked with Brian, calling the transplant "a temporary inconvenience for permanent improvement."

Finally the skyline of Baltimore appeared before them. Brian turned off the highway and drove past endless rows of tenement houses. He detoured for a look at the newly completed Inner Harbor development along the waterfront, with its numerous shops and restaurants and the twenty-eight-story pentagonal Baltimore World Trade Center. "Mommy, look at the big boat!" Ellie exclaimed, pointing at the U.S.F. *Constellation,* first launched in Baltimore in 1797 and now permanently on display. Sally promised Ellie that they would come back and visit the tall ship as soon as they had a chance.

Following Diane's directions, they continued on toward the Johns Hopkins Medical Center, which was located in a poor section of the city. The Oncology Center was a five-story, red-brick monolith rising in the midst of the medical complex. Opened in 1976, it had been the first of twenty regional comprehensive cancer centers in the United States created by the 1971 National Cancer Act and had been constructed at a cost of nineteen million dollars in federal, state, and private funds. The facility was divided into four fourteen-bed units: Two-North and Three-North were for solid tumors, Two-South was for leukemia, and Three-South housed the Bone Marrow Transplant Unit. There were also ten research laboratories, many of them devoted to basic research on bone-marrow transplantation or its therapeutic applications. The sleek modern building, housing its state-of-the-art medical technology, was in sharp contrast to the surrounding urban decay. With some alarm, Sally noticed that armed guards were stationed at all entrances of the hospital to check identification.

Directly adjacent to the Oncology Center stood the old hospital building, with its handsome dome and spires; it in turn was located across the street from the Sheraton Johns Hopkins Motel. Brian parked in the motel lot, unloaded the bags from the trunk, and went inside to register. The woman at the desk noted Ellie's sparse hair and puffy face but did not seem surprised; many cancer patients stayed at the Sheraton. Brian carried their bags to the room, which was blandly decorated in typical motel style. It had a color TV and a window looking out on the swimming pool in back.

By the time they had unpacked, they had only ten minutes to get to their 1:00 P.M. appointment with Diane Marks. They walked across the street, up the steps, through the rotunda of the old hospital building with its huge marble statue of Jesus, and along an enclosed walkway to the Oncology Center. The corridor was bustling with doctors and nurses all hurrying to their various destinations, and every few seconds the intercom paged another name. Feeling lost, the Murphys went over to the information desk and were directed to the Transplant Unit.

As they emerged from the elevator on the third floor, they noted a visitors' lounge on their left, and straight ahead a set of double doors leading to the Unit. Sally peered through the windows in the doors down the long corridor, with its white linoleum floor gleaming in the light of the ceiling lamps. She saw a few nurses walking up and down, and then she caught sight of a teenage boy in pajamas, his head completely bald and the lower half of his face covered by a blue surgical mask, walking slowly down the corridor and wheeling his IV pole along beside him. Four bottles hanging from the top of the pole were connected to various tubes feeding into his body. He was bent over with fatigue but kept plodding along determinedly, waving at people inside the rooms along the corridor. Then he turned out of sight behind the nurses' station.

Could this be the Transplant Unit? Sally wondered. She had expected something more futuristic and confining, like the seven-bed unit at Memorial that Nelson had described to her: a series of large laminar-airflow rooms, like sterile incubators, from which the patients never emerged. But this unit was surprisingly ordinary—it looked just like a regular private medical ward.

Just then a young black woman emerged into the corridor and came out

169

to greet them. "Are you the Murphys?" she asked with a cheerful smile. "Hi, I'm Diane. Why don't you come into my office?" She gave Ellie and Beth pats on the head and turned to lead the way.

Once inside the small room a few doors down the corridor, she gestured the Murphys to sit on the couch. The office was rather cramped, since it was shared by the two transplant coordinators and the physician's assistants. In addition to the couch, there were two armchairs, a coffee table, three desks piled high with papers and patient charts, and a computer terminal. A few large travel posters decorated the walls, and Diane had pinned up some amusing sayings over her desk: "People who think they know everything are particularly aggravating to those of us who do." "A neat desk is a sign of a sick mind." "Doing a good job around here is like wetting your pants in a dark suit . . . you get a warm feeling but no one notices."

Diane began by telling the Murphys that the evaluation period would take two or three days and involve a battery of tests for both Ellie and Beth, as well as blood tests for Brian and Sally so that blood types and tissue types could be determined. If Ellie passed all the tests and the family chose to go through with the transplant, they would have to remain in the Baltimore area for at least one hundred days. Ellie would be an inpatient for four or five weeks and treated for the rest of the time as an outpatient. Because of possible complications of the procedure, however, she might be hospitalized for as long as three months. Diane referred all technical questions about the transplant itself to Dr. Krueger, the attending on duty that month, who would be meeting with them later on.

Sally wanted to know about the isolation procedure, since she had read an article about bone-marrow transplants that had stated that the patients were all kept in sterile rooms and that everything brought into the room, including toys and food, had to be sterilized as well. She was surprised when Diane told her that Hopkins required only masks and hand-washing, and not caps, gowns, or surgical gloves. In fact, as soon as patients were out of immediate danger of infection, they were encouraged to leave their rooms and walk "laps" around the nurses' station. Sally remembered the patient she had seen and nodded. She asked why the isolation procedures at Memorial Sloan-Kettering were so much stricter. Diane explained that each transplant center did things somewhat differently, often for historical reasons. The unit at Memorial, for instance, had been set up initially to treat children with combined immune-deficiency disease, who required a totally germ-free environment in order to survive. Because increasing numbers of leukemic patients were being transplanted in remission, however, the length of time when their absolute poly count was below 800 was actually quite short, so that strict isolation was rarely necessary. Sally also asked about visiting hours, which were from 8:00 A.M. to 11:00 P.M., although parents of young children like Ellie were allowed to sleep over occasionally.

During the question-and-answer session, Ellie and Beth seemed unusually calm and muted because of the unfamiliar surroundings. Afterward, Diane took the Murphys on a tour of the Unit. On the door of each room, the patient's name was spelled out in large letters cut from colored construction paper, often accompanied by drawings or get-well cards. Through the open doorways Sally saw that some of the patients looked extremely sick, but others were dressed in their street clothes and appeared fairly strong. The loud, agonized sound of retching came from one room, and in another a heart monitor beeped. One young man, bald and with an unsightly red rash on his face due to a profusion of cold sores, was playing a banjo in his room. The pleasant country music seeped out into the corridor, and passing nurses smiled. Sally was impressed by the courage of these young patients, who seemed to be keeping their spirits up in spite of near-constant discomfort.

Diane led them over to the nurses' station, where some residents were busily studying patient charts, and introduced Ellie to a few of the doctors. She quickly did the same for Beth, lest she become jealous of all the attention her sister was getting. Then they returned to the office and Diane paged Dr. Krueger. A few minutes later the attending appeared. He was a tall, soft-spoken, rather somber man, with a drooping mustache. Since the office was too busy for them to talk, he took Brian and Sally into the visitors' lounge while Beth and Ellie stayed behind with Diane. She entertained them by letting them play with her computer terminal, which they kept calling "this funny typewriter."

The lounge was a small, sunny room with a large window looking out onto the façade of the old hospital building. Two comfortable couches were arranged in an L, with a round coffee table between them that was amply stocked with old issues of *National Geographic* and news magazines. A television, perched on a high shelf jutting from the wall, was tuned to a religious program, and Krueger reached up and switched it off. Then he sat down on the couch across from the Murphys.

"I've discussed Ellie's case with Dr. Nelson," Krueger began, "and he agrees that in view of the prognosis of conventional therapy for ALL after relapse, Ellie is a reasonable candidate for a bone-marrow transplant. We can't make the decision for you, though; we can only present the facts. You should be aware that although marrow transplantation for acute leukemia is effective, it is not one hundred percent effective by any means, and potentially fatal complications can occur."

171

"What does the transplant consist of?" Brian asked.

"Well, if Ellie is in good shape and you do decide to go ahead, she will first be given an intensive eight-day treatment regimen to eradicate any residual leukemic cells that might be hidden away in her tissues and to destroy her existing marrow to make way for the graft. Our current protocol specifies four days of chemotherapy with the very powerful drug Cytoxan, followed by four half-hour exposures to total-body irradiation. Once this regimen has been completed, we will proceed immediately with the transplant."

"Is it true that Ellie will not have to be operated on?" Brian asked.

Krueger smiled. "Yes. Actually it is the donor child who gets the operation. When many people first hear about transplants, they are familiar with bone-marrow aspirations, so they assume that we suck the marrow out of the donor's bones and inject it back into the patient's bones. In fact, it's nothing as bad as that. Enough marrow to give Ellie a fresh start on blood-cell production will be drawn from Beth's hips under general anesthesia in the operating room. We will then filter the marrow and infuse it intravenously into Ellie's arm, as we would a unit of blood. Since the marrow cells have a special affinity for the cavities inside the bones, they are able to travel there from the bloodstream and take up residence, multiplying and producing new blood cells. So as far as Ellie is concerned, the transplant is not surgery—it's little more than a blood transfusion. If the grafted marrow is not rejected, it will begin to generate new blood cells in two or three weeks."

Brian was disturbed that one of his healthy children would have to be operated on. "What's the risk to Beth?" he asked.

"Minimal, less than with an appendectomy," Krueger replied. "Bone-marrow harvesting is a very simple procedure requiring little surgical skill—which is why physicians like myself can do it instead of surgeons. It's like a bone-marrow aspiration from the hip, except that we make lots of aspirations, more than one hundred, all through two small holes in the skin over the hipbones. Since no incision is made, the risk of infection is low and the marrow itself regenerates in a very short time. Other than having a very sore behind for a few days, our donors have few problems and generally leave the hospital the day after the operation. There is, of course, the remote possibility of a life-threatening reaction to general anesthesia, but that is really infinitesimal—about one in ten thousand."

Brian did not know how to deal with those numbers. One in ten thousand? But what if Beth were that one?

"Will the procedure be painful for Ellie?" Sally asked.

"I wouldn't say painful," Krueger replied. "Unpleasant, yes. The first month or so after the transplant, when the blood counts are very low, the patient is usually very uncomfortable with nausea from the chemotherapy and radiation and often with infections and mouth ulcers, in spite of all the precautions that are taken. Some patients have it easier than others, but for all of them the transplant is nauseating and frightening. As I've explained, the actual transplant is very simple: suck out some bone marrow from the donor and infuse it into the recipient. Very straightforward. But keeping the patient well after the transplant can be enormously difficult. In fact, it's probably the most challenging management problem in all of clinical medicine today. Since we have ten years of experience in this business, though, we are usually able to predict problems and try to prevent them before they happen. Anyway, let's have Ellie admitted. Once she is set up in her room, one of the residents, Lynn Schwartz, will come in to do an admitting history and physical. Her tests will start tomorrow morning, and Beth will also begin testing in the Outpatient Clinic. Tomorrow afternoon, the fellow, Dr. Wade Peters, will meet with you to describe the transplant procedure in greater detail and go over the informed-consent sheets with you to answer any questions you might have. If any other questions or problems come up over the next few days while you are considering the transplant, please do not hesitate to ask Peters or me."

The Murphys got up to go.

"Oh, one more thing," Krueger said. "Let me just add that there are two parties involved in this decision: your family and our whole enterprise. If you're religious, then there's a third party as well. In any case, cooperation is essential. If this decision is a one-sided one, the transplant will be awfully tough. Should you decide to go ahead with the procedure, I hope we'll be able to work well together to make it a success."

The Murphys nodded, thanked him, and left the lounge. After they had gone, Krueger sat alone for a while. For him, attending was a full-time, twenty-four-hour-a-day job, and he relished an occasional few minutes alone to gather his thoughts. Every time he was on duty for his annual six-week rotation he found himself getting totally involved. His thoughts were constantly with his patients; even away from the ward he was pondering how to manipulate their medical management so that they had the best possible prognosis. He had learned to build up certain emotional defenses, but they did not equip him for the shock of relapse or of a patient not doing well.

Once, when he had been working in general oncology, there had been a leukemic who had relapsed two weeks before Christmas. Krueger knew how much the family was looking forward to spending the holiday together, so he had said, "Okay, have a good Christmas. We'll start the chemotherapy after the holiday." As it happened, the boy had gone rapidly downhill and died. After that painful experience, Krueger had become more pragmatic. There was always a holiday or a birthday. His hard line sometimes seemed callous to families, but someone had to maintain objectivity.

For the six weeks each year Krueger was on the Transplant Unit, he did not contribute much to his family life. He tried to shift gears when he got home but found it very difficult. When his wife wanted to go out to a party he usually declined, saying he was tired. It was very hard to tolerate small talk or to chuckle at inane jokes when one of his patients was dying. He knew he could be an absolute bore with people who were not living through the same thing. When he left the Unit after six weeks, he always felt a certain amount of guilt over "abandoning" his patients, but he knew that his effectiveness was wearing down from the strain and that his emotional strength was near depletion.

Nancy Curtis, the primary-care nurse assigned to Ellie on the day shift, helped the child get settled into Room 335, directly across from the nurses' station on Three-South. The room had been thoroughly scrubbed and disinfected by Housekeeping, and the white linoleum floor stripped and rewaxed so that it gleamed. It was a fairly large room, with a bed, bureau, bathroom and shower, a telephone on a bedside table, and an overhead color TV. A sink was located beside the door so that visitors could scrub their hands before entering. The single window looked out onto the hospital parking garage.

After helping Sally unpack Ellie's suitcase, Nancy fastened an ID bracelet around the child's wrist. Ellie had brought along her favorite dolls and stuffed animals, which Nancy helped arrange in a row on top of the bureau.

Nancy was one of the twenty or so nurses who worked on the Unit. At any one time, she was responsible for the daytime nursing care of three patients. She conferred often with the other nurses and technicians who took care of "her" patients and with the nurses' assistants who did routine hygiene and care. The Transplant Unit was an intensive-care facility, and each twenty-four-hour period was divided up into three nursing shifts. Nurses on the day shift, from 7:00 A.M. to 3:00 P.M., were responsible for administering all medications, giving the patients a bath or shower, and preparing them for whatever tests were to be done that day. The major responsibility on the evening shift, from 3:00 P.M. to 11:00 P.M., was administering blood products. Nurses on the night shift, from 11:00 P.M. to 7:00 A.M., gave chemotherapy and caught up with any activities that had been passed over during the day.

Nancy was one of the few nurses who had been on the Transplant Unit ever since it opened in 1976. She had come to the Oncology Center at age twenty-one, right out of an undergraduate nursing program, very flattered that Johns Hopkins wanted to hire her. At that time she was not sure in what field she wanted to specialize; in nursing school, students were advised to get a general background first. But the director of nursing at the Oncology Center had turned out to be very dynamic and had sold her on bone-marrow transplantation. Nancy had soon learned that the Transplant Unit was an extraordinarily stressful place. During her first few years there, marrow transplantation had a very high failure rate, since nearly all of their patients were being transplanted in relapse or in end-stage disease.

A transplant attending had once observed that all of the nurses on the Transplant Unit had certain personality traits in common: they were very easygoing, adaptable to changing and adverse conditions, and able to obtain gratification from their work. They learned to get their rewards in ways different from those of the nurses on most other hospital units. Although not all of Nancy's patients went home, she could find meaning and gratification in the fact that a patient who had formerly been bedridden could now walk a whole lap around the nurses' station, or in improvements such as a 2.0 rather than a 1.6 on a patient's pulmonary-function test.

Those nurses who were not able to adapt left quickly, after a month or two, whereas those who remained stayed on for at least a year. Six or seven of the nurses on the Unit had begun their jobs together two and a half years earlier, providing continuity and experience in the nursing staff that had proved to be a stabilizing force for the service. Nevertheless, the high turnover rate meant that most of the nurses were young—twenty-one or twenty-two—and for many of them this was their first working assignment. As a result, they made mistakes: they did not get the patients out of bed often enough, or they had trouble starting IV's.

Many of these younger nurses quickly became "burnt out," particularly after a string of deaths or even the isolated death of a patient with whom their involvement had been particularly intense. They became depressed and self-doubting, thus requiring a good deal of support by all segments of the staff. When morale was at a low point, Saunders would call a meeting of the entire nursing staff and try to give them the big picture of what they were trying to accomplish, complete with graphs and statistics, emphasizing that some bad results were inevitable.

In addition, a psychological support group for the nursing staff met once a week for about an hour. Run by a nurse from Staff Development who had a master's degree in psychology, the meetings usually focused on the crisis of having to confront death time and time again, and the personal feelings of guilt and inadequacy experienced by the younger nurses. When a patient died, the whole meaning of the nurses' efforts was often called into question.

Sometimes even the veteran nurses like Nancy faced emotional exhaustion. Two years before, she had become very close to a boy of seventeen who was dying of complications of the transplant. She was on the night shift with him when he died. Afterward she had wept, and the boy's mother had comforted her. "Be sure to tell the other nurses tomorrow that they have our thanks," the woman had said.

"How can you say that, now that your son is dead?" Nancy had asked.

"Because you gave us a few more months," the woman had answered quietly but with conviction.

That experience had made a deep impression on Nancy. She had decided that although a marrow transplant was something she would never want to endure herself, patients should definitely have the right to do it if they wished. The transplant was their last chance—they were literally fighting for their lives—and she admired their courage.

Nancy was pleased that she had been assigned to take care of Ellen Murphy, since she enjoyed working with young children. The Transplant Unit was the only service in the hospital that was both pediatric and adult, and while Nancy enjoyed the variety, some of the nurses consciously avoided assignments to the younger patients. Taking care of an unhappy, uncooperative, or violent child could be very frustrating, but Nancy had discovered that most children were remarkably resilient, both medically and emotionally. They tended to have fewer bad side-effects from the chemotherapy and radiation and often bounced back faster from emotional upsets. She remembered the words of a pediatric resident she had worked with, spoken only half in jest: "When kids are sick they grow up, and when adults are sick they act like kids." The only really hard part was when the children did not do well. Sometimes Nancy found the irony unbearable: the leukemic children came to the Unit in remission and healthy, and the transplant was supposed to be such a wonderful thing, curing any dormant traces of the disease. Yet the procedure could make a child so sick. There was nothing more excruciating for Nancy than to watch one of these children die.

When Ellie was in bed in her pajamas, Sally let her watch TV until the doctor came. Ellie liked her room because it was directly across from the nurses' station, giving her a good view from her bed of all the action. She could watch the doctors and nurses coming and going, and the nurses could look in on her often.

A half hour later, Dr. Lynn Schwartz came in, introduced herself as the

176

resident who had been assigned to Ellie, and began to take a history and physical. She was new to the floor, having begun her rotation on the first of the month. Three first-year residents rotated through the Transplant Unit every month, dividing up the fourteen transplant patients so that each was responsible for four or five. In addition, each resident was on call every third night, so that the three house officers became familiar with all the patients.

Lynn had gotten married a few months earlier to a man she had met in medical school; her husband was working in Boston for the summer but planned to join her in Baltimore in the fall. Because the Transplant Unit was considered the most demanding rotation, she had chosen to do it over the summer to get it out of the way before her husband arrived. She was living with her parents in suburban Baltimore and commuting to the hospital to save money. Although this arrangement had been working well, the continual stress she was under on the Transplant Unit had begun to precipitate terrible arguments with her mother. Lynn found the work challenging and often overwhelming, especially when she was expected to make critical medical decisions on only a few hours' sleep. No one seemed to understand how exhausted she was after a night on the Unit, being wakened repeatedly from a deep sleep on the cot in the On-Call Room by the shrill beep of her electronic pager, as one patient after another spiked a fever.

When Lynn had learned that she would be admitting a six-year-old, she had groaned, remembering the obstinate brats she had encountered as an intern during her Pediatrics rotation. She had skimmed the medical summary sent by Dr. Nelson and then found her way to the child's room, preparing herself for the worst.

As it happened, she was pleasantly surprised. Ellen Murphy seemed apprehensive but well behaved, and except for her thin hair and slight steroid-induced plumpness, she looked healthy. Lynn introduced herself to the parents and then proceeded to take a history, jotting down notes on the admitting form attached to her clipboard. Her report read:

Admitting Resident: Dr. Lynn Schwartz; *Admitting Fellow:* Dr. Wade Peters; *Attending Physician:* Dr. James Krueger.

Informant: Dr. Nelson's preadmission note and the parents of the patient.

Chief Complaint: This is the first Johns Hopkins Hospital admission for this six-year-old white female, with ALL in remission, for bone-marrow transplantation from her sister.

History of Present Illness: The patient's acute lymphoblastic leukemia was diagnosed in September of 1978, presenting as malaise, fever, and bruising.

Remission was induced with vincristine, prednisone, and L-asparaginase. She was given intrathecal methotrexate and cranial irradiation for central-nervous-system prophylaxis. She was maintained on oral 6-MP and methotrexate with pulses of vincristine and prednisone.

She relapsed in April of 1980, and this was in the bone marrow only. She was reinduced with vincristine, prednisone, L-asparaginase, and daunomycin. She was consolidated with IV and intrathecal methotrexate.

Past Medical History: Initial hospitalization in September 1978, for diagnosis of ALL and initial induction. Second hospitalization in August 1979, for liver biopsy due to elevated liver-function tests while on maintenance chemotherapy. Third hospitalization in November 1979, due to complications of chicken pox infection. Immunizations: Up to date. Growth and Development: The patient was a seven-pound, five-ounce product of a full-term gestation to a twenty-four-year-old Para 1-0-0-1 [one pregnancy, no miscarriages, no abortions, one birth]. This was a normal spontaneous vaginal delivery, with a normal neonatal course, and normal developmental milestones.

Review of Systems: Positive for occasional headaches which were relieved by Tylenol.

Family History: Positive for heart disease, cancer, stroke, hypertension, and hay fever. Negative for leukemia, diabetes mellitus, seizures, and asthma.

Social History: The hometown is Menlo Park, New Jersey. Her father is a sales manager for a medical-equipment company. Her mother is a housewife. Their religion is Catholic.

Physical Examination: The temperature is 37.0, pulse rate 80, respirations 20, blood pressure 120/70. General: She is an alert, active, well-developed white female, in no acute distress. Skin shows no petechiae. Tympanic membranes are motile, with clear landmarks, and pupils are equal, round, reactive to light and accommodation. The extraocular movements are full. The throat is clear and moist. Her teeth have no obvious caries or noted tenderness. The optic fundi show disks that are sharp, with no hemorrhages or exudates. The neck is supple, with no masses. There are no palpable nodes. The chest examination is clear, equal, and unlabored. Cardiac: Normal S1 and S2, with no murmur or gallop. Femoral and brachial pulses are 2+ symmetric. Abdomen: Soft, active bowel sounds, no organ swelling, no masses palpable. Extremities: Full range of movement in all joints, no muscle wasting. Neurologic: She is oriented times three [person, time, place], has good strength and tone in her arms and legs. Her pain and touch reflexes are intact and symmetric. Her gait is within normal limits.

Impression is one of a six-year-old girl with ALL in remission, for bone-marrow transplant, who is otherwise healthy.

It never failed to amaze Lynn that a child with a chronic and potentially fatal disease could look so well between relapses.

20 Informed Consent

On Monday morning, June 2, the testing began. At 7:00 A.M., blood was drawn from Ellie's arm for complete cell counts, a "chemzyme" series (a set of twelve different blood analyses), clotting studies, and an immunological work-up. Then she was wheeled all over the hospital for X-rays, a CAT scan, an EKG, a neurological consult including an EEG, and a bone-marrow aspiration. Although Ellie's white count was depressed to 2,300 because of her maintenance chemotherapy, there were no blasts in her marrow; the remission was holding. Later on that morning, Brian, Sally, and Beth went to the Outpatient Department, where blood was drawn from all of them for HLA typing. Then Beth was given a complete physical, an EKG, and a chest X-ray.

Beth could not understand why they were doing so many strange things to her when she didn't even feel sick. In the back of her mind she began to wonder if she had the same illness Ellie had, only they weren't telling her.

After a lunch of crab cakes, the local specialty, the Murphys met with Peters in his office. The oncology fellow was a good-looking man of twenty-eight with curly brown hair, a cropped mustache, and intense brown eyes. He had gone to medical school at Hopkins, done his internship and residency at Massachusetts General Hospital in Boston, and then returned to Hopkins for a two-year fellowship in medical oncology. Peters had chosen this area of specialization because he liked the intellectual challenge of a dynamic, research-oriented field. During his three-month rotation through the Transplant Unit, he advised the house staff and was on call twenty-four hours a day in case difficult problems arose. He and Krueger went on morning rounds with the residents and consulted every afternoon. Peters found his work on the Unit demanding but always interesting, and he still felt he was learning a substantial amount of new information.

The senior medical staff was now sufficiently experienced with the details of bone-marrow transplantation so that when the new house staff came on board at the beginning of each month, the attending on duty could brief them on what to expect during each stage of the post-transplant period. Unlike many of the residents, who often seemed to feel they were incapable of making a mistake, Peters knew that he was not a miracle worker. When he could not do enough about a serious complication, his patients got sick and died. It was always an emotional jolt when that happened, and in a sense it was a defeat, but Peters's even-tempered attitude enabled him to get through such times without feeling overwhelming guilt or despair. "Not everybody makes it, by a long shot," he would tell new residents, "but you have to balance the other side of the coin." At times Peters would hide behind the walls of his intellectualism, forcing his rationality to fend off his emotions, and then he appeared cold or arrogant.

In spite of Peters's well-developed defenses, there was one incident during the preceding month that had managed to get under his skin. A little girl, Marsha, had developed a serious viral infection after her transplant that had destroyed her marrow and created ulcers in her gut. Only a few days later, she had suddenly gone into septic shock and died, and there had been nothing they could do to save her. Afterward, her mother had been very angry and bitter. "You killed my child!" she had accused Peters. That had been unfair and hard to take, but he had not argued with her. Although he knew it was her grief that made her lash out in that way, the incident continued to haunt him.

Peters introduced himself to the Murphys, immediately sensing a lack of rapport between the parents and a great deal of anxiety. He handed them a copy of the informed-consent waiver and prepared to go over it line by line. The irony of informed consent was that the transplant inevitably sounded far worse on paper than it actually was. Every possible complication had to be mentioned, more than even the most unfortunate patient could be expected to suffer. Peters tried to explain all of the risks and hazards in as much depth as possible, yet he did not want to overload the family with so many details that he would scare them unnecessarily. If people read all the possible side effects of aspirin in the *Physician's Desk Reference,* they would be convinced to leave headaches untreated.

Peters began by discussing the toxic side effects associated with the intensive chemotherapy and total-body irradiation Ellie would receive to prepare her for the transplant. These treatments could induce severe nausea and vomiting, sterility, weakness, increased susceptibility to infection, and total hair loss after two weeks (although her hair would begin to grow back one month later). Following the transplant Ellie's blood counts would be very low for a few weeks, putting her at risk of a life-threatening bacterial or fungal infection. Finally, after the graft took and the marrow came back, there were still more potential hazards, including the danger that the grafted cells might reject the host. . . .

"Wait a minute," Brian interrupted. "Isn't it Ellie who would do the rejecting?"

"No, I said it right," Peters replied with a smile. "Rejection of the marrow graft by the host is rarely a problem because the host's immune system is suppressed by the chemotherapy and radiation. What can cause problems are the mature lymphocytes that get transplanted along with the donor's marrow, since marrow is inevitably mixed with some peripheral blood. Because we can match up the HLA antigens of nonidentical siblings but not all their different types of minor tissue antigens, it's largely a matter of chance how good the match turns out to be. If the match is not very good, the donor lymphocytes 'contaminating' the marrow will recognize the host's tissues as foreign and attack them. This is called 'graft-versus-host disease,' or GVHD, and it's the greatest hurdle to successful transplantation between nonidentical siblings. In most HLA-matched transplants—about seventy percent—we see some GVHD; it's life threatening in about twenty percent. Fortunately, we're now beginning to get a better handle on how to control and even prevent it."

Peters went on to discuss the additional problems created by the red-cell incompatibility between Beth, who had type A blood, and Ellie, who had type O. Because of this difference, if Beth's marrow, containing substantial quantities of red cells, were directly transfused into Ellie, a severe and probably fatal reaction would result. Beth's mismatched red cells would therefore have to be removed from the extracted marrow prior to the transplant; this would be done by spinning the marrow in a blood processor to separate out the various blood cells by weight. Since the red cells, packed with hemoglobin, are heaviest, they would sink to the bottom, so that the marrow cells could be skimmed off the top like a layer of cream. These purified marrow cells would then be transfused into Ellie.

Peters cautioned, however, that the separation process was not perfect, and it was still possible that the purified marrow would contain significant numbers of mismatched red cells. Administration of the marrow might therefore give rise to a transfusion reaction, including fever, hives, labored breathing, and kidney damage. In addition, the process of separating out the red cells might damage the marrow cells, resulting in failure of the graft. Peters assured the Murphys that although he was required to inform them of these risks, all necessary precautions would be taken to prevent and minimize the adverse effects of the separation procedure and the subsequent transfusion. Because red-cell incompatibility constituted a special case of the current transplant protocol, however, an additional informed-consent waiver would have to be signed.

When Peters had gone through this litany of risks, Brian took a deep breath and let it out slowly. "Okay, all things considered," he said, "what are Ellie's chances if we go ahead with the transplant?"

"I would say her chances of surviving the transplant and achieving a remission are around fifty percent," Peters replied. "If she survives for two years after the transplant without a recurrence, chances are that she will be cured. A few odd patients relapse after that, but the great majority make it through the next four or five years. We can't yet talk about ten- or fifteen-year survival because we just don't have the numbers—it's all so new."

There was a silence. Although Nelson had told the Murphys repeatedly that there were no guarantees with the transplant, the odds struck Sally like a thunderbolt. It was as if she had never heard them before. It was not a lapse of memory—just that the mind protects itself from intolerable facts by blotting them out. Each time she heard the truth, it was overwhelming.

Brian was obviously thinking the same thing, for he said, "Fifty-percent survival may sound good to you, as a professional, but for a parent it's hard to accept. Is it really no higher than that?"

"Consider the alternative," Peters said. "The chances that chemotherapy alone will produce a cure after a child has relapsed are less than ten percent."

"With the transplant, though, you're taking a child who's reasonably well and exposing her to huge risks," Brian countered.

"Yes, on the grounds that her ultimate chances of survival are better if we take that risk," Peters replied. "I'd like to make it easy for you, but I can't. Recommending a marrow transplant has become much harder than it used to be, when every patient transplanted was in relapse or end-stage disease. Now the procedure is being done when the patient is in first or second remission and apparently healthy. I understand your reluctance to start another hazardous course of therapy now that things seem to be going so well. But you should realize that because Ellie has relapsed once, the odds are high that she will relapse again, probably within six to eight months. I'll be the first to admit that the transplant is a huge gamble: basically, we're asking you to wager your child's life for the chance to prolong it. If you do opt for the transplant, you should do so knowing that for a minimum of one hundred days, Ellie will be at extremely high risk of running into some major-league problems, and that the quality of life during that period will not be good. We don't know if the transplant is going to work, we don't know that she is not going to develop GVHD, which is potentially fatal, and we don't even know that once the transplant is a success, the leukemia won't come back. But the odds with chemotherapy are so slim that we think it's probably worthwhile taking the experimental route."

Sally glanced at her husband, who was staring gloomily straight ahead, and then back to Peters. She found the young doctor very cold and cerebral. Did he really have to go into such morbid detail about all the terrible things that could happen? Should she believe Peters, when her heart told her that Ellie was surely cured? "Can't we just wait a little longer?" she asked. "Ellie feels so well now, and she looks so healthy. She doesn't even seem sick anymore. After all, her first remission lasted a year and a half. We don't want to burn our bridges behind us."

Peters shrugged. "You could wait until she relapses and then attempt the transplant in third remission. But a third remission will be harder to achieve and will not last long, since the leukemic cells will have become resistant to multiple agents. Here at Hopkins, we've transplanted a few patients in third or fourth remission, but the results have not been nearly as good as in first or second—about thirty percent survival or less. Plus, if Ellie should develop a drug-resistant relapse and be unable to get back into remission, she would no longer be eligible for a transplant."

Sally sighed. "I don't know. Maybe if we did it now, it would put too much stress on Beth and the baby."

"I don't think that's the real issue," Peters replied. "You may not want to go ahead with the transplant, and I would understand that—there's no hard and fast evidence that this is the only way to go. But you should sit down and try not to fool yourself with irrelevant issues. Try to be rational about this decision, although I know it's very hard."

Peters sensed that Mrs. Murphy was repressing an enormous amount of emotion. Right now her self-control facilitated his task in that he did not have to deal with her rage and sadness. But her use of denial, when carried to the extreme of blocking out the truth, would cause major difficulties later on. She was not seeing clearly what was happening to her child. Peters had known other parents who had nothing to fall back on when their child died, since their lives had become centered around both their child and their denial.

"Let's move on to the last consent waiver," Peters said, turning to the single-spaced form titled "Donor Consent for Participation in Bone-Marrow Transplantation." He went on to enumerate the risks to the donor child associated with the marrow-harvesting operation. Some states, such as Pennsylvania and Massachusetts, considered it a conflict of interest for parents to give informed consent for both the transplant donor and recipient, and required a court process to ensure that a minor child was not coerced into being a donor. A lawyer appointed by the Family Court represented the donor child at a hearing and made sure that the child's rights were being protected and that the parents were not sacrificing one sibling for the other. Maryland, however, did not require such a legal process.

Although Peters felt some qualms about subjecting the donor to an operation and anesthesia from which that child would derive no medical benefit, he had rarely encountered reluctance on the part of a brother or sister to donate bone marrow. In fact, the transplant was often emotionally enriching for the donor child and the family as a whole. It seemed to draw the family together in confronting the crisis, creating a sense of unity that overcame the petty irritations of sibling rivalry and family conflict so apparent during earlier periods of strain. The situation was very different with kidney transplants, since in that case the child was donating an organ that would not regenerate and hence was making a permanent sacrifice. It was well known that children who donated a kidney to a sibling often mourned their lost organ and became angry and depressed. Bone-marrow donors, on the other hand, usually considered marrow to be the same as blood and were willing to give it away, confident that it would grow back.

Peters had encountered only one difficult case in this respect during his fellowship rotation: a set of identical twins in which the potential donor did not want to have anything to do with his sick brother. Both children were minors, and the parents had finally persuaded the donor child to cooperate. Peters did not know if that was right or wrong, but they had gone ahead with the transplant anyway. Fortunately it had not been necessary to drag the child into the operating room kicking and screaming; that would have been traumatic for both the staff and the family. If anything had gone wrong under those circumstances, they would have had a crisis on their hands.

Brian finished reading over the donor consent form and handed it to Sally. "How long will you give us to make up our minds?" he asked.

"Ideally, once Ellie has been evaluated and put on the waiting list, you would have as much time as you need to decide," Peters said. "Practically speaking, though, the next transplant protocol is scheduled to begin this coming Thursday, so if you want to go ahead right away, I'll need to have those signed waivers by Wednesday morning at the latest. If you choose instead to postpone your decision, Ellie will have to give up her bed to the next person on the list."

The Murphys were taken aback. "My God, do you need a decision so soon?" Brian asked.

"I'm afraid so," Peters replied. "The problem is that we reserve the operating room months in advance for the marrow harvests. Because our protocol specifies eight days of preparation before the transplant takes place, that means that our schedule has to be quite rigid: we begin the protocol on a Thursday, and do the transplant eight days later, on the following Friday."

"I see," Brian said, shaking his head. "What if we decide to postpone the decision and then choose to do the transplant at a later date?"

"In that case, you will have to wait for the first available bed, which may take anywhere from a week to over a month. That's assuming that Ellie remains in remission and that no one with a better prognosis moves ahead of her on the waiting list." Seeing the Murphys' obvious concern, Peters handed them the waivers. "Look, read these over carefully and think hard about the decision. If any more questions come up, please call me. I'd be grateful if you can let me know, either way, by Wednesday morning."

Feeling shell-shocked, the Murphys thanked him and got up to go.

On Tuesday, the tests continued. Ellie had an echocardiogram, another chest X-ray, pulmonary-function tests, and skin tests to detect previous exposure to a variety of viruses. In the afternoon, she went to the Wilmer Building for an eye exam, returning to her room for an arterial stick to determine the concentrations of oxygen and carbon dioxide in her blood. Nutritional tests were begun to evaluate how well her intestines were absorbing nutrients. At 2:30 P.M. she had a spinal tap, and methotrexate was injected into her spinal fluid to kill off any stray leukemic cells that might be lurking there. To Ellie, the tests and examinations seemed endless; just when she thought the ordeal must finally be over, the poking and probing began again.

While all this was going on, Brian and Sally continued to debate the pros and cons of the transplant. They had been talking in increasingly circular arguments all day, and still had not made a decision. Tuesday night, after Ellie had drifted off to sleep, they returned to their room at the Sheraton and continued their discussion, lowering their voices so as not to wake Beth. Brian picked up the copy of the consent form and read it over for what seemed like the hundredth time:

We, Sally Murphy (mother) and Brian Murphy (father), consent to the intravenous administration of bone-marrow cells to our child, Ellen Murphy, who suffers from acute lymphoblastic leukemia.

We understand that this mode of therapy, which we know is experimental, is desirable because of the high probability that our child's present remission will not last, and of the high likelihood that he/she will eventually succumb to the complications of the disease, i.e., bleeding or infection. We understand that some patients with leukemia who have undergone high-dose anti-leukemic drug therapy, total-body X-ray treatment, and bone-marrow transplantation have achieved unexpected prolonged remissions. In the hope of achieving such a remission in our child, we consent to undertake the risks of this treatment. We understand that our child's chance of surviving this treatment is increased if transplantation is performed when he/she is in remission and relatively good health.

We understand that in order to prepare our child for transplant, four large doses of the antileukemic drug Cytoxan will be given. The reason for this is to kill the greatest possible number of leukemic cells which presently exist in our child's body.

We further understand that in order to prevent our child from "rejecting" the transplanted marrow and in the hope of killing even more leukemic cells,

185

four doses of total body X-ray treatment will be given. The combined dose is large (1,200 rads) and will kill the bone marrow. In order for our child to survive, he/she must accept the marrow graft.

The side effects of Cytoxan and total-body irradiation and the side effects of the marrow transplant itself have been explained to us and include: initial nausea and vomiting, transient fluid retention, cystitis (bladder irritation and blood in urine), loss of hair, possible myocardiopathy (damage to the heart), bone-marrow aplasia with attendant infections and hemorrhagic (bleeding) risks, potential graft-versus-host disease with attendant dermatitis (skin rash), diarrhea and liver disease, interstitial pneumonitis (a severe form of pneumonia), immune insufficiency (susceptibility to certain infections), sterility, and the possibility of cataracts (clouding of the eye lens).

The possible benefit of this procedure is a long-term remission or even cure of our child's leukemia. We understand that the chances of this favorable result occurring are presently not known but probably lie between 25 and 50 percent. We understand that the proposed chemotherapy and total-body irradiation followed by transplantation offers our child an opportunity for control of his/her disease which is comparable to or better than that provided by other treatment regimens.

We understand that this is a research-oriented procedure and we consent to the use of any blood, tissue, or other body fluid removed from our child for the purpose of diagnosis, teaching, or research.

We further understand that neither failure to join nor withdrawal of our child from participation in this study will prejudice the availability of medical care for our child at this medical center.

Brian put down the sheet. "Think how terrible it would be if she went through all this agony and it didn't work," he said. "That's what I can't accept."

Sally bit her lip. "But if we don't go through with the transplant and she dies, how could we ever forgive ourselves for not trying everything possible?"

Brian pointed at the consent form. "Did you read that thing? Look at that list of side effects and possible complications! Even if she makes it, she might end up some kind of cripple, or worse. If we packed a lifetime of happiness into the next six months, or however long she has left—would that be failing her?"

There was a silence, and then Sally said, "Yes, it would, Brian. God is offering her this chance for a normal life, and what right do we have to deprive her of it? Ellie's always been a fighter, and she would want to battle the disease to the end. Giving up now would be like throwing away everything we've struggled for."

Brian held his head in his hands, as if it were too heavy for his shoulders to bear. After a long pause, he let out a weary-sounding "All right." With a deep breath, he gave in. "But promise me one thing: if the situation becomes hopeless, she won't have to suffer needlessly."

"I promise." Sally closed her eyes and wept quietly. Although she had finally accepted Peters's assertion that Ellie was not yet cured and that her days of remission were probably numbered, she fell back on her blind faith that none of the terrible complications listed on the waiver form would happen to Ellie. The child had suffered enough, and if there was any justice in the world, she would survive the transplant unharmed. "You know," Sally said aloud to Brian, "somehow I think she's going to make it. If we have enough faith, God won't let us down." Through her sadness she began to feel her strength return, knowing how desperately Ellie would need her.

The next morning, Wednesday, June 4, the Murphys arrived at Peters's office with their decision. The fellow tried to play devil's advocate, forcing them to confront the risks of the transplant before signing. Even with the facts in black and white before them, many parents seemed to deny that anything could possibly go wrong. He wanted to make sure that both Mr. and Mrs. Murphy were committed to the transplant 100 percent, because if one of them was not, going ahead would be very destructive.

"Are you making this decision deliberately enough to know that if the transplant doesn't work, you'll be able to get through hard times without feeling that you made a bad decision?" he asked them.

Sally nodded. "I believe we're doing the right thing. It's in God's hands now."

"Can you accept His will, whatever it turns out to be?" Peters pursued.

Although they both said yes, Peters was aware that Mrs. Murphy's hand trembled as she signed the forms, and her husband seemed almost numb, signing automatically without appearing to absorb the implications of his act. As Peters watched them, he thought to himself that the Murphys would never really know if they had made the right decision. If Ellie survived the transplant and continued to do well, they would wonder if she could have done well without it. And if she did not do well, they would probably regret their decision. It was a strange situation: things could only go wrong.

21 Orientation

Now that the decision was made, the Murphys felt as if a great weight had been lifted from their shoulders. For the rest of this Wednesday morning,

Sally sat in the room with Ellie while Brian went sightseeing with Beth at the Inner Harbor. Soon after they left, a technician came up from Radiation Therapy to take a variety of measurements of Ellie's body, including height, weight, chest circumference at the nipples and navel, and the thickness of her chest and abdomen, so that the appropriate dose of total-body irradiation (TBI) could be calculated.

Fifteen minutes later, Dr. Krueger came in to speak to Sally. They went out into the corridor, leaving Ellie absorbed in a TV show. Sally liked the fact that Krueger had made an effort to come to her, without her having to seek him out. Already she trusted him; he never sugar-coated anything, was very frank about problems, and unlike most of the other doctors, who seemed to lapse almost unconsciously into medical jargon, he knew how to talk on her level.

Krueger rarely wasted time in getting to the point. "Ellie's chemotherapy will begin at four-thirty tomorrow afternoon," he said, "and if she's like most people it will make her very nauseated. Later on she may develop ulcers of the mouth or the gastrointestinal tract that will make it impossible for her to eat or drink. To prevent her from becoming weak and malnourished, we'd like to give her intravenous nutritional support through what's called a central line. It's a thin plastic tube, or catheter, a third the width of regular IV tubing, that is inserted into a large vein in the chest and pushed close to the heart. With a young child like Ellie, the insertion is done in the operating room under general anesthesia. The line should be able to stay in place for a month or longer, until she is able to eat solid food again."

"You mean she won't be able to eat a thing for an entire month?"

"Well, not enough to keep her from losing weight. With the central line, we'll be able to infuse a special mixture of nutrients called hyperalimentation fluid that contains all of the carbohydrates, vitamins, minerals, and amino acids that Ellie needs to maintain her weight and to grow at a normal rate for a girl her age. Although hyperalimentation is not a curative therapy in itself, we've found that it's essential to the success of the transplant."

Sally did not like the idea of a plastic tube being inserted into her daughter's chest. "Why can't Ellie get the nutrient solution through a regular IV?" she asked.

"The hyperalimentation fluid is too concentrated to administer through a regular vein in the arm," the doctor replied. "If we did, sclerosis—inflammation and scarring of the vein—would set in pretty quickly. Instead, we insert the catheter into the large subclavian vein, beneath the collarbone, which feeds into the heart. Since this vein is very large and the

188

blood inside it is moving rapidly, the hyperalimentation fluid is diluted before it can irritate the vessel walls. The hyperal is pumped through the central line into the bloodstream at a controlled rate twenty-four hours a day. In this way, we can adjust the nutrient mixture to meet Ellie's changing nutritional needs.

"Repeated peripheral IV's also hurt and are hard to maintain," he went on. "For this reason, we now recommend inserting two central lines in young children, one for administering hyperal and another, larger one for drawing blood and for infusing electrolytes, blood products, and anti-biotics. With a second central line, we hardly ever need to start a peripheral IV, which spares the patients a lot of discomfort and gives their veins a chance to heal. So we feel strongly that the benefits of the central lines more than outweigh the risks."

"What are the risks?" Sally asked, feeling a now-familiar numbness coming on.

"Well, the catheters must be implanted surgically, and although it's a simple procedure that takes less than an hour, we have to use general anesthesia in young children. If Ellie's platelet count is low, there may be some prolonged bleeding, but that's unlikely in her present condition. Since the catheters will be left in place for several weeks, there's a risk of infection, but the dressings will be changed daily and the insertion sites kept scrupulously clean to minimize this possibility. As I said before, the alternative to the central lines is the use of numerous peripheral IV's, which would have to be changed frequently and involve a much greater risk of sclerosis or infection. This way we can avoid the pain, bruising, and scarring associated with repeated sticks."

After a moment's thought, Sally said, "All right. I trust your judgment, doctor. I know you're doing what you feel is best for Ellie."

"Thanks. There's no question that hyperalimentation has made a big difference in our success rate, and it's also made the whole process much easier for the patient and family. When I started in this business in the early 1970s, we didn't hyperaliment at all and it was a constant battle to get patients to eat, particularly young children. They were miserably sick and had bad mouth sores, so they weren't getting nourished and were just melting away. We were afraid that they were going to die of starvation, and that put tremendous pressure on parents to force their kids to eat and drink. Besides that, the patients' arms and legs were terribly bruised and scarred from all the punctures. The central lines have taken a lot of pain and tension out of the procedure. Now we only have to battle with young children to get them to take their oral antibiotics, which taste awful. Those kids have real power over us—they don't have to open their mouths!"

They laughed together. Then Krueger took out a simple form that read:

CONSENT FOR CENTRAL LINE INSERTION

Indications: Deep venous access for hyperalimentation, medications, blood transfusions, and drawing blood.

Major risks: Bleeding, infection, adverse reaction to general anesthesia.

Alternatives: Peripheral venous support.

Sally signed the form and Krueger thanked her. "Some orderlies will come to take Ellie to the operating room shortly after eight tomorrow morning," he said. "I'll look in afterward to make sure everything's okay."

Brian and Beth returned after lunch for a one o'clock appointment with the social worker, Gail Siegel, to discuss finances and living arrangements. Beth watched TV with Ellie and played with dolls while their parents went to Gail's office, which was located next to the visitors' lounge.

As cancer specialists had come to recognize the importance of emotional coping, they had increasingly incorporated psychiatrists and social workers into oncology treatment teams to work with the entire family, not just the patient. For many years this had not been the case; pediatric oncologists had overlooked the emotional impact of catastrophic illness, partly because they lacked psychological expertise and partly because they needed to erect emotional defenses against their own feelings of vulnerability and mortality. Although Gail did not feel that she was yet considered a full-fledged member of the transplant team, she did attend rounds and census meetings. She saw all of the families extensively before the transplant, and if problems developed later on, she was always available to talk. She also tried to check in with the families every few days just to see how things were going.

Brian's current concerns were very practical: he was worried about the enormous cost of the transplant and how much their insurance would leave unpaid. Gail reassured him that the Transplant Unit would not let them get into a position where they would have to sell their house or car to pay the bills. The Murphys' insurance contract with an independent Major Medical company provided 80 percent payment up to a maximum level and then switched to 100 percent. Because the transplant was such a costly procedure, Gail said, they would most likely reach the full-reimbursement level. She stressed that the Unit physicians accepted insurance payments, whatever coverage provided, as their full fees. In addition, families who were in desperate financial straits were eligible for Medicaid.

190

Gail warned that the most significant strain on their resources would come from small, out-of-pocket expenses including housing, restaurant meals, parking in the hospital garage, and transportation from New Jersey. Combined, these costs could total as much as fifty dollars a day, and none of them were covered by health insurance. Added up over the three months Ellie would have to be in Baltimore, they could wipe out the family's savings. Gail advised the Murphys to save every receipt, since any out-of-pocket expenses related to essential medical care were tax deductible.

"One of you will have to stay in the Baltimore area for at least a hundred days, so housing is a major consideration," she went on. "Unfortunately, our housing options are fairly limited, and cost can be a problem."

Sally imagined that a lot of people could not afford to live in a strange city for three months. It was like managing two homes, and most people nowadays could barely afford one. "What would you recommend?" she asked.

"Well, let's go over the possibilities," Gail began. She counted them out on her fingers: "There's the Sheraton, where you're staying now, but it's very expensive, especially for a stay of three months."

"It's out of the question," Brian said. "That place could break us in one month."

"Well, there's also inexpensive housing available for oncology families in Reed Hall, right across the street from the hospital," Gail continued. "It's like a dormitory and there's not much privacy. Eight families share two four-room suites, including a living room, kitchen, and bath. We'd like to provide more space and privacy for families, but we can't afford to expand the program at this time with our current contributions and fees. Given the limitations of the place, the families really make the best of it."

Brian shook his head. "That kind of arrangement really doesn't appeal to me," he said. "For one thing, I'll just be coming down on weekends, and while I'm here, I know we'll need time alone." He paused, and then added, "I also don't like the idea of sharing facilities and cleaning up after other people. Aren't there any other choices?"

"I could help you apply for grants from the American Cancer Society or the Leukemia Society to help cover your living costs at the motel," Gail suggested. "But they usually last for only a month or so."

The Murphys thought for a while; then Sally had an idea. "Doesn't your Uncle Joe have a trailer he's not using?" she asked Brian. "Maybe we could borrow it and stay at a campsite or a trailer park near Baltimore. That would be private and not too expensive, if there's a place nearby. Do you know of any, Mrs. Siegel?"

"Please call me Gail," the social worker said. "I'm pretty sure there's a trailer park in Woodbine, about a forty-five-minute drive from here. I have a friend who used to go there in the summer. If you like, I could call her and get directions for you. In the meantime, I can find out if there's one closer by."

"Thanks, that really sounds best," Brian said. "I'll call my uncle and find out if the trailer is a real possibility."

"Fine," Gail replied. "I'll be in to talk to Beth and Ellie about the transplant in about an hour."

When Gail arrived at Ellie's room, Brian told her that he had already been in touch with his uncle, who would be more than happy to lend them the trailer; Joe had even offered to tow it down to Woodbine for them from New Jersey, since a big car was required. The Murphys were clearly relieved that one major problem had been solved.

Gail sat down on the edge of the bed beside Ellie, and Brian, Sally, and Beth pulled up chairs in a semicircle. The social worker's difficult task of explaining the transplant procedure in simple terms was facilitated somewhat by the fact that Ellie was already familiar with the effects of chemotherapy and radiation.

"You know, Ellie, that you have a problem with your blood," Gail began. "Do you know what's wrong?"

Ellie nodded gravely. "I'm sick, but if I get chemo I won't have it anymore."

"That's right, Ellie. You were sick before, and then you got sick again. The reason is that there are some bad cells in your bone marrow—the stuff inside your bones that makes your blood. The chemo makes the bad cells go away, but every once in a while they come back and make you sick again. We want to make the bad cells go away forever by giving you some very strong treatments. Beginning tomorrow, you will get some special chemo. The chemo will make you tired and sick to your stomach, and all your hair will fall out again, but it will grow back like it did before. Maybe it will be a different color this time, Ellie. Which color hair do you want?"

"Guess which color," the child countered.

"That's what Gail asked you," Sally admonished her.

"No, you guess," Ellie insisted.

"All right," Gail said. "Blonde? Black? There's not much left. Red? You want red hair?"

Ellie smiled and nodded.

"What a funny girl! You'd probably look good with red hair, though. Anyway, after the chemo, you'll get some radiation, like an X-ray. It won't hurt, but you'll have to lie still under a big machine for a long time. When that's over with, the doctors will give you some of Beth's bone marrow, which is good and healthy. We hope that your sister's good cells will grow inside you and start making lots of nice baby cells, so you won't be sick anymore."

Ellie looked apprehensive. "Will they put Beth's cells inside me with a needle?" she asked.

"No, Ellie," Gail replied. "It won't be anything like a bone-marrow test. We'll give it to you through an IV, just like red cells or platelets, so it won't hurt. After you get the marrow cells, they'll need time to grow, just like when you plant seeds in a garden. So you'll have to stay in the hospital for quite a long time, and for a while you'll feel worse than you did before. Your mouth will get very sore, and you'll have to stay in the room all day and drink some bad-tasting medicine. Everyone who comes to see you will have to wear a mask, so you won't catch any germs. It won't be much fun being in the hospital, but we hope that when the transplant is over the bad cells will have gone away forever and you won't get sick ever again."

"So I won't need any more chemo and bone marrows?" Ellie asked.

"That's right, as long as everything turns out okay," Gail replied. She was reluctant to simply reassure Ellie that the transplant would be a success, since she had seen some children do beautifully and others die of infection or develop chronic GVHD.

During this discussion, Beth had grown increasingly fidgety. Her first wish had naturally been to help her sister, but now she was beginning to have second thoughts. She had been to the clinic in New York once when Ellie had her bone-marrow test and had heard her sister's screams and cries from inside the examination room. Now they were going to do the same thing to her, and she was scared. If they took away her good cells, would she then get sick like Ellie? Were they taking chances with her so that Ellie could live? "Will the transplant hurt?" she asked nervously.

"No, Beth," Gail reassured her. "You won't feel a thing. They'll put you to sleep before the operation, and by the time you wake up it will all be over."

Gail remembered to mention that Beth would wake up, since she had learned the hard way that children took what she told them very literally. She had once forgotten to tell a six-year-old donor that he would wake up after the operation; it had never occurred to her before to say so. Only later did she find out that the child had been convinced he was going to be killed for his brother's sake. No one had been aware of his terror until he was on his way home from the hospital and said to his mother, "Oh, I'm so glad they woke me up!" The experience had been traumatic for everyone, including Gail.

Beth felt reassured somewhat about the screaming, but she was still very frightened. "Will my bone marrow grow back?" she asked.

"Oh, yes, Beth," Gail told her. "The doctors won't take out *all* your bone marrow, just a little bit of it. Since the marrow cells grow very quickly, the amount that is removed will be replaced in a very short time. When you wake up from the operation you'll probably feel sick to your stomach and your hips will be sore for a while; it may even be hard to walk for a day or two. But you should be able to leave the hospital the very next day."

Beth looked very serious and sat up straight in her chair. "I'm gonna get up and walk right after the operation," she said confidently.

Gail laughed. "I'd like to see that! Does anyone want to place bets?"

"Don't be so sure she won't do it," Sally said with a smile. "Beth's a tough cookie."

"I changed my mind, I'm not gonna walk," Beth said, pausing for effect. "I'm gonna run!" She chortled at her own joke. Even Ellie was laughing now.

"I can believe it," Gail said. "Anyway, Beth, the doctors say you're in tip-top shape, all ready for the transplant. It will be nine days from now, on Friday, June thirteenth."

Beth suddenly grimaced.

Sally was alarmed. "What's the matter this time?"

"I don't want any operation on Friday the thirteenth!" Beth moaned.

Sally caught her breath; she had not realized the significance of the date. Meanwhile Gail came to the rescue. "Some people think Friday the thirteenth is the luckiest day of the year," she said soothingly. "And I'm afraid we don't have much choice. We just can't afford to wait another week."

Sally tried to console her child. "It's only a number," she said, giving Beth a hug. "Like Gail said, it's good luck, not bad luck." Beth cheered up, but Sally was privately upset as well. It was easy to be superstitious, particularly when one of her healthy children was about to undergo surgery.

Brian looked at his watch. "It's getting late, and Beth and I should be hitting the road, since she has school tomorrow. Thank you, Mrs. Siegel, for all your help."

"You're quite welcome. Please keep me up to date on your living arrangements. If you ever need me, I'm here for you, but you've got to let me know. By the way, Mrs. Murphy, I would also suggest that you speak with some of the other mothers, particularly the ones who have been here for a while. They should be able to give you a better perspective on the transplant procedure, having gone through it themselves. Just go sit in the lounge for ten or fifteen minutes while a dressing is being changed or when you need a short breather. The mothers all go there to talk, and most people here are open and friendly. Even families from very different backgrounds become close because they're all going through the same thing; the experience that's being shared is more powerful than the differences. People try to help one another get through. I'm sure Ellie will be making some new friends, too.''

Gail said good-bye, and Sally walked her out of the room. "I really should talk to some of the other mothers," Sally reflected aloud. "I guess I've been reluctant up to now because I was afraid of hearing too many horror stories. If another child didn't do well—I'm not sure how I'd react.''

"Well, in any transplant center, when you're talking about statistics you're averaging the results over a four- or five-year period," Gail explained. "During that time, there are going to be some patients who do very well and a bunch who don't. If your child is in the hospital at a time when a lot of other kids aren't doing well, it can be very scary. But it's important to remember that each patient is different, and just because the person in the next room is having problems doesn't mean that Ellie will, too.''

Sally nodded and smiled, although her stomach was churning and her palms were damp with sweat. "Thanks, Gail. I think I'll take your advice,'' she said.

"Good. And please come see me again.''

Gail went back to her office and sat at her desk for a while, thinking about what this family would go through in the next few months. It was impossible to provide enough emotional support for such an ordeal; they would be in constant psychic pain. She was amazed that most people in this situation did not go crazy or give up. It was a great testimony to the strength and resilience of the human mind.

Gail often marveled at the way so many of the mothers spent eight to ten hours a day with their sick child. They rarely talked but just sat in the room and read, knitted, or watched TV, leaving only briefly for meals or to chat in the visitors' lounge for a few minutes. The fathers came in on weekends or, when they had sick leave or vacation time, during the week. Gail sensed that the fathers, as a group, tended to withdraw a little, knowing that the mothers would be there anyway. Still, the fathers who could provide care for their child were a source of immeasurable relief for their wives, and she hoped to encourage more of them to become actively involved.

During her two years on the Transplant Unit, Gail had observed that parents reacted to the overwhelming stress of the transplant by exaggerating their normal coping styles. If a mother tended to be intellectual, she would read everything she could find on bone-marrow transplantation and become a real expert on the subject. If a father usually coped by taking charge of a situation, he would insist on multiple consultations with specialists, call up the hospital board of directors to register a complaint, or even travel to distant transplant centers to see how things were done elsewhere. Parents whose coping mechanisms were more primitive and who believed in "miracle cures" were known to withdraw their child from therapy and seek out a Laetrile clinic or a practitioner selling some other unproven treatment. Others became angry and even threatening, openly blaming the staff for causing the child pain.

How well young children like Ellie accepted the transplant procedure was largely determined by their parents' behavior. The children understood in their own way that what was being done to them was in their best interest, but they picked up a lot of cues from their parents about how to deal with the illness. If the parents were firm believers in what they were doing and were able to maintain discipline and provide entertainment, the child's emotional course would be reasonably smooth. Particularly helpful were the solid bedrock of a strong, mutually supportive relationship and the availability of emotional resources such as grandparents or close friends.

The parents who had trouble supporting the child were often not entirely convinced they had made the right decision and, in many cases, had a weak marriage plagued by conflicts and communication problems. These parents had trouble disciplining the child, who was allowed to become miserable and manipulative. This kind of behavior had the further effect of angering the staff and deepening the rift in the parents' relationship. The worst situation from the child's standpoint was when divorced or separated parents who had been living apart for some time were brought back together by the child's hospitalization. Inevitably, all the rancor and hate that had caused the marriage to fail would reappear. Each parent would blame the other for the illness, and that could be very disruptive to the child.

When parents were totally unable to cope with the disease or the transplant, they mourned the child prematurely in order to protect themselves from further loss, a syndrome known as "fear of reinvestment." After the mourning period they considered the child "dead" and cut off virtually all contact. This situation was disastrous for the child, who was left with no parental support. Later on, when the child really died, the parents would feel enormously guilty for not having lent support during the terminal phase and for having let the child die alone.

Since most of the patients on Three-South were adolescents and young adults, Gail dealt primarily with their very special problems. It was essential to the nature of intensive care that the patient regress to a passive state, but adolescents usually felt great anxiety about losing the recent gains they had made toward independence. Now they suddenly found themselves living in a fishbowl, monitored twenty-four hours a day and given absolutely no privacy or sense of autonomy. Small wonder that they searched desperately for ways to exercise control, and the result was usually detrimental to their medical treatment. They were very stubborn, insisting that they did not need their parents or anyone else; some refused to eat, to get out of bed, to take their medications, or to see their parents. A few devised manipulative rituals, such as making everyone leave the room when they received their chemotherapy. One patient rebelled by making hundreds of long-distance telephone calls, running up a bill of several thousand dollars; others became abusive or violent, swearing or throwing things at the nurses. Teenagers were also at a very self-conscious time of life and were devastated by unsightly changes in their physical appearance such as hair loss, cold sores, rashes, or fluid retention. Gail tried to help them accept these changes and to set realistic goals for achievement, since most of them were acutely aware that their time remaining could be limited and precious.

Although Gail had majored in English in college, she no longer felt her old urge to read tragic novels or see Shakespeare plays. On the rare nights she went out to a movie with her husband, she preferred something escapist such as a thriller or a light comedy. All the human drama she could ever want was right here on the ward.

22 Central Line

Since Ellie had passed all her tests and her parents had opted to go ahead with the procedure, the pretransplant regimen was scheduled to begin on Thursday, June 5. All of the details of the regimen—drugs, doses, times of administration, and management of toxicities and complications—were specified by a written protocol, designated JH-79-15, which had been activated in March 1979. The eleven-page document also described the background and objectives of the transplant study, the limitations placed on patient and donor selection, and the plan of treatment and evaluation. Although the major function of the protocol was to serve as a guide for the doctors to follow, the written document was also needed to secure approval for the Transplant Unit's activities from the hospital's Clinical Investigation Committee: a group of doctors, lawyers, and clergymen from outside the transplant field who examined all clinical research protocols to determine if they were both reasonable and ethical. The committee usually wanted to make sure that the protocol would answer some important questions, yield unambiguous and statistically significant results, and provide adequate informed consent.

Unlike the situation with chemotherapy protocols, no multi-institutional studies were underway to compare different approaches to marrow transplantation; there were simply not enough transplant centers or patients to make randomized studies worthwhile. Nevertheless, each of the major transplant centers wrote its own protocols (which differed slightly in the details of the preparatory regimen and the management of the patient after the transplant) so that the effectiveness of alternative approaches could be roughly compared. The relationship among the major transplant centers was a curious hybrid of competition and cooperation. The field was so small that all of the leading investigators knew one another personally and often exchanged anecdotal data over the phone. Yet at the same time they were competing for the same patients and government research funds.

In spite of their somewhat divergent approaches, all of the transplant teams were seeking the same basic goal: to minimize the side effects of marrow transplantation and still get good results. The field had progressed to the point where there were now long-term survivors, six and seven years out, so that the transplant groups were not only interested in preventing recurrences of leukemia but in enabling these patients to live essentially normal lives. That goal was still a long way off, however. Although the incidence of serious complications from the procedure had declined somewhat because most transplants were now being done in remission rather than relapse, there were still major problems to overcome. One of the objectives of protocol JH-79-15, for instance, was to reduce the incidence of interstitial pneumonitis—a serious form of pneumonia induced by radiation damage to the lungs—by spreading the dose of total-body irradiation out over four days and shielding the lungs for one exposure, instead of giving the radiation in a single massive dose.

At seven-thirty Thursday morning, Nancy came in to give Ellie some medication in preparation for her minor surgery. "You're going to get an IV in your chest this morning, Ellie, instead of in your arm," she explained gently. "It's a special IV that will stay in the whole time you're in the hospital, so we won't have to stick you so much. We'll be able to feed you with it, so that even though you don't feel like eating much, you won't get skinny."

"No! I don't want another IV!" Ellie moaned, but the sedative was already taking effect: she was too groggy to fight hard.

"Come on now, Ellie, be good," Sally said, holding on to her child's hand and hoping the orderlies would come soon. They appeared a few minutes later and wheeled the dozing child away.

In the operating room, Ellie was anesthetized and transferred to the operating table. The charge nurse positioned her on her back with her legs elevated slightly so that the blood would flow toward her head and enlarge the subclavian vein, making it easier for the surgeon to find. She then placed a small rolled towel between Ellie's shoulder blades, so as to better expose the right collarbone, and turned the unconscious child's head to the opposite side.

When Ellie's shoulder, neck, and chest had been prepped with antiseptic and draped with sterile towels, a surgical resident came in to do the insertion. The scrub nurse handed him a syringe with a long aspiration needle attached to it. After feeling for landmarks with his rubber-gloved fingertips, the surgeon slid the needle in just below the child's right collarbone, probing blindly for the large subclavian vein while applying gentle suction on the syringe. A few seconds later there was a sudden surge of dark blood into the syringe, indicating that the vein had been found. Leaving the needle in place, the surgeon disconnected the syringe, and the charge nurse immediately pressed down hard on Ellie's belly. The purpose of this forced expiration, or Valsalva maneuver, was to prevent air from entering the catheter during insertion and forming dangerous bubbles in the blood.

Working quickly now, the surgeon threaded an eight-inch sterile catheter through the open needle, feeding the flexible, spaghettilike tube into the vein until the plastic hub at the end of the catheter was flush with the hub of the needle. With the catheter inserted, the child was allowed to breathe normally again. Finally, the surgeon removed the needle, leaving the tubing in place. He sutured the puncture site to prevent the catheter from being dislodged accidentally, applied antibacterial cream, and covered it with a sterile dressing of gauze and tape. In order to make sure the catheter did not clot off, the charge nurse hooked it up to an IV set and began to infuse saline solution.

The surgeon then proceeded to implant the second central line. It was a Brobiac catheter, larger in diameter than the hyperalimentation line since it would be used for administering fluids and medications and for drawing blood. After the charge nurse had prepped Ellie's neck and left shoulder, the surgeon made an incision with his scalpel at the base of the child's neck and located the external jugular vein descending from the head. He inserted one end of the catheter into the vein and then, clamping the other end in a long forceps, tunneled it under the skin and down over Ellie's sternum, so that it exited through a small incision near her left nipple. A Dacron cuff

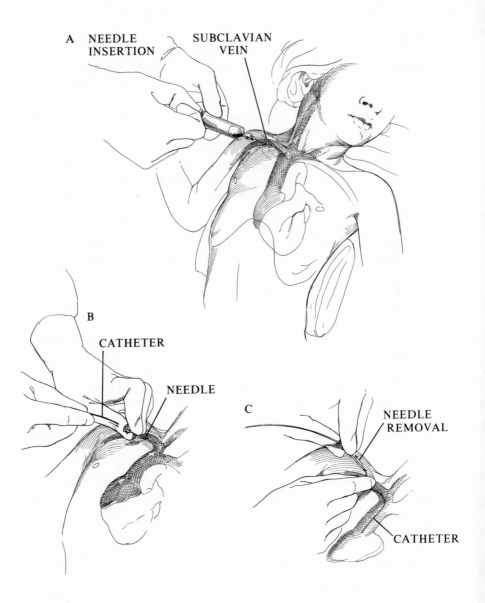

A NEEDLE INSERTION — SUBCLAVIAN VEIN

B — CATHETER — NEEDLE

C — NEEDLE REMOVAL — CATHETER

Insertion of a central line is done with the patient lying on her back, with a pillow between her shoulders to expose the clavicle. A needle attached to a syringe is first inserted into the subclavian vein; a spurt of blood into the syringe indicates that the vein has been found (A). Leaving the needle in place, the syringe is removed and pressure is then applied to the patient's chest to prevent air from being sucked in through the open needle. Next, a catheter is fed through the needle and into the vein, where it is pushed close to the heart (B). Finally, the needle is removed (C), the catheter is sutured to the skin, and a sterile dressing is applied. *Original drawing by Carol Donner.*

attached to the catheter remained beneath the exit site. Since the cuff adhered to the skin and would not be rejected by the body, tissue would grow around it, anchoring the catheter and making it less likely to pull out or become infected. Finally the cut-down and exit sites were sutured and dressed. In order to make sure that the Brobiac catheter stayed open, the charge nurse flushed it with six cc's of saline solution containing heparin and then filled the sealed tubing with more heparin solution, effectively "locking" it. The catheter would have to be flushed twice a day for as long as it was not used, to prevent it from clotting off.

The operation over, Ellie was wheeled out to the recovery room, where she awoke partially, and was then taken directly to Radiology, so that an X-ray could be done to confirm the proper placement of the hyperalimentation line in her right subclavian vein. The silastic catheter was opaque to X-rays and hence showed up clearly on the film. After Ellie was returned to her room, Nancy did an electrocardiogram to make sure that the catheter was not disturbing the child's heart.

Ellie slept for a few hours until the effects of the anesthetic wore off. When she awoke, she was still somewhat groggy and anxious, and the cut-down site bothered her, requiring an analgesic. Sally read to her for a while but the child's attention span was short. She soon lost interest in the story and, inspired by a set of handmade get-well cards from her first-grade classmates, became engrossed in a coloring book.

Sally glanced at her watch. It was after 2:00 P.M., and the Cytoxan chemotherapy was scheduled to begin in less than three hours. When that happened, there could be no turning back; they would have to go through with the transplant. Watching Ellie labor over the coloring book, Sally found it incredible that her seemingly healthy child was about to undergo a procedure in which she could die or become seriously disabled. "If only it were me lying there and not one of my children!" she thought. She urgently wanted to talk to someone, but the nurses had no time for prolonged conversations.

Telling Ellie she would be right back, Sally walked out to Gail's office, but the social worker was not in. Desperate, she went over to the nearby visitors' lounge to sit alone and gather her thoughts for a few minutes. Catching sight of two women talking on the couch, she changed her mind, quickening her pace as she passed the open door. Instead she went down to the hospital chapel to pray. Brian would be returning on Saturday morning, and she missed him more now than she had in a long time. She did get emotional support from Barbara and Cindy, who called often to find out how things were going, but it was not the same as having someone actually there with her.

At 4:30 P.M., Liz Ochs, Ellie's primary-care nurse on the evening shift, came in with a small bottle of Cytoxan solution, which she hooked up to Ellie's Brobiac catheter while Sally watched anxiously. The nurse unclamped the tubing and the innocuous-looking solution began to drip slowly into the central line. Liz calibrated the flow so that it would take about an hour for this dose to be administered. She glanced at her watch and marked down the time on Ellie's chart.

Liz was well aware that high-dose Cytoxan chemotherapy was an extreme treatment, exceeding all safe limits of toxicity, and that getting Ellie through the next four days without serious side effects would be a delicate balancing act. Cytoxan (generic name, cyclophosphamide) was one of the most potent drugs in the anticancer arsenal. Derived in the 1950s from mustard gas, a chemical-warfare agent, the drug worked by attacking the nuclei of rapidly dividing cells, rendering the cells incapable of replication and ultimately eliminating them. Although cancer cells and bone-marrow cells were highly sensitive to the drug, it could also damage rapidly growing normal tissues such as the lining of the mouth and gut, the skin and hair follicles, and vital organs such as the bladder, liver, kidneys, and heart.

Because of the drug's numerous toxicities, extensive precautions had to be taken. For six hours after each intravenous administration, dangerous metabolites of the drug would accumulate in Ellie's urine. If not adequately diluted, they could crystallize out and irritate the lining of the bladder, causing inflammation and bleeding. In order to avoid this serious complication, known as hemorrhagic cystitis, Ellie would have to receive large amounts of intravenous fluids and to void frequently, eliminating the toxic metabolites quickly in her urine.

Potentially even more serious than the risk of bladder disease was the drug's toxicity to the heart muscle. Because of this side effect, any prospective transplant recipient who had a heart condition was automatically disqualified. Every morning during the four days of chemotherapy, Ellie would receive an electrocardiogram in order to detect any incipient damage to her heart; a decrease in voltage would be a significant and ominous sign. Frequent samples of her blood and urine would also be taken for analysis, since elevated levels of certain enzymes in the blood, such as CPK (creatine phosphokinase), would also indicate cardiac toxicity.

The infusion was complete by 5:40 P.M. Soon afterward Ellie began to feel nauseated, and she vomited into the plastic basin that Sally held for her. At six-fifteen, Liz began an infusion of normal saline solution in order to provide sufficient hydration to ensure a urine output greater than four ounces per hour over the next twenty-four hours. In addition, the diuretic drug furosemide was added to the stock IV solution to enhance further the flow of urine.

Ellie's nausea had worsened considerably by six-thirty. Liz gave her an intravenous injection of Thorazine, a potent tranquilizer that suppressed the vomiting reflex. Although the drug made Ellie extremely dazed and uncoordinated, her vomiting did stop and she finally sank into a restful sleep. Because of the diuretic in her IV solution, Ellie would wake about every two hours during the night with the urge to void. If she had recovered enough from the Thorazine, the night nurse would help her to the bathroom; otherwise she would have to use the bedpan.

Sally finally left about 10:00 P.M., stopping for a solitary dinner in the hospital cafeteria. Diane Marks had warned her that the hospital area was dangerous at night and that she should not leave the Oncology Center alone after 6:00 P.M. Sally followed Diane's suggestion and stopped at the security desk by the front door. A tall, dour member of the University Police was called in to escort her across the street to the Sheraton.

This fortress mentality, combined with the rising June heat, made Sally's isolation and claustrophobia even more intense. All day she had managed to keep up her cheerfulness with Ellie, holding her anxiety and grief at bay. But now that she was alone she let the tears come, weeping for quite a while into what had been a freshly starched pillow. When she became too exhausted to cry, she began praying. "God never gives you more than you can handle," she told herself, but she wondered how much longer she could continue this way. Although she tried not to dwell on her other children, she missed them terribly, particularly little Amy. She thought of calling home for the second time that evening, but the kids would be asleep by now.

Sally tried to read a novel she had bought in the hospital gift shop, but she soon found herself going over the same paragraph several times without comprehending. Giving up, she turned on the TV, if only because it provided the illusion of human company. She kept telling herself that the transplant would be a cure and that everything would work out fine with just a little more patience. Otherwise, nothing made any sense at all.

23 The Lounge

Saturday morning, June 7, Brian Murphy drove down to Baltimore, reviewing in his mind the strains of the past few days. It had been hard to be so far away from the hospital, not knowing precisely what was happening to Ellie. He spoke to Sally every evening on the phone and got a daily progress report, but he suspected that she was not telling him everything. Amy had also been a burden. Although Beth was coping fairly well with her sister's transplant and her own prospective role as marrow donor, Amy was too young to understand what was happening; she knew only that her mother was gone. Despite her grandmother's coddling, she had crying fits and could not be comforted.

It had admittedly been a great help that Brian's parents had moved temporarily from their Staten Island home to Menlo Park to look after the two girls and help with the cooking and cleaning. Even so, Brian was finding it increasingly difficult to get along with his mother. The elder Mrs. Murphy found fault in every aspect of Ellie's treatment. Why had they taken her to Baltimore when there were perfectly good hospitals in New York? Why were they persisting in giving her conventional therapy, when the drugs and radiation had already failed to cure her and had side effects that were "worse than the disease"? She thought that Brian should bring Ellie home from Baltimore immediately and send her to a doctor on Long Island who specialized in "holistic" therapies: megavitamin regimens, organic diets, coffee enemas, and the like. When she persisted in her criticism in spite of all his patient explanations, he found himself getting so angry that he shouted at her to shut up. At.that point he decided that it would be better to avoid the subject entirely.

At work, he had been preoccupied and depressed, and it was only the fear of losing his job that had forced him out of his daze and back to work. He could not even afford to take a day off to rest his nerves; he was saving all his accumulated sick leave and vacation for later on after the transplant, in the event a serious complication developed and he had to spend several days in a row in Baltimore.

From what Sally had told him, Brian expected Ellie to look bad, but it was still a shock to see her. A week before, she had been happy and healthy—but for her slightly sparse hair, you would have thought her a normal child. Now she looked nauseated and washed out, bent over the yellow basin into which she had just vomited. A cluster of IV bottles dangled like strange fruit from the metal tree beside the bed, feeding plastic tubes into her chest. Brian remembered his mother's ravings about the horrors of chemotherapy and felt a twinge of guilt. Ellie was going through this agony because he and Sally had signed the consent form; the choice had not been hers.

Eager to find out for himself how Ellie was doing, Brian sought out Dr. Krueger. The attending reassured him that the protocol was proceeding as planned, without serious problems so far. Ellie had now completed two days of Cytoxan and would be receiving her third dose that afternoon. Her white count had dropped sharply to 2,700 and her side effects included possible cystitis: she had pain while voiding and a trace amount of blood had been detected in her urine. The medical team was maintaining vigorous hydration and administering diuretics in an effort to prevent any exacerbation of this problem.

Ellie rested in bed all morning. The chemo made her feel terrible and there was no reprieve from her discomfort. The more she vomited the weaker she became, and although the Thorazine suppressed the nausea somewhat, it made her feel dazed and heavy. She had no desire to do anything but lie in bed and watch TV. Her eyes were so sensitive that she could not even bear to have the bedside lamp on, so the family spent the day with the blinds drawn against the sunlight, in a gloomy twilight relieved only by the blue glow from the TV screen.

"When am I going home?" Ellie kept asking. She wanted to be having a real summer, playing with her friends and doing fun things, instead of being cooped up in an awful hospital.

Sally tried to explain to Ellie that she would have to stay in the hospital for a very long time, more than a month, but she knew that the child did not have a very good sense of time. To her, a month seemed like an eternity.

When Ellie refused to touch anything on her lunch tray, the nutritionist decided that it was time to begin hyperalimentation, which would provide the child with 2,300 calories per day—enough to maintain her body weight and even grow. As soon as the bottle of hyperal solution arrived from the pharmacy, the nutritionist connected it to Ellie's silastic catheter. From now on this central line would be used only for hyperalimentation and kept sealed off from the outside, since the high concentration of glucose in the nutrient solution would make it a fertile breeding ground for bacteria.

The nutritionist connected the silastic catheter to a battery-powered infusion pump known as an Imed: a boxlike device with dials and switches that was clamped to the IV pole. She set the dials and switched on the pump; a red light began to blink. The Imed would deliver a constant, regulated amount of the nutrient solution through the catheter twenty-four hours a day. The device also contained an electric eye that monitored the flow rate of the solution and could detect the presence of air bubbles, blocks, or kinks in the line. If any of these problems developed or the batteries were low, a beeping alarm would go off.

Careful watch would have to be paid to the rate of infusion in order to prevent fluid overload. The nurses kept input-and-output (I & O) records listing Ellie's daily consumption and excretion of fluids. If her weight increased or her total fluid input greatly exceeded her output, she would be given diuretics to bring her fluid balance back to normal. In addition, the ingredients of the hyperalimentation solution would be carefully adjusted to meet Ellie's needs as they developed. The nutritionist maintained detailed flow-sheets for each patient on which she recorded weight changes, electrolyte balance (the proportions of water and inorganic salts), blood sugar, blood urea nitrogen (a measure of kidney function), and the levels of various essential minerals.

That afternoon, with Nancy's encouragement, Ellie and Sally did a few "laps" around the nurses' station. Sally pushed Ellie's IV pole, with its clinking bottles and blinking Imed, and Ellie held on to her mother with one hand and her plastic basin with the other, in case she got sick. A few other patients were doing laps, and although the halls were wide, so much equipment was parked in them that traffic jams occasionally developed.

As they walked past the doors of patient rooms, Sally was confronted repeatedly with the brutal realities she had been struggling to deny. Passing one doorway, she saw a young man in bed covered from head to toe with red, scaling skin. That must be GVHD, she thought to herself, terrified that Ellie might develop the same complication. In another room, a black teenager was retching horribly, his body racked by dry heaves. Further on, a heart monitor was beeping. Sally looked in, expecting to see an elderly patient, and was shocked to see a young girl on a respirator. It seemed to her the cruelest irony: children growing and maturing at the same time that they were dying.

Ellie seemed not to notice the horrors that surrounded her. She waved and smiled at the other patients doing laps, and one of them, a twelve-year-old black boy named Gregory Sikes, flashed her a brilliant grin. Gregory was the unchallenged champion of the Unit as far as laps were concerned, often doing more than five hundred in a single day. He came from a family of "born-again" Southern Baptists from rural Georgia who were constantly handing out religious pamphlets to whoever would take them. According to Gregory's parents, at the age of nine he had experienced a religious revelation and had proceeded to convert the entire family. Whatever the reason, Gregory clearly had an intense will to live. He would do laps continually all morning, up and down the corridors, even though he was often bent over with stomach cramps. Sally enjoyed watching him: his drive and persistence were an inspiration to everyone on the floor. Gregory made her believe that maybe if one's will was strong enough, it would be sufficient to get one through anything.

The afternoon passed extremely slowly. Instead of the five doctors on service during the week, there was only one resident, and fewer nurses as well. The ward seemed deserted. "I just hope Ellie never gets really sick on a

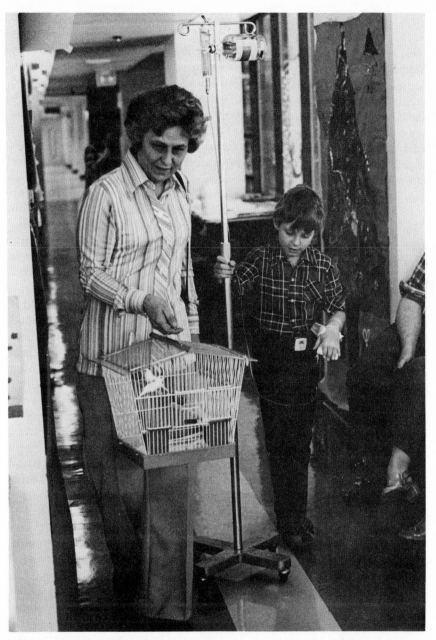

Child doing laps around the ward with an IV pole is accompanied by a hospital volunteer. Exercise is essential to maintain the muscle tone and lung capacity of patients undergoing chemotherapy or bone-marrow transplantation. *Photo courtesy of the American Cancer Society.*

weekend," Sally commented to Brian, "because nobody's here." The hours dragged by. There was little good programing on TV and it was impossible to read because the light in the room was so dim. Ellie was nauseated and irritable, and Brian was going stir-crazy in that small, dark, oppressive space. It was like being in a prison cell or a sailboat becalmed at sea. He sat in a corner and stared straight ahead for long minutes like a senile old man. Sally missed his customary light banter and tried to bring him out of his depression, without success. She could see it disturbed Ellie to see her father so withdrawn.

After Ellie's third dose of Cytoxan on Saturday, her white count fell to 2,000 and her hematocrit plummeted to 25 from a near-normal value of 36 the day before. A transfusion of packed red cells was hung at 4:50 P.M. At six, Ellie's supper tray was brought in, although she had not touched any of the past four meals. Reluctant to see the food go to waste, Sally picked at it guiltily while Ellie vomited up a thin, watery gruel into the plastic bowl between her knees.

Sunday was another long day. In the morning Sally went to Mass, held at the Oncology Center auditorium. At the end of the service the priest stood by the door as people filed out and introduced himself to the unfamiliar faces, including Sally. He wanted to know if there was anything he could do, and she mentioned that maybe he could come up and visit with Ellie when he had a chance. The priest said he would be happy to.

When she returned to the room, Brian was still quiet and withdrawn. After an hour of trying to start a conversation with him and being answered with only grunts or silences, Sally gave up and went out to sit in the lounge, desperate for a responsive person to talk with.

As she had hoped, the lounge was not empty. Two women sat on the couch, talking in low tones, while the TV droned in the background. Sally sat down in the armchair across from the couch and, although they recognized one another by sight, formal introductions were made. The younger of the two women, Mrs. Willis, looked to be in her early thirties, with a round, pasty, haggard face, lined beyond her years. She had short, mousy hair and a soft, plaintive twang to her voice—a Carolina accent that seemed further slowed and muted by strain. The other woman, Mrs. Cox, was in her late forties, with graying dark hair, sharper features, and a deeply lined forehead. She had a Southern accent as well, but it was harder and more nasal, with an angry edge to it.

Sally presented her "credentials" in order to let the two women know she was the mother of a patient and not just a visitor—that she shared the common bond of suffering. "We got here just a few days ago, and I haven't been out of the room much," she explained. "My daughter Ellie's getting her Cytoxan now, and her transplant is scheduled for next Friday."

"What does she have?" Mrs. Willis asked.

"ALL. She was in first remission for a year and a half and doing so well that we were sure she was cured. Then out of the blue she relapsed, and our doctor told us that a bone-marrow transplant was her best hope. They say if the first remission fails, chances are slim that chemotherapy will be a cure."

Mrs. Willis shook her head. "You have to be ready for anything; it's so damn unpredictable. My son Keith—he's sixteen—has aplastic anemia. He can go to sleep feeling great and wake up in the morning feeling terrible. You just have to live from day to day."

"What exactly is aplastic anemia?" Sally asked.

"It's not cancer, like leukemia," Mrs. Willis said quickly. "It's just when the bone marrow stops making new blood cells. They don't know why it happens. Keith had it when he was a baby and it went away by itself, but it started coming back when he was fourteen, and it kept getting worse and worse. Finally they told us a transplant would be his only hope. Fortunately his sister was a good match."

Although she had just met this woman, Sally felt herself quickly becoming caught up in her life story. "So how's he doing now?" she asked. "Has he had his transplant?"

"About a month ago," Mrs. Willis replied. "Things could be better. He had a real good take the first week, but the second week his counts were the same, and by the third week they had started to fall again. We had some more bad news yesterday."

Sally felt her stomach tense up. "What happened?"

"Keith's bone-marrow test wasn't good at all. There was hardly anything there. They figure that either the marrow is completely destroyed or it's not evenly distributed inside the bone and they just got a bad sample. So they're going to repeat the bone marrow tomorrow."

"I've got a lot of prayer groups going back home," Mrs. Cox said. "I'm going to make sure they put Keith's name on the list."

"Thank you," Mrs. Willis said softly. "We've had a lot of people up here praying for him. I think he's getting kind of tired of all those people praying in the room. He says he doesn't believe in it anymore."

"Oh, he'll be all right," Mrs. Cox said. "We have to have faith in the good Lord. Why, Brad Stevens was a long time coming, real slow coming. Each person's different, but seeing Brad do so well the second time around was real encouraging to me."

Mrs. Willis nodded sadly. "I asked Dr. Krueger about Brad's case. Apparently he just got Cytoxan the first time, and the marrow didn't take, so they added radiation treatments the second time around. That's why he did so well with the second transplant. But they've already given Keith radiation and they can't do it again. He can only get Cytoxan. So that already goes against him. I just hope the test tomorrow looks better and they won't have to do another transplant. But if his marrow has gone to nothing, they won't have any choice. They want to use my ten-year-old as a donor this time. It's hard . . . the idea of starting all over again."

"Maybe another donor will do the trick," Mrs. Cox offered.

"Yes, there's still hope, I know. It's just that his chances are less this way. You see, with the second transplant, he can get more infections. That's why I think they're trying to hold off on it as long as they can." Mrs. Willis paused, her eyes abstracted. "You know what's strange?"

"What?" Sally asked.

"You'd think to look at him that he's doing real well. I mean, he really looks healthy. He was up and walking around today."

"That's right," Mrs. Cox said. "He looks real good."

"Yeah," Mrs. Willis mused. "That's the strange thing. How's Bob today?"

Mrs. Cox's face darkened and the lines in her brow seemed to deepen. "Oh, I think he's a little better. He's still on the respirator, but all it's doing is giving him some oxygen. He can breathe on his own now."

"That's really good."

"Well, he was feeling a little bit stronger for a couple of days, so they turned off the respirator yesterday. It was off all day. He had a tube up his nose giving him oxygen, but he was doing everything himself. They were going to take out the tube this morning, but when I got here after breakfast he was back on the respirator—they turned it back on during the night. So I don't know. They told me they want him to start walking again. His muscles have gotten so weak from just lying there so long that it's hard for him to walk. The physical therapist is going to help him next week, and the nurses have been trying to cheer him up."

Sally wanted desperately to say something positive, to help dissipate the gloom that had settled over the conversation. "Maybe the transplant will cure him," she said.

Mrs. Cox looked up at her, startled, and then slowly shook her head. "It's been a hundred days since the transplant, and Bob is critical right now," she murmured.

Mrs. Willis sat forward earnestly on the edge of the couch and took Mrs. Cox's hand. "You've done everything you could," she said. "The disease isn't your fault. Anyone can get leukemia—there's no reason for it." She paused. "Let me tell you something. When Keith was born, the doctors took us into a little room and told us he had only six months to live. They said you don't survive with only one percent of your white cells. But he's sixteen now. He did it, all on his own. And now, God willing, he has a chance to beat this completely. So never give up."

Mrs. Cox looked down at her bony hands, clenched in her lap. "It's up to God. If Bob doesn't make it, I would feel terrible because I'd miss him, but I know he'd be in the hands of the Lord."

"I'll pray for him," Sally murmured, close to tears. She felt an intense compassion for these two women; they had all been brought here by the same incomprehensible twist of fate.

There was a silence, and then Mrs. Cox let out a long sigh and stood up. "I'd better be getting back to the room," she said. "The resident has probably left by now, and Bob will be wondering where I've been all this time." She backed slowly toward the door, obviously reluctant to leave. "I'm gonna get him up and around even if it hurts," she added. "The nurses insist on it. They won't settle for him staying in that bed. Maybe later on I'll get him out in the hall so you can see us together. He's looking good today."

"Great," Mrs. Willis said. "I'll see y'all then."

"Well, bye now," Mrs. Cox said. "Nice meeting you, Mrs. Murphy, and good luck with your daughter's transplant."

After Mrs. Cox had left, Sally and Mrs. Willis sat in silence for a while. "Poor woman," Mrs. Willis said suddenly. "Her son came very close last night. One of the doctors told me that he was like Lazarus, arisen from the dead."

"Gosh, I hope he makes it," Sally said.

"Yeah."

Feeling awkward, Sally picked up an old *National Geographic* and leafed through it absently. She thought about Keith and Bob. All of the patients on the floor went through such suffering that it seemed only fair that every one of them would get well and go home. It was a hard truth to accept that about half of them were not going to make it.

In spite of her feelings of compassion, however, Sally felt a separateness. Mrs. Willis and Mrs. Cox were too different from her in their Southern ways for her to be totally comfortable with them. She also needed to distance herself from the life-threatening complications that Keith and Bob had developed. Identifying with them too closely would mean confronting the fact that Ellie, too, could do poorly and even die. And she had to believe that Ellie would be a miracle child, breezing through the transplant and the hundred days afterward with none of the usual problems.

After a few minutes, Sally put down the magazine and glanced at her watch. She excused herself politely and went back to the room.

At 4:00 P.M., Brian left to drive back to Menlo Park. Sally walked him to the elevator, wanting somehow to reach out to him; there was so much that had remained unsaid. But he was remote, preoccupied, weary; the distance between them seemed unbridgeable. "I'll be back on Thursday with Beth," he told her. "Have a good week." A quick kiss, and then the elevator doors slid shut. She was almost relieved to see him go.

24 Countdown

On the evening of Sunday, June 8, Ellie received her final dose of Cytoxan. Her four-day course of total-body irradiation (TBI) was scheduled to begin the following day.

Extending the TBI over four days was a fairly recent innovation, done in the hope of maximizing the antileukemic effect of the radiation while minimizing its toxic effects on normal tissues. The original transplant regimen developed by E. Donnall Thomas had specified a single dose of 1,000 rads. Subsequent laboratory experiments on animals revealed, however, that if the radiation was fractionated—divided into a series of shorter exposures over a period of days—the normal cells in the lungs, liver, and other organs were able to repair themselves significantly faster than were the leukemic cells, resulting in a better antileukemic effect with less damage to healthy tissues. Accordingly, the major transplant centers developed their own TBI fractionation schemes. For example, Sloan-Kettering irradiated patients for a few minutes three times a day over a period of several days, whereas Hopkins gave single, longer exposures on each of four consecutive days. The various centers had also begun shielding the lungs during some exposures to reduce further the incidence of lung damage.

At two o'clock Monday morning, the nurse woke Ellie to take her vital signs and weight and make sure she went to the bathroom. Ellie was still receiving a large volume of fluid through her Brobiac catheter and attempting to void every few hours with great difficulty. Nauseated by the Cytoxan and disoriented by the sedatives, she found it exhausting to climb out of bed to be weighed, with her central lines threatening to tangle. Nonetheless, this routine had to be repeated several times during the night.

At 7:00 A.M., the resident came in to draw blood, which was done by attaching a syringe directly to the hub of the Brobiac catheter, flushing it afterward with heparin solution. He also took surveillance cultures of Ellie's throat and groin. The child fell back asleep until eight-thirty, when a breakfast tray was brought in even though she was still too sick to eat any solid foods. Sally arrived at nine, and the rest of the day passed uneventfully: mostly TV and games, with a few laps around the nurses' station in the afternoon when Ellie's nausea had eased somewhat. At 5:00 P.M., an hour before the TBI was to begin, Liz Ochs gave Ellie some phenobarbital pills to sedate her. While they were waiting for the orderlies to arrive, Sally told Ellie what she would be getting, since she doubted that the child remembered the cranial irradiation she had received a year and a half before. The radiation would be like getting an X-ray, she explained, only Ellie would have to lie still for a long time, alone in a big room. But Mommy would be watching her on a TV screen nearby and there would be a speaker system so that they could talk back and forth.

At six-fifteen, two orderlies arrived and transferred Ellie onto a stretcher, along with her IV bottles. She held tightly to her favorite doll, Polly. Liz tied a surgical mask on the child's face so that she would not be exposed to bacteria during her trip downstairs, and Ellie asked if Polly could have a mask, too.

"Is Polly going to get some radiation, Ellie?" Liz asked.

"Yes, she wants to stay with me."

"Isn't she lucky to be getting a transplant like you? Then she won't need any more needles, either," Liz said, tying a mask over the doll's face. Ellie nodded and held Polly close to her chest.

The orderlies strapped her to the stretcher and covered her up to her chin with a light green sheet. As they maneuvered the stretcher out of the room, Sally took hold of Ellie's hand and kept pace with the orderlies, moving down the hall and into the waiting elevator.

Emerging at the basement level, they went past the reception desk into the Radiation Therapy Department. The door of the TBI chamber was open, and the orderlies pushed the stretcher inside, asking Sally to wait. By this time, Ellie's eyes were drooping heavily from the sedative. The windowless room was dominated by the giant, gleaming fuselage of the linear accelerator, supported on a hinged gantry above the metal table.

Dr. Charles Wolff, the chief radiation therapist, came over and introduced himself to Sally, noting that she appeared very anxious. He had observed that parents and older patients were generally much more upset by TBI than young children, who, although frightened, seemed to accept their first treatment without undue concern. Perhaps it was because the children were unaware of all the possible side effects. He explained to Sally that Ellie would be irradiated for fifteen minutes lying on her back and then for another fifteen minutes on her stomach, receiving a total midline dose of 300 rads at a dose rate of 10 rads per minute. "Young children tolerate the radiation well, much better than older patients," he reassured her. "Kids are very resilient because they have young tissues with a tremendous regenerative capacity."

"What happens if she moves?" Sally asked. "Will that mess up the radiation?"

"No, the field is large enough that it doesn't matter."

Inside the chamber, Ellie was placed on the table on her back and strapped down. One of the technicians pushed a button on a wall panel and, with a loud whirring, the huge machine swiveled into place over the table. With the aid of projected cross-hairs, the accelerator was aligned over the child's body. Then the radiotherapy nurse injected 5 cc's of Thorazine into Ellie's stock IV solution and adjusted the flow so that it would run slowly throughout the exposure, allowing the child to sleep and lessening some of the inevitable nausea afterward. "Okay, we're ready," she said.

The room quickly emptied, leaving Ellie alone under a pale beam of light that would make her visible on the TV monitor. The 4½-inch-thick door rumbled shut, sealing off the chamber within massive walls of lead and concrete.

Seated at the console outside, a technician started the timing device and a digital dial began to count out the seconds with a sharp clicking sound. Sally stared at the ghostly black-and-white image of her solitary child, still clutching her doll, motionless under the massive machine. "She looks so tiny," Sally murmured. "Just like a little baby." Pushing down the button on the intercom, she said into the mike, "You're doing real well, Ellie. Keep it up."

When the machine had switched on, some white horizontal streaks had appeared on the TV monitor, apparently due to electrical interference from the accelerator. Although Sally knew that the beam of X-rays was invisible, those white streaks made her think of a giant ray-gun, firing lethal bursts of radiation at her defenseless child. The scene was reminiscent of an execution: the victim strapped helplessly inside a sealed chamber beneath an enormous machine, while the grim act was witnessed dispassionately on closed-circuit TV. Indeed, there was some truth to the analogy: after four treatments, Ellie would have received enough radiation to kill her if she were not to be "rescued" by a transplant of her sister's marrow.

The minutes passed slowly, accompanied by the clicking of the digital timer. Dr. Wolff stared fixedly at the screen, concerned that if Ellie vomited in her highly sedated state she might choke on her vomit and suffocate. He was prepared to stop the treatment at the first sign of trouble.

Finally a buzzer sounded, indicating that the first fifteen minutes were up. The heavy door slid back and the technicians entered the chamber, turned Ellie over, and realigned her with the machine. Groggy from the medications, she let them do what they would, without protest. Then the door slid back once more and the timer began its staccato count, as insistent and precise as an electronic metronome.

In spite of all the sophisticated equipment that surrounded them, Sally felt that there was something medieval about the whole process. Here they were purging a sick child with poisons and lethal rays, much as early physicians had treated fever with leeches and blood letting, and migraine headaches by drilling holes in people's skulls. However sophisticated, the weapons of modern cancer therapy were also crude—a sign of massive ignorance. If only Ellie had been born a century from now! Sally thought.

When Ellie finally returned to her room, she retched uncontrollably, shivering and groaning on her bed. Sally wiped the vomitus off the child's face and changed her into clean pajamas, while Liz replaced the IV bottles. For the next twenty-four hours, Ellie would have to receive a liter of IV fluid containing sodium carbonate every four hours. The purpose of all this hydration was to maintain a brisk flow of alkaline urine during the period of maximum marrow-cell destruction, thereby preventing a dangerous buildup of uric acid in the kidney tubules. The intravenous fluids would be continued until Ellie was able to drink a liter of fluid every twenty-four hours.

Over the next three days, the countdown continued, accompanied by a gradual decline in Ellie's blood counts. The radiation and chemotherapy were killing off the rapidly dividing precursor cells in her bone marrow, so that no fresh blood cells were being made. Although the mature, nondividing blood cells now circulating in her bloodstream were less sensitive to radiation and would remain viable for another week or so, the lack of replacements meant that Ellie would soon enter a period of aplasia—a severe deficiency of blood cells of all types—until the marrow graft took and began producing new blood cells on its own. By Tuesday, June 10, Ellie's white count had dropped to 1,700.

During Ellie's third TBI treatment on Wednesday, her lungs were shielded from the radiation by lead plates. The plates, cut out to conform to the contour of the lungs, were positioned on her chest according to reference lines drawn on her skin. An X-ray film was placed under her and exposed by the beam so that the correct placement of the shielding could be verified. Ellie managed to sleep through the third treatment entirely, and her nausea afterward subsided quickly.

Brian and Beth arrived in Baltimore on Thursday, June 12, the final day of the pretransplant regimen. Although Beth was nervous about the transplant, she felt proud of her role as older sister and marrow donor. She had explained the transplant to a few of her close friends and they had responded with admiration and encouragement. Brian was also in good spirits, cheered by a moving demonstration of support he had received the day before. He had told a few of his close associates at work about the transplant, and when they had asked him how much it would cost, he had said what the doctors had estimated: between $40,000 and $100,000, although insurance would probably cover most of it. His colleagues had been stunned. A week later Jack Ellison, one of his fellow sales managers, had handed him a check for $1,000 which had been raised through an office fund. When Brian began to protest, Ellison had shushed him up. "Listen, you're going to need that money for something," he had said. "When you dip into the well and nothing's there, it can get pretty grim. Let's face it, Brian, you have enough to worry about." This impressive display of concern and support had lifted Brian's spirits, and he was more optimistic now about the transplant than he had been in a long time. During the car ride down to Baltimore, he even managed to joke with Beth about how she would be up and running the day after the operation.

On their arrival, he checked into the Sheraton; they planned to move out to the trailer after the transplant. Brian dropped his bags off at the room and then took Beth across the street to the Oncology Center to be admitted. She was placed in one of the donor rooms, which happened to be located right next to Ellie. While Beth changed into pajamas and had her admitting physical done, Brian and Sally shuttled back and forth between the two rooms.

Beth was elated by all the attention she was getting and enjoyed playing with the remote-control TV suspended above her bed. She hated having her blood drawn again, though, and when the novelty of the TV had worn off, she began to think that being in the hospital might not be as much fun as she had hoped. She was also troubled by the fact that she and Ellie were a "match." Did that mean that she was likely to get Ellie's sickness, too? Whenever she felt an ache or a pain she was convinced that she was coming down with leukemia, and she only relaxed when the "symptom" went away.

As soon as the admitting process was over, Dr. Krueger came into Beth's room to speak to both parents. "Ellie's done very well with her chemotherapy and radiation and has no major problems to speak of," he said. "She goes into the transplant in very good shape. Beth, I'm pleased to say, is in excellent health."

Krueger was nonetheless concerned that Beth might become ill at the last minute, prior to the transplant, but after Ellie had received her final, lethal dose of TBI that evening. This catastrophe had actually happened twice before at Hopkins. In the first case, the donor had developed a fever a few days before the transplant, but an alternate HLA-identical sibling had fortunately been available. In the second case, no other donor existed, and a decision had been made to go ahead with the transplant even though the risk of infecting the recipient was high. Krueger would have liked to keep Beth "under glass" until the operation was completed.

He described to the family the nature of the marrow-harvesting procedure, which had been scheduled for ten o'clock the next morning, making sure Beth understood that she would be in no way responsible for the success or failure of the transplant. Her marrow was healthy—that was a known fact—and if it did not work for Ellie, the reason was that the disease had interfered and not that Beth's marrow had been defective. Krueger found it necessary to stress this point because of the tendency of marrow donors to feel personally responsible for the outcome of the procedure.

Krueger also tried to dispel another common misconception. After the transplant, Ellie's blood type would change to that of her sister, and since Beth was allergic to dust and pollen, Ellie, too, would become allergic. No other physical or psychological traits would be passed along, however. Some people seemed to think that because the blood was so pervasive, the recipient child would adopt many characteristics of the donor. This myth caused particular concern when the donor and recipient were of the opposite sex. Krueger assured the Murphys that the different genetic identity of Beth's marrow cells would have absolutely no effect on Ellie's appearance or personality.

The Murphy family spent much of the evening before the transplant sitting with Ellie and talking. Although her spirits were high, she was exhausted; she had received the final dose of TBI that evening and the eight days of intensive treatments had worn her down. She went to sleep early, and Brian and Sally moved into Beth's room for a while.

"Tomorrow's the big day," Sally said.

"Yeah," Beth said, taking a deep breath. "I'm pretty scared."

"You're going to do fine," Sally reassured her. "Daddy and I are both very proud of you."

Beth beamed. "They're going to make Ellie all better, right, Mommy? Then we can play together when she gets out."

Sally nodded, smiling. She could not afford to let herself think that far ahead.

25 Beth's Gift

On the morning of Friday, June 13, Beth was awakened at seven-fifteen for routine temperature and blood-pressure readings. She was very apprehensive and restless and could not manage to fall back to sleep. She wondered where her parents were and got annoyed when the nurse told her she would not be allowed to eat breakfast. By the time her parents arrived, she was hungry and irritable. First she wanted to watch TV, but grew bored in a few minutes. Then she decided to do a few laps around the nurses' station, but Nancy told her to stay in bed because they would soon be giving her some medicine to make her drowsy and did not want her falling down and hurting herself. Beth became angry about having to stay in bed and started to cry. "I'm hungry!" she whined. Nancy gave her a preoperative injection of phenobarbital, but instead of acting as a sedative, the drug seemed to make Beth even more hyperactive, as sometimes happens in young children.

There was a delay over in Surgery, and the resident told them that the orderlies would not be up for Beth until around nine-thirty. While they were waiting, Sally went next door to see Ellie. The child was very weak and pale, but her excitement was obvious. Sally helped her out of bed and they walked slowly over to the window. All that could be seen from the room was the drab concrete façade of the parking garage, aglow in the morning sunlight, but Ellie stared at it longingly for several minutes before returning to bed.

It was not until a quarter to ten that the orderlies arrived to take Beth to Surgery. Sally followed the stretcher down to the main floor in the elevator and, her mouth dry and stomach churning, bent down and kissed her daughter's forehead. "Everything will be fine," she said. "We're all rooting for you, Beth. Don't be afraid." Beth smiled and nodded, but her eyes were glistening with tears.

The bone-marrow harvests were done by three rotating teams, each made up of an attending and a physician's assistant (P.A.). Four or five transplants were done every month. Nick Billings, one of the three P.A.'s who worked on the Transplant Unit, would be assisting with the procedure that morning.

At 9:50 A.M., Billings checked the surgery schedule posted in Diane Marks's office and saw that the harvest that morning was listed for 10:00 A.M. in O.R. #1. Realizing he was almost late, he hurried over to the main hospital building and took the elevator to the surgical floor. Across from the elevator as he emerged was a glassed-in entranceway with a sign forbidding admittance to unauthorized personnel. A heavyset woman behind the reception desk nodded to him familiarly and handed him a slip of paper with a locker combination written on it. He thanked her and walked down the hall into the locker room, where he changed into a green-cotton scrub suit: baggy pants with a string belt, a collarless tunic threadbare from too much washing, a hair cover, shoe covers, and a disposable surgical mask.

Emerging from the locker room, he turned right down a long white-tiled corridor, flanked on either side by a dozen operating rooms in which procedures were already underway. O.R. #1 was at the end of the corridor on the right-hand side. A sign on the door read ISOLATION: STAY OUT. Billings knew that the sign was there to minimize traffic during the operation; the extracted bone marrow would remain in an open beaker and it was essential to minimize the risk of contamination.

Billings went into an alcove adjacent to the O.R. and walked over to the sink. With a presoaped brush, he scrubbed his hands and forearms and then rinsed well. Raising his wet arms, flexed at the elbows and held away from his chest, he backed into the green-tiled operating room. Ron McIver, the charge nurse, handed him a sterile towel. Billings dried off and then picked up a corner of a folded surgical gown, let it fall open, and put his arms through the sleeves, while Ron tied it in back. Finally he pulled on a pair of sterile surgical gloves, being careful not to touch the outside of the gloves with his bare hands. The rest of the surgical team was already gowned up and busy at various tasks: the attending, Dr. Wood; the nurse-anesthetist, Trudy Logan, with a nursing student under her supervision; and the technician, Luke Jones.

Beth Murphy lay face-up on the stretcher, looking bewildered as Trudy Logan prepared to induce her into anesthesia. Trudy was a registered nurse who had completed an additional two-year course in anesthesia and hence was qualified to work on routine operations that did not require an MD anesthesiologist. She had already placed a blood-pressure cuff on Beth's arm and affixed two recording leads to her chest; an electronic beep from the monitor signaled Beth's regular heartbeat.

The team carefully transferred Beth onto the operating table. Then Trudy filled a small syringe with sodium pentothal and injected it into the tubing of Beth's IV. Holding the child's hand, she said, "Now I want you to count to ten for me, Beth."

Beth smiled and started, "One . . . two . . . three . . . fo—" Then she was asleep. When the child's vital signs had been checked and recorded, Trudy injected a few cc's of curare into the IV, to be followed a few minutes later by succinylcholine. Both drugs were muscle relaxants and served to prevent Beth's throat from going into spasm when the breathing tube was inserted. Trudy placed a rubber mask over the child's open mouth, giving her 100 percent oxygen for a few minutes, and then suctioned out her throat to rid it of secretions. Next, she slid the plastic endotracheal tube down Beth's throat and taped the exposed piece of tubing to her chin to hold it in place. This done, she attached the gas supply to the end of the breathing tube and began to feed a mixture of 60 percent gas anesthetic (halothane, cyclopropene, and nitrous oxide) and 40 percent oxygen into the child's lungs to keep her unconscious throughout the procedure. Each individual in the room now had a specific contribution to make; for the next three hours they would participate in the highest form of teamwork.

A few minutes later, Beth was fully anesthetized; when Trudy touched her eyelid, the blinking reflex was absent. Since Beth would be positioned face-down on the operating table for the procedure, the nurse-anesthetist applied ointment around the child's eyes and taped her eyelids shut to prevent them from opening inadvertently, allowing her corneas to be scratched or to dry out. The heart monitor was beeping smoothly. Ron McIver orchestrated the process of turning Beth over on the table, instructing Billings and Dr. Wood on how to proceed. They had to maneuver her flaccid limbs into position, taking care that each movement was within the normal range so as to avoid wrenching a joint or a muscle. It was easy to injure an unconscious patient.

They positioned Beth face-down in a spread-eagled position, with her arms extended at forty-five-degree angles on either side of her head. Then Dr. Wood exposed her back, small and pale in the glow of the overhead lights. He and Billings proceeded to scrub the skin over Beth's lower back and hips with a gauze sponge soaked in antiseptic soap and held with a pair of tongs. Next the coating of soap was removed with alcohol, and Wood painted on yellow-brown Betadine over and around Beth's hips. This done, Billings covered her with sterile drapes except for a rectangular area in the small of her back, clamping the drapes in place with towel clips.

Meanwhile, at the foot of the operating table, Luke opened up a bone-marrow sterile kit and spread out the contents on a tray: two scalpels, several aspiration needles, six glass syringes, six specimen tubes, two large stainless-steel beakers, and several strainers. Luke fit one of the beakers into a metal stand that would prevent it from being knocked over accidentally. He then poured 50 milliliters of a solution of heparin and tissue-culture medium into each of the two beakers.

Wood and Billings stood on opposite sides of the operating table, looking down at the exposed rectangle of skin. "She's a small child, and I hope we can get enough marrow," the attending said. "At least the hip crest is easily accessible, so the aspirations shouldn't be difficult." Sometimes they had donors with a lot of fat tissue over the hips, which made it hard to reach the bone.

"Scalpel," Wood said, and Luke handed it to him. The attending made two tiny X-shaped incisions, one over the crest of each hip, and soaked up the oozing blood with a gauze sponge. All of the aspirations would be made through these two incisions, so that there would not be unnecessary scars.

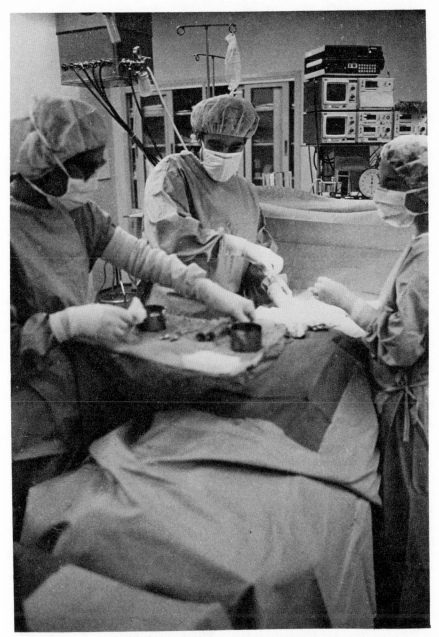

Operating room scene shows a bone-marrow harvest in progress. Two physicians take aspirations from the donor's hip crests, while a technician assists with the procedure. Sterile drapes cover the donor's body, leaving only the hips exposed. *Photo by Frederic T. Serota, Children's Hospital of Philadelphia.*

"Aspiration needle." The long needle contained a thin metal rod, or stylet, which fit snugly inside the bore and prevented the needle from collapsing as it penetrated bone. The stylet was attached in turn to a heavy steel handle. Wood made sure that the small metal prong on the hub of the needle was locked into the deep notch on the handle, so that the needle would not become dislodged during insertion. He then pushed the needle through the small incision closest to him, penetrating fat and muscle and finally the crest of the pelvic bone. The outer layer of bone was hard and required some force to enter. When the resistance lessened, he knew that he had reached the spongy marrow. He unlocked the handle from the hub of the needle and withdrew the stylet, leaving the hollow needle in place. Meanwhile Billings forced a needle into the opposite hip.

"Syringe." Luke rinsed out one of the large glass syringes in the smaller beaker of heparin solution and handed it to Wood, who attached the syringe to the implanted needle. Rotating syringe and needle continuously, he pulled back on the plunger, drawing about 3 cubic centimeters of dark red marrow into the syringe. It looked just like blood, although richer and thicker.

Since the marrow was highly permeated with tiny blood vessels, continued aspiration from a single site would yield mostly blood and few additional marrow cells. Accordingly, Wood stopped applying suction after a few seconds, moved the needle forward a few millimeters, and aspirated again. After four aspirations at different depths and angles, he withdrew the needle and syringe together from Beth's hip. He then handed them to Luke, who squirted the extracted marrow into the metal beaker, rinsed the syringe, and returned it to the tray. Wood sponged away the oozing blood from the puncture site, picked up a clean stylus and aspiration needle, and began again, just as Billings was finishing up his first aspiration from the other hip.

It was hardly a delicate procedure; people untrained in surgery could learn it quickly and perform it well. In fact, the technique soon reduced itself to a mechanical sequence of motions: *force needle into bone, remove stylet, attach syringe, aspirate, remove syringe and needle, pass syringe to Luke, sponge away blood, begin again.* This methodical, monotonous work was accompanied by distinctive sounds: the rhythmic beeping of the heart monitor, the whooshing and bubbling of the thick marrow being squirted into the beaker, the squeaking of the glass syringes being rinsed.

"Christ, this kid has hard bones," Wood exclaimed.

Billings nodded. "Once you're inside you can get a good pull."

The attending turned his attention to the anesthetists. "How's she doing?" he asked.

Trudy Logan looked up, still listening to her stethoscope as she took Beth's blood pressure. "Fine," she answered. "Pressure's good, pulse good." Some phlegm had accumulated in Beth's throat around the breathing tube, and Trudy suctioned it out to keep the passageway clear. The unconscious child was taking long, slow breaths of the gas mixture.

Satisfied, Wood returned to his labor, while he and Billings chatted idly. He withdrew the stylet, attached a syringe, and sucked up more of the crimson marrow.

After a while, the attending turned to Luke and asked how much marrow had accumulated. Luke measured the depth of the suspension in the beaker with a metal ruler: almost 100 cc's. "Could you send off a specimen from the pot?" Wood asked McIver. "A tuberculin syringe would be fine. You can take it to the front desk and ask them to call the Hematology Lab; somebody will come and pick it up."

A specimen was necessary because the richness of the marrow varied greatly from one donor to the next; some donors gave a large number of marrow cells per pull, whereas others gave few marrow cells and mostly blood. Wood liked to joke that the marrow-cell count was directly related to "how many Wheaties you eat for breakfast every morning." The Hematology Lab would determine the average number of nucleated marrow cells per cubic centimeter of Beth's aspirate. This count would then indicate the total volume of marrow that they would have to extract.

After the specimen had been sent off, they went on working in silence. All of a sudden, the beeping of the heart monitor accelerated. Apparently Beth was beginning to come out of anesthesia and was having pain. Trudy Logan looked concerned and checked the child's blood pressure. She then whispered to the student-anesthetist, who quickly drew some morphine into a hypodermic and injected it into the tubing of the IV. He increased the flow for a few seconds, so that it would run in quickly, and moments later Beth's pulse slowed to normal. The student looked relieved. "Is everything okay?" Wood asked, and Trudy nodded.

Several minutes later the results of the marrow-cell count came over the intercom: 36 million nucleated cells per cubic centimeter of aspirate. Wood calculated quickly in his head. Since blood was mixed in with the marrow, he first had to subtract Beth's white count, which was 6.3 million cells per cc—that left about 30 million marrow cells per cc. He knew that they needed at least 300 million marrow cells per kilogram of a recipient's weight to get a good graft. To achieve that number with Beth's marrow, they would need 10 cc's of aspirate for each of Ellie's 25 kilos, or a total of 250 cc's. At 3 cc's of aspirate per pull, there was still a long way to go.

After a while Wood asked, "What do we have now, Luke?"

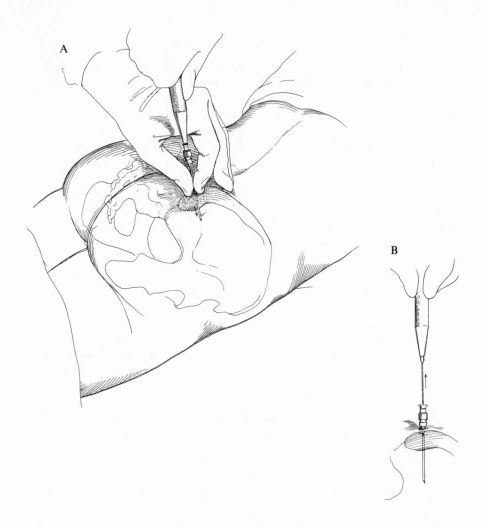

Bone-marrow transplant procedure is outlined in this series of drawings. First the physician forces a hollow aspiration needle into the crest of the donor's pelvic bone (A). The handle and stylet are withdrawn, leaving the hollow needle in place (B). A syringe is attached to the needle and 3 cc's of marrow are sucked out. During the aspiration, the tip of the needle is moved through the marrow space in order to harvest the maximum amount of marrow cells with the minimum amount of blood (C). The aspirated marrow is discharged into a metal beaker containing a solution of heparin anticoagulant (D). Once 200 to 300 cc's of marrow have been extracted from the donor by multiple aspirations, the marrow suspension is passed through three strainers of increasingly fine mesh to remove bone chips, fat globules, and other large particles (E). The strained marrow is then passed through two screened syringes of even finer mesh to break up large clumps of cells (F). This suspension is then placed in a plastic blood bag and (if no further processing is required) taken immediately to the bedside of the transplant recipient. There the donor's bone marrow is infused into the recipient's bloodstream through the central line (G). *Original drawing by Carol Donner.*

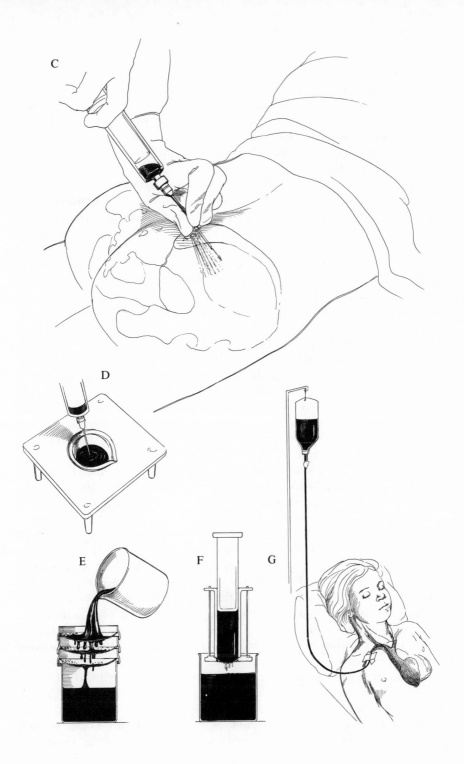

The technician measured the pot. "Just over 200 cc's."

Wood nodded. "Okay, that means we'll have to do the anterior hip crests. We need to get a little extra anyway because we'll be losing some marrow when it's processed to remove the red cells."

Since they were no longer obtaining much marrow per pull from the back crests of the pelvis, they now had to stop, turn Beth over, and prep and drape the front of her hipbones, a process that took a good twenty minutes. Then they continued aspirating until a total of 300 cc's had been extracted. That was a considerable quantity for a child Beth's size, and the operation had been going on for two and a half laborious hours. Wood guessed that they had done about a hundred aspirations.

"Let's give Beth her unit of blood, so she'll feel better about going home tomorrow," he said. A week earlier, Beth had donated a unit of her own blood, which had been stored in the hospital blood bank. It would now be retrieved and given back to her. The advantage of giving Beth her own blood was that it avoided the dangers of a random-donor transfusion, such as hepatitis and allergic reactions.

The nurse-anesthetist ordered the blood over the intercom, and a few minutes later it arrived. Trudy hung it from the IV pole and plugged it into Beth's line. While Billings bandaged the aspiration sites, Trudy switched from anesthetic gas to oxygen in order to bring Beth slowly back to consciousness. Then she slid the tube out of Beth's throat and removed the tape from her eyelids. "Beth, take a deep breath," she said in the child's ear. "Your operation is over." But Beth remained unconscious.

While Dr. Wood jotted down some notes on the procedure, Trudy, the student, Luke, and Nick helped transfer Beth from the operating table onto a stretcher, which had just been wheeled in. Ron McIver supervised to make sure no damage was done. "Hold her head," he warned. "All right. Ready, set, one, two, three, lift!" Beth was raised up and then lowered gently onto the stretcher. When the IV pole had been transferred as well, she was wheeled out of the O.R. and into the recovery room. Wood asked Ron to call upstairs and tell the Murphys that Beth had done beautifully and would be in the recovery room for the next hour or so.

In the meantime, Nick and Luke immediately began to process the thick, dark-red suspension of marrow. First, it was poured into a second beaker through three strainers of increasingly finer division. Little pieces of skin, bone chips, and globules of fat were caught in the screens and left behind. The straining process was repeated with two cut-off 20-milliliter syringes that were covered at the cut end with a fine stainless-steel mesh. Billings poured the suspension into the barrel of the syringe until fat globules and clumps of cells blocked the flow; he then inserted the plunger of the syringe and worked it slowly up and down a few times to break up the clumps. By

226

the time the marrow suspension had been passed through the finest screen, it consisted almost entirely of single cells.

The straining and screening was essential for obtaining an accurate final cell count, but it had another, more important function. It eliminated large particles or clumps of cells that, when infused into Ellie's bloodstream, might block a blood vessel in the brain or lung, with serious consequences.

When the screening was finished, Billings covered the beaker containing the processed marrow suspension with a sterile towel. "Okay," Dr. Wood said, "we need a large plastic transfusion bag, one 50-milliliter syringe, two pieces of extension tubing, a stopcock, and a 16-gauge needle." McIver obtained these items from the supply cabinet, and Billings attached the tubing to the blood bag and used the syringe to transfer the marrow suspension into the bag. Having mixed the suspension well, he drew off two small samples with a syringe for final cell counts, bacterial and viral cultures, and a "colony-forming assay": a test that would indicate how well the marrow cells would grow in their new host. Finally, Billings wrapped the transfusion bag in a towel and placed it in a metal basket, so that if he accidentally dropped it, the bag would not break open, spilling or contaminating the precious marrow. He then hand-carried it to the Hemophoresis Lab, where the marrow would be spun in a blood processor to remove Beth's mismatched red cells. It was nearly 2:00 P.M. by the time he handed the marrow to the chief hemophoresis technician.

At two-fifteen, Nancy came into Ellie's room and began setting up oxygen and suction equipment. She obtained appropriate doses of the emergency drugs Benadryl, epinephrine, and Solu-Medrol and placed them in envelopes at the bedside. A 20 percent solution of mannitol, a sugar-alcohol diuretic, was also prepared; should Ellie begin to show signs of a transfusion reaction, the mannitol would be infused, rapidly increasing her urine flow so as to clear the red-cell breakdown products from her body without damaging her kidneys.

Meanwhile, the Murphys waited anxiously, trying to distract themselves from the drama at hand by watching an "I Love Lucy" rerun on TV. Ellie was too excited for the show to hold her interest; she kept asking Nancy when the bone marrow would get there. The nurse patiently repeated that it would not be much longer.

Indeed, Dr. Wood came in a few minutes later, wearing a surgical mask. On hearing that Ellie's white count was still above 1,000, he removed the mask. "Beth is awake now and doing fine," he said. "She told me she still has plans to go dancing at the Inner Harbor tonight."

Brian laughed. "That is, if she can walk. I imagine she'll be sore for a while."

Sally shook her head. "That girl is something else, let me tell you."

"Is the bone marrow coming soon?" Ellie asked, shifting her attention away from Nancy.

"It's still being processed, but the first batch is almost ready," Wood replied. "Dr. Peters will be bringing it up in ten or fifteen minutes. We'll have to keep a close watch on you, Ellie, during the transfusion, although I don't foresee any major problems. Still, we've got to take all the necessary precautions."

At a quarter to three, Peters arrived with the first batch of purified marrow. It was a small bag containing 102 cc's of the purest sample of marrow cells, from which the red cells had been removed. Formerly scarlet, it was now a dull yellow color, like corn syrup. Brian, who had been expecting something more exotic looking, felt slightly let down, but it was still amazing.

Peters hung the bag of marrow from the metal tree beside the bed. He then sorted through the tangle of plastic tubes hanging from the IV stand and finally connected the bag to Ellie's Brobiac catheter without any of the usual in-line filters. Except for that and all of the emergency equipment in the room, it looked like a routine transfusion. "This bag has the purest marrow, so I'll give it to you first," Peters said to Ellie. Turning to her parents, he added, "Any adverse reaction that develops will be apparent within an hour. If we don't see a reaction, I'll send down for the second bag, which has a few more red cells in it. We could purify it more, but we'd lose many more of the marrow cells in the process."

Nancy took Ellie's vital signs and recorded them on her flow-sheet. When she had finished, Peters unclamped the central line and a slow-moving yellow ribbon made its way down the tubing and into Ellie's chest. Ellie felt strange: a part of her sister was becoming herself.

Nancy continued to record Ellie's vital signs every fifteen minutes for the first hour, while everyone watched and waited. Peters knew what to look for: the first signs of a transfusion reaction would be a throbbing headache, severe back pain, shortness of breath, and a flushed face. If these indications occurred, he would stop the infusion immediately and administer mannitol through the IV for five full minutes. Even so, major complications might later develop, the most serious being kidney failure.

There were other potential problems to watch out for as well. First, an excessive rate of marrow infusion would cause a rapid increase in the volume of Ellie's blood, resulting in high blood pressure and even heart failure. To minimize this danger, a diuretic was given at the same time as the marrow. Second, there was the risk that clumps of marrow cells might temporarily block capillaries in the lungs, making breathing difficult. If this happened, pure oxygen from the tank would be administered until the emboli cleared. Finally, there was the unlikely possibility that the marrow had been contaminated with bacteria or viruses and would introduce an infection into Ellie's system.

Other than a mild feverish reaction and a slight headache, however, the transfusion went along smoothly with no apparent side effects. At three-fifteen, while the first bag of marrow was still flowing into Ellie, Beth was wheeled back to her room. She was still groggy and nauseated from the anesthesia and felt a throbbing ache in her buttocks. She also had to go to the bathroom urgently, but the nurse refused to let her out of bed. Finally the nurse brought her a bedpan and showed her how to use it.

When Beth saw her parents, she was relieved and happy that it was over. Dr. Krueger also came in to see her. "You did a great job," he said. "How do you feel?"

"All right," Beth replied, in spite of her nausea. "Can I go home tomorrow?"

Krueger smiled. "That depends on how you're doing. They took a lot of marrow out of you today. This evening, if you're up to it, you should try exercising your legs. We like to get our donors up on their feet five or six hours after surgery."

Several other doctors and nurses came in to congratulate Beth. Although she enjoyed their praise, she did not feel what she had done was so wonderful. Ellie was her sister, which made giving up some of her bone marrow less than a chore; she knew that Ellie would have done the same for her. Now her only major concern was that the transplant be a success. She called her sister on the phone, and each asked how the other was doing. Both said "fine," even though Ellie had a headache and Beth was nauseated and sore.

By a quarter to four, the first bag of marrow was just about empty. An hour had now passed since the infusion began, and Ellie still looked fine. Sally was surprised that everything was going so smoothly. Just to make sure, Nancy did an electrocardiogram and then a pulmonary-function test that measured Ellie's forced vital capacity (FVC). She fitted a paper mouthpiece onto a simple instrument and told Ellie to fill her lungs with air and blow into the tube as hard as she could. The force of her exhalation drove a mechanical pen, tracing a line that was proportional to the volume of air she had expelled. Ellie's FVC was normal, indicating that the bronchioles in her lungs were not being constricted by an allergic reaction.

Since all was well, Peters sent down to Hemophoresis for the second bag of purified marrow. This bag was smaller than the first, containing only 97 cc's, and slightly pinker due to the higher concentration of red cells. Since Ellie had shown no adverse reaction to the first batch, he was not overly concerned. The second bag was hung at 4:00 P.M., and a half hour later it had been infused without any noticeable side effects. Ellie had received enough of her sister's marrow to give her a good start on blood-cell production. There was nothing for the family to do now but wait and hope.

Peters told the Murphys that the next few days were known as the "honeymoon" period. Ellie would feel fairly good, since she would no longer be suffering from the acute nausea caused by chemotherapy and radiation, and her aplasia would not yet be severe. Within a week, however, she would begin to feel the full impact of the massive doses of treatment she had been receiving. Her blood counts would drop precipitously, ulcers would develop in her mouth and GI tract, and her hair would fall out completely. Infections and fever would also be likely. This difficult phase would last for another week or two until the graft took and began producing significant quantities of blood cells of all types.

Until Ellie's counts returned, she would receive liberal transfusions in order to keep her hematocrit above 25 at all times and her platelet count above 20,000. Although her low poly count would render her susceptible to bacterial and fungal infections, if she accepted the graft there would be no reason to anticipate any major problems. Fevers were practically inevitable, but the use of multiple-antibiotic regimens and protective isolation had lowered the mortality rate due to early infections from 40 percent in 1975 to less than 5 percent in 1980. In most cases, infections became dangerous only when there was a breakdown in the procedure, such as a failure of the marrow to grow. Other major difficulties, such as graft-versus-host disease, did not usually develop until between days twenty and fifty post-transplant, so Peters told Brian to go back to work. He promised to inform him as soon as there was any sign of trouble.

By five-thirty that evening, Beth's nausea had diminished sufficiently for her to attempt to walk. Brian and Sally helped her out of bed and supported her as she took a few tentative steps. She was not in great pain but could only step on the balls of her feet. It was as if both legs had been in a cast for a long time, making it difficult to put full weight on her heels. She was soon exhausted from her effort, and Sally sat her down in a wheelchair and steered her in to visit Ellie. The two sisters chatted for a while, but Beth could not answer any of Ellie's questions about the operation, explaining that she had been out from start to finish. They exchanged good-nights and Beth returned to her room to find the dinner she had ordered that morning waiting on her bed tray. Although it contained many of her favorite foods, including ice cream, she still felt too nauseated to give it a try.

Beth slept very well that night, although she woke once before dawn feeling very frightened and alone, wishing her parents were closer by. She

230

quickly fell back to sleep. When she woke again it was morning and she was comforted to see her parents already in the room. She was feeling much better and could not wait to get the IV out of her arm and go home. Since Ellie was sleeping late, the Murphys spent most of the morning exercising Beth's legs. Sally helped her out of bed and walked her very slowly along the side railings and then out into the corridor. They stopped for a little rest and then Sally lifted her up again and had her walk some more.

In the meantime, Brian tried to get Beth discharged. Krueger was supposed to be there by 1:00 P.M. to sign the discharge papers, but he was busy in the clinic and it was after two before he arrived. He prescribed iron pills for Beth, saying that it would take between two weeks and a month for her marrow to regenerate completely and that she should avoid strenuous exercise for at least a week. She was to have a blood test at a local hospital in a month's time to make sure her marrow was recovering well.

When the IV had been pulled and Beth was packed up, she and Brian stopped in to say their good-byes to Ellie. Beth promised to call in a few days. Although she would have Monday off from school to recuperate further, by Tuesday she would be back to normal routines, unchanged except for the four small scars on her hips and the less tangible effects of the transplant experience on her emotional development.

26 Isolation

The daily blood counts had enormous significance for all of the patients and families on Three-South. The bloods were drawn at 7:00 A.M., and by eleven-thirty or twelve noon the parents would converge on the front desk of the nurses' station to find out the latest results. The counts quickly became the general topic of conversation. When parents met in the hall or in the lounge, they would always ask, "What were your son's (or daughter's or spouse's) counts today?"

The numbers could really make or break Sally's day. As soon as she found out, she would call Brian at work and Cindy Lewis at home from the phone in Ellie's room. Brian had begun writing Ellie's daily counts on the wall calendar beside his desk at work so that he could follow trends, and Sally did the same on a pocket calendar.

Over the weekend, Ellie's counts continued to drop slowly and she slept for long periods, although she still felt reasonably well. By Sunday, June 15, two days after the transplant, her white count had fallen to 892 and her platelet count to 79,000, less than half of what it had been at the time of the procedure. The decline in counts was a good sign, Sally thought; it meant that the existing bone marrow had been destroyed, making way for the grafted marrow cells to grow. But in spite of Krueger's reassurances, she was almost frantic with anxiety over whether the graft would take. For the first week, there was no sense even asking the doctor anything; it was just too early to know. They were awaiting a sentence of life or death, and there was absolutely nothing she could do about it.

Ellie had also begun receiving intravenous injections of low-dose methotrexate every other day in an effort to prevent or decrease the severity of a possible attack of GVHD by killing off a fraction of the mature lymphocytes transplanted along with Beth's marrow. Unfortunately, the chemotherapy had the side effect of lowering still further Ellie's absolute poly count: the proportion of her white cells able to fight off invading bacteria and fungi. By Sunday her poly count had shrunk to fewer than 500 per cubic millimeter, making her highly vulnerable to infection.

On Sunday afternoon, therefore, a pink card went up on Ellie's door that read PROTECTIVE ISOLATION: MASKS MUST BE WORN AT ALL TIMES. Although visitors had once been required to suit up completely in surgical gowns, masks, hair covers, gloves, and booties, the isolation procedure had recently been reduced to just masks and thorough hand-washing with no apparent increase in the incidence of infections. Still, the masks had to be changed every half hour to avoid losing their effectiveness, and close physical contact between patients and visitors was kept to a minimum. In addition, all of the patient rooms on Three-South were equipped with high-efficiency air filters that generated twenty-eight air exchanges per hour and could remove contaminants as small as bacteria. The curtain of warm, filtered air wafted gently over Ellie's bed, blowing away microbes that might otherwise have floated into contact with her.

It bothered Ellie that she could not make out her mother's expressions behind the surgical mask. Even worse, she could never escape from the fact that she was seriously ill; there seemed to be no end to the constant poking and probing and questioning. Although she was technically in "isolation," she was hardly ever alone. Someone was in her room nearly every minute of the day or night: nurses, residents taking blood or cultures, doctors on rounds, specialists coming in for consultations, respiratory therapists, IV therapists, nutritionists, housekeeping personnel. Occasionally, when Nancy felt that Ellie was getting overwhelmed by the traffic in and out of her room, she put up a sign on the door that read NO ONE CAN ENTER—MUST SEE NURSE in order to give Ellie a little time to herself. Although the nurses and visitors made every effort to bring the child all sorts of new games and toys, her attention span was short. She often stared out at the sunlight and thought of all the fun she was missing, how it was summer and she could have been making trips to the beach with her friends and their families.

For Sally, isolation was a state of constant crisis. Potentially lethal germs seemed to lurk in every corner, and she could not let anything get by unnoticed. She knew that the slightest infection could rapidly spiral out of control: a small cut could open the way to a bacterial invasion throughout the body, and a cold could turn overnight into pneumonia. Sally harnessed her nervous energy by helping Ellie perform the daily routines of personal hygiene that were so essential if infection was to be kept at bay. She carefully brushed out the child's shedding hair, kept her nails pared, and helped clean her teeth and gums with "toothettes"—little sponges on a stick—since with Ellie's low platelet count, a toothbrush would have caused profuse bleeding. Every morning Ellie was expected to take a shower, an excellent means of removing skin bacteria, although it was often a battle to get her out of bed. Nancy covered the central-line dressings with a plastic wrap to keep them dry, and then Ellie sat on a stool beneath the shower while her mother washed her back, since she was too weak to stand for more than a few minutes. Sally also applied lotion to Ellie's skin to keep it from getting dry and irritated. With all the precautions Sally was taking in her constant vigil against infection, it made her very angry when a few arrogant residents, apparently convinced they were germ free, came in with unwashed hands or with their masks untied.

More dangerous than the possibility of infection from without, however, was the threat posed by the microbes harbored within Ellie's own body. When her immune system had been intact, the millions of bacterial flora that inhabited her skin, nose, mouth, and gut had done no more mischief than to cause an occasional boil, dental cavity, or stomach cramp. The bacteria inhabiting her intestine had, in fact, served a useful function, facilitating digestion and manufacturing vitamin K, an essential nutrient. But now that Ellie's poly count had dropped so low, these normally benign bacteria could become virulent, multiplying out of control and causing serious infections.

It was therefore essential to wipe out the bacterial flora before they had a chance to cause disease. This was done through a combination of several oral antibiotics known collectively as "bowel prep." Since these drugs were not absorbed into the bloodstream, they could be given in large enough doses to essentially sterilize Ellie's mouth and GI tract. The bowel prep was given three times a day, at 10:00 A.M., 2:00 P.M., and 6:00 P.M. Young children like Ellie received the antibiotics in liquid form rather than pills, with each dose consisting of 15 cc's (about a half ounce) of liquid. The bowel prep was extremely foul tasting, however, and Ellie quickly developed stalling tactics to avoid taking her medicine. As soon as she caught sight of Nancy coming in with the liquid antibiotics, she had a sudden urge to urinate. "I have to pee," she said. "Wait till I pee." When she finally returned from the bathroom and climbed back into bed, she continued with: "I'm not ready, I'm not ready. I have to get set."

Since she really had to be forced to take the drugs, it was not a pleasant time for her, the staff, or Sally, but there was no alternative; no amount of reasoning or cajoling could change the fact that the stuff tasted horrible and was absolutely necessary until Ellie's white count was back over 1,000 with a healthy percentage of polys. Nancy finally had to insist: "Look, Ellie, do you want to take it yourself in the cup, or shall I give it to you in the syringe?"

"In the cup," Ellie replied.

By the third day, her strategies had become more elaborate. Before Nancy gave her the bowel prep, Ellie said, "I need some cherry with it." The cherry syrup helped disguise the flavor of the drug somewhat, but it still had a bitter aftertaste.

Still patient, Nancy poured the drug into a cup, mixed in some cherry syrup, stirred it, and drew up 10 cc's of the mixture into a syringe. "Okay, this is it," she said. "Open up."

"I need something to drink first."

"Here's some ginger ale," Sally said. "Take a sip."

"No!" Ellie whined. "I want some Hawaiian Punch."

Nancy sighed wearily. "Do you promise that you'll take your medicine if I get you some Hawaiian Punch?"

Ellie nodded, and the nurse left the room. She returned a few minutes later with a can of Tahitian Treat. "We don't have any more Hawaiian Punch, but this stuff is almost the same," she said.

"No! I want Hawaiian Punch."

"I'm sorry, Ellie," Nancy said firmly, "but you'll have to make do with what we have. We've wasted enough time already. Come on now, open up."

Ellie shook her head. "I have to hop first," she said.

"What?" the nurse asked, incredulous.

"I have to hop on one leg before I can take it."

Nancy shook her head. "Ellie, it's not funny anymore. Come on, open up." She forced the syringe between the child's lips.

Finally subdued, Ellie gave in. She held her nose, took a sip of ginger ale and a sip of punch, and then opened her lips only wide enough to let the syringe in. "Only give me down to number four," she said, referring to the numbers on the side of the syringe. As the fluid went in, Ellie grimaced horribly and gagged, becoming so agitated that she began to vomit.

"Oh, Ellie!" Sally exclaimed. "Why can't you just be a good girl and take your medicine?"

"If you throw up, you'll just have to take it again later," Nancy warned. "No!"

"Yes! Now open up wide, and no more funny business." The nurse's voice was sharp and authoritarian. Despite all of Ellie's tears and protests, Nancy made her swallow the entire contents of the syringe, even though she kept down only half of it.

Ellie also had to take an antifungal drug, nystatin, which she was told to swish in her mouth and then swallow. Fortunately the nystatin did not taste as bad as the bowel prep, although Ellie still put up a fight. The drug was needed because the antibiotics in the bowel prep disrupted the balance between bacteria and fungi in the "ecosystem" of the body. Normally, disease-causing fungi such as *Candida* and *Aspergillus* grew in the GI tract and the mouth, but they were crowded out by the more numerous bacterial flora and hence their numbers were too small to cause disease. When the bowel prep wiped out the normal flora, however, it left the field wide open for fungal superinfections.

It soon got to a point where it took up to an hour for Ellie to take her medicines, and the nurses were losing their patience and composure. Finally Sally developed an effective strategy, threatening to stop reading bedtime stories to Ellie if she failed to take her medicines without a fuss. For a time, this threat proved surprisingly effective.

Ellie's fluid restriction caused another area of tension. Although she had not eaten solid food since a week before the transplant, her weight was being kept stable by the 2,300 calories she was receiving daily in her hyperalimentation fluid. Since she had also been given large volumes of fluids during the pretransplant protocol, Peters worried that the excess fluid might accumulate in her radiation-weakened lungs, causing pulmonary edema. He therefore decided to treat her with diuretics and to restrict her oral intake of fluids to a liter per day. Ellie often complained of thirst and begged her mother for water. Sally felt in a bind each time; she wanted Ellie to be comfortable, but she knew she should follow Peters's instructions.

Other battles arose over getting out of bed. The nursing staff urged Ellie to exercise at least once a day, in addition to her morning shower. When the child refused, Nancy would insist. "I know you're feeling sick, but that's the best time to get out of bed," she would say. Ellie also exercised her lungs by blowing into an "incentive spirometer," a small, hand-held plastic toy with a little ball inside that bobbed up and down when she exhaled.

On Tuesday, June 17, Ellie developed uncontrollable diarrhea, most likely a side effect of her bowel prep. It embarrassed her, and she tried to clean herself without telling her mother or the nurse. She did not do a thorough job, however, and an irritation similar to a diaper rash developed on her buttocks. By Wednesday, the rash seemed to be getting worse, in spite of numerous sitz baths and the application of dry heat to the spot with a portable hair-dryer. Ellie began to complain about the soreness and cried a few times.

At ten o'clock on Wednesday, soon after Sally arrived, the doctors went on rounds, and a group of white-coated personnel filed into Ellie's room, surgical masks concealing the lower half of their faces. "Good morning, Ellie," Dr. Krueger said cheerfully. "I brought everyone in to wake you up this morning. How are you doing?"

"Okay," Ellie said shyly.

"I see you didn't eat any of your breakfast. Still feeling sick to your stomach?"

Ellie nodded.

"It's her throat," Sally broke in. "It's so bad she can barely swallow."

Krueger selected a flashlight from the electrically powered set of instruments hanging on a wall unit beside the bed. "Okay, Ellie, let's take a quick look at the back of your throat. Open real wide now, wide as you can."

Using a tongue depressor, he checked the inside of the child's mouth for redness, white patches, or ulcers. There seemed to be some redness at the back of her tongue, and he pressed down to get a better look.

Ellie gagged and then groaned in pain.

"Was it your tongue that hurt when I pressed on it?" Krueger asked. "Or was it down in your throat?"

"My tongue," Ellie moaned.

Krueger straightened up with a sigh. Turning to Peters, he said, "It's unclear whether this is viral or some ulceration due to the chemotherapy. It's not clearly vesicular. I think it's chemical, but we'll have to rely on cultures. Let's do them daily for the time being."

"Can't you give her something for it?" Sally asked. "She's very uncomfortable."

Peters shook his head. "We'll have to follow it for a few days to see what develops, since we don't know yet what's causing it."

"But it's just going to get worse," Sally said, exasperated. "How can you just let her lie there and go through this?"

"I'm sorry," Peters said firmly. "We'll treat her as soon as we get the results of the cultures."

Sally was angry: by the time they started treating the symptoms, Ellie's sore throat would be so bad that it would take that much longer to cure. But she controlled her temper, afraid of alienating the doctors.

After taking a throat swab, Krueger continued his examination. He listened to Ellie's chest and heart, and peered into her eyes and ears. "Ellie, does your bottom hurt today?" he asked. When she nodded, he said, "Okay, let's take a quick look."

He helped her turn over on her side and pulled down her pajamas. "Oh, boy," he murmured. The skin surrounding the anus was bright red and there were three raw, oozing spots. Krueger was particularly concerned because this area was a potential source of infection. "I'm going to take a perianal swab," he said. "I'm surprised she hasn't yet spiked a fever."

Peters nodded. "It's practically inevitable. Do you think we should start IV antibiotics?"

"Yes, that would be a good idea. Let's put her on intravenous ticarcillin and gentamicin every six hours and then see what the cultures tell us." Krueger pulled the child's pajama bottoms back up and covered her with the blankets. "Okay, Ellie, hang in there, and make sure you keep taking those sitz baths. I'll look in this afternoon," he added to Sally.

A half hour later, Nancy came in and hung the first bottle of antibiotics, connecting it to Ellie's Brobiac catheter.

By Thursday, June 19, six days after the transplant, the "honeymoon" was completely over. Ellie's white count was down to zero, her platelets were at 24,000, and ulcers had begun to appear in her mouth. She also developed a large cold sore on her lip, due to a herpes simplex virus that had been latent in her body for many years and was now being allowed to flourish while her immune defenses were down.

Ellie felt totally miserable. Her throat now hurt so much that she was unable to swallow liquids, and a white mucus accumulated so thickly in her mouth that she would sometimes gag on it. She went into the bathroom and tried to brush it off her tongue with toothettes, without much success; Nancy encouraged her to try mouthwash, which helped a little. Even so, it was now virtually impossible for her to swallow her bowel prep or nystatin.

Ellie could not understand why she had been fine before she had come to the hospital and now she ached all over. Weren't hospitals supposed to make you get better? She felt very confused and more than a little betrayed by both her parents and the doctors. Increasingly she withdrew into herself, first refusing to talk to Krueger, then the residents, and later, as she became more deeply depressed, the nurses and even her mother.

Sally wondered if Ellie's suffering would ever end. Although Ellie had all the physical pain, Sally identified with her completely. She remembered that Krueger had told them at the outset that the transplant was going to be very stressful and that Ellie would go through a lot, but she had never imagined it would be this bad. She kept asking herself: Is this going to work? Will it be a cure? Otherwise she doubted she could keep pushing.

That evening, after leaving the hospital, Sally checked out of the Sheraton and drove to the trailer park in Woodbine. As Brian's uncle had promised, he had towed the trailer down to the campground and registered it in their name; it had already been there a few days. Sally followed Gail's directions to the place, getting lost once. By the time she arrived, she had been on the road nearly an hour and darkness had fallen. She turned into the driveway and stopped at the main office, where the superintendent gave her the key Brian's uncle had left and directed her to the trailer.

She parked nearby and let herself in with the key. The trailer was a thirty-foot Monitor, much more luxurious and spacious than she had expected. There was a living room, bedroom, cooking area, and bath. It was a real home away from home, far more private and comfortable than the hotel room. Completing her brief tour, Sally carried her bags into the bedroom and began to unpack.

It was so quiet outside that it frightened her: nothing but the eerie, high-pitched drone of crickets and the occasional patter of squirrels running across the metal roof. She thought of calling home, but the nearest pay phone was up at the main building and she felt too drained and exhausted to drive back.

When her clothes were put away, she turned on the portable black-and-white TV in the bedroom. The noise and tinsel of a variety show were somehow comforting, a defense against the forbidding silence and darkness outdoors. She was already having second thoughts about the trailer; maybe staying out here wasn't such a good idea after all. It would be a pleasant refuge from the hot, muggy city when Ellie was an outpatient, and very private when Brian came down on weekends, but she was afraid that the isolation during the week would drive her crazy. . . .

The TV failed to distract her; she thought guiltily of her other children, particularly Amy, who must feel terribly abandoned. God, how she missed that child! But her mind kept returning to Ellie, alone in her hospital room, kept awake by the open sores in her mouth and on her buttocks, attended only by the nurses who came in every few hours to check her vital signs or change her IV bottles, and no doubt haunted by imaginary monsters looming out of the darkness. . . .

"I have a job to do here," Sally thought, "and Ellie needs me more than anyone."

She undressed and slid between the cold, starched sheets. Leaving the TV on low in the darkened room to keep her company, she closed her eyes, awaiting the brief oblivion that sleep would bring.

27 Hemophoresis

On Friday, June 20, a week after the transplant, the long decline in Ellie's white count unexpectedly reversed itself; when Sally went to the nurses' station to get the information, she was told that the white count was 66. Elated, she rushed into Ellie's room with the good news. She then sat down and called Brian's office. He was not available, so she left a message and called her in-laws at home.

Beth was thrilled and proud when she learned that Ellie's counts were coming back. The procedure had brought about a new sense of closeness between the two sisters, almost like the intense emotional ties between identical twins. The grandparents also rejoiced with an elation they had not felt before. Even Brian's mother admitted that the transplant might have not been such a bad idea after all.

The bubble did not wait long to burst, however. That afternoon, Dr. Krueger came in with some ominous news: Ellie's stool surveillance culture had contained *Pseudomonas aeruginosa,* a rod-shaped bacterium that could cause serious infections in patients with an impaired immune system. Ellie was still without fever, but in view of her positive stool culture and the fact that her poly count was still less than 100, it was highly probable that the bacteria had already infected one of the open sores near her anus. If the *Pseudomonas* invaded her bloodstream, her chances of survival would be poor. Krueger's plan of attack was therefore to prevent the localized infection from spreading internally by means of aggressive antibiotic therapy.

The problem was that some strains of *Pseudomonas* were resistant to all but the newest antibiotics. Krueger found the increasing resistance of disease-causing bacteria to antibiotics a truly frightening trend. The more these drugs were utilized to combat infections, the more the processes of natural selection favored the emergence of resistant bacterial strains, each endowed with a subtle biochemical alteration that enabled it to thrive in the presence of previously lethal drugs. Pharmaceutical companies were therefore engaged in a perpetual race against nature to devise new antibiotics before disease-causing bacteria became resistant to the old ones. It was a thin tightrope indeed, Krueger realized, that kept them all suspended above the abyss. Since gentamicin and ticarcillin in combination were effective against many but not all strains of *Pseudomonas*, Krueger decided to keep Ellie on them. If she spiked a fever within the next twenty-four hours, however, he would discontinue the gentamicin and replace it with a newer antibiotic of the same family.

By six o'clock Saturday morning, Krueger's prediction had become a reality: Ellie's temperature was 101°. During the prerounds conference, which was held at eight-thirty in the house staff lounge adjacent to the nurses' station, the medical team discussed her case. They decided to discontinue Ellie's gentamicin, which was apparently ineffective, and switch her to another antibiotic, amikacin, while maintaining her on ticarcillin. Since the antibiotics would not work well in the absence of sufficient polys to clear away the killed and injured bacteria, they elected to supplement the drugs with white-cell transfusions, beginning that night.

When Sally arrived at Three-South later on that morning, she received a double shock. Not only was there the news of Ellie's fever, but she was told that the child's white count was back to zero. All the elation and hope of the previous day suddenly collapsed into ashes. Stunned, Sally sought out Dr. Krueger for an explanation. He told her that they were not yet sure that the *Pseudomonas* bacteria in Ellie's stool were the source of her infection, but that in any case she was being treated intensively with antibiotics and would be cultured daily in an effort to determine the organism responsible. As for her disappearing white count, that was nothing unusual; there was always a considerable fluctuation in the counts when the grafted marrow began to function. "For the first week or so it's like a roller-coaster, up and down," he said. "It's much too early to worry that something's gone wrong."

"But why does it vary so much?" Sally asked. "Yesterday her white count was 66, and today it's back to zero."

"Two reasons," Krueger replied. "First, Ellie's been getting small doses of methotrexate on alternate days to prevent the development of GVHD, and that has an impact on the bone marrow. Second, when the marrow is just starting to come back, the production of blood cells is not yet uniform. The counts may be high one day and down the next. Hang in there for a few more days, and I think we'll begin to see a more convincing recovery."

Throughout the day, Ellie's fever made her weepy and irritable. Sally bathed her with a solution of hydrogen peroxide and placed cool compresses on her forehead and pulse points; the child's skin was so sensitive that she could not tolerate the cold anywhere else. When Nancy came in to change Ellie's central-line dressings, Sally took a breather in the lounge and spoke to Mrs. Willis, who told her that Keith had developed a high fever after his transplant that had lasted a week. "They all go through more or less the same thing," she said. Just hearing that other patients had survived fevers made Sally a bit less anxious.

That night, the white-cell transfusions were begun. Ellie was premedicated with an intravenous injection of Benadryl and a large oral dose of Tylenol. The white cells were hung at 2:50 A.M. and the infusion lasted until 5:20. Although a mild allergic reaction to the white cells caused Ellie to spike a fever of 103°, she managed to sleep much of the night.

By the next morning, Sunday, June 22, Ellie's white count was up again, to 77. Even more significant was the presence in the blood smear of immature, nucleated red cells, called reticulocytes. In a healthy person, these cells are extremely rare in the circulating blood, comprising about 1 percent of the blood-cell population, but when a patient is severely anemic or recovering from a marrow transplant, the marrow discharges its immature red cells prematurely into the blood before they have had a chance to manufacture their hemoglobin or lose their nuclei. The presence of reticulocytes in Ellie's blood indicated to Krueger that her body had peaceably accepted the graft of Beth's marrow and that the new blood-forming tissue was beginning to function. He therefore felt comfortable offering the optimistic prediction that although Ellie's white count was still very low, it would begin to climb rapidly over the next several days.

Ellie's fever continued unabated, however, accompanied by a rapid decline in her platelet count, which fell to less than 9,000 by Sunday. Scattered petechiae appeared on Ellie's ankles and shoulders, and blood began to ooze from her gums. Alarmed, Krueger ordered eight units of platelets for transfusion. He suspected that Ellie's bacterial infection was responsible for her low platelet count, even as her marrow was recovering. It had been found that aggregates of bacterial organisms could damage the inner walls of blood vessels, either by sticking to them or producing toxins that in some way exposed the vessel lining to the flowing blood. These sites then attracted platelets, causing them to clump together in large numbers, and filling up small vessels with clots. In the process, both platelets and clotting factors in the blood were rapidly consumed, reducing the patient's ability to repair leaky capillaries and hence increasing the chances of spontaneous hemorrhaging.

Krueger encouraged Sally to donate platelets, since there would be less risk to Ellie of exposure to blood-carried viruses such as hepatitis and cytomegalovirus (CMV) if parents, rather than random donors, were used. Happy to learn that there was something tangible she could do to help Ellie directly, Sally called the Hemophoresis Center early Monday morning. She made an appointment for 2:00 P.M. that afternoon, assuming that the

241

donation would take fifteen minutes or so, as it did with whole-blood donations.

Shortly before two, Sally took the elevator down to the basement level and followed the signs to the Hemophoresis Center. After weaving through a maze of corridors, she found the right door and walked into a small reception area. Directly ahead was a small honeycomb of cubicles, where a group of technicians in white coats were talking and sipping coffee. Off to the left was the donor room proper, with six blood processors and stretchers arranged in two rows. The processors were white boxlike units the size of a child's desk, topped with a vertical slab containing contoured spaces for IV bottles and a serpentine array of channels and clamps that looked like the innards of a movie projector. In one corner, a hospital maintenance man was hooked up to a processor with IV's in both his arms. Muzak was playing softly and a color TV mounted high up on the back wall was operating without sound. Sally was mystified.

Just then, one of the technicians caught sight of Sally and came over. She was young, not more than twenty-three, with short brown hair and an attractive smile. "Do you have an appointment?" she asked.

"Yes, Sally Murphy, two P.M."

"Good. Have you ever donated platelets before?"

"No, just blood."

"Okay, fine. Come with me, please. By the way, my name is Lisa." The technician led Sally to a small partitioned-off cubicle and filled out a registration form. Sally mentioned that she was the parent of a patient on Three-South, so Lisa checked the computer file for her HLA and blood types. She then took a brief medical history, listing the criteria that could disqualify Sally from donating: a history of significant illness, high blood pressure, severe allergies, asthma, hepatitis, kidney problems, or diabetes. Sally had none of these. Lisa took down her height and weight, measured her vital signs, and then did a finger-stick for counts and hemoglobin levels, sending the blood sample immediately to the lab. While they waited for the results, Sally asked how much time the donation would take. "Is it any more than fifteen minutes?" she asked. "I don't want to leave my daughter alone too long."

Lisa looked surprised. "Didn't anyone tell you? A platelet run takes between two and a half and three hours."

"What? My God, I had no idea," Sally exclaimed. "I don't even think I could sit still for that long."

"Oh, don't worry about that," Lisa replied with a smile. "You'll be lying down the whole time, just relaxing."

A technician came in with the print-out of Sally's blood tests. Lisa perused the slip quickly: the counts were well within acceptable limits.

"Everything looks fine," she said. "Shall we begin?" She led Sally into the donor room and directed her to lie down on the stretcher in front of one of the futuristic machines. "Make yourself comfortable," she said. "You're going to be here for a while."

Sally lay down nervously on the stretcher, facing away from the machine, while Lisa explained the basics of the procedure. "The problem with obtaining white cells or platelets is that together they make up less than one percent of the volume of the blood," she began. "There's only one white cell for every six hundred red cells and one platelet for every fifteen red cells. So purifying white cells or platelets from whole blood is like panning tons of mud to obtain a few flecks of gold. The advantage of this machine—a continuous-flow blood processor—is that it can process several pints of blood from a single donor at one sitting, extracting the platelets and returning everything else to the donor. Although it takes a long time, more than ninety-five percent of the original blood volume is returned, so you won't feel the weakness you may have felt after donating whole blood."

Sally nodded, wondering how she would entertain herself for the next two and a half hours. Since she would not have the use of her arms, reading would be impossible, and if she wanted to watch TV she would have to use earphones. Anxious, she watched as Lisa took down a sterilized plastic centrifuge bowl from a shelf, unwrapped it, and placed it into the waiting cavity beneath the heavy Plexiglas top of the blood processor. The technician then unwrapped another sterile package and took out a long piece of plastic tubing with numerous connectors, valves, and transfusion bags attached to it; this she stripped into the various slots and channels in the face of the machine, clamping the tubing in place between metal disks that would serve as peristaltic pumps to push the blood through.

When the apparatus was set up, Lisa rubbed alcohol on the insides of Sally's elbows and inserted large intravenous needles into both arms. The needles stung as they went in, making Sally wince. Immediately blood from her right vein began to flow down the tubing into a small bag, or holding reservoir; an anticoagulant mixed with the exiting blood to keep it from clotting. Meanwhile the IV in Sally's left arm delivered a slow drip of normal saline, which would keep the line open until her blood, minus platelets, was ready to be reinfused.

Lisa pressed a button on the console and the centrifuge bowl began to spin, rapidly accelerating to a speed of forty-eight hundred revolutions per minute. Next she switched on one of the peristaltic pumps, which began to feed blood from the holding reservoir into the spinning bowl. The blood entered a valve at the top of the bowl, passed through a channel down the central core, and flowed across the bottom of the bowl and up the sides.

The bowl took about ten minutes to fill. As it did so, the powerful

243

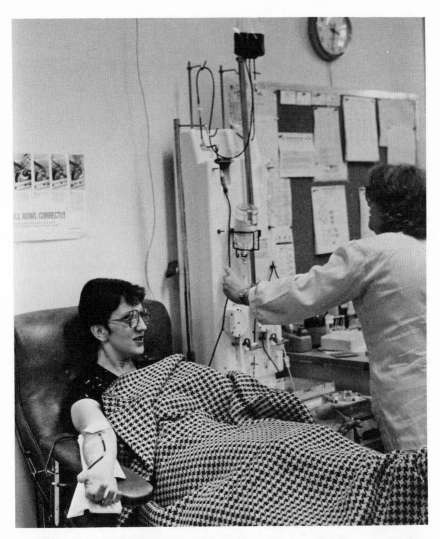

Hemophoresis is a method for obtaining concentrated platelets or white cells from healthy donors for transfusion into leukemic patients with low blood counts. The donor shown here has intravenous needles in both arms. Blood flows from her left arm into a continuous-flow blood processor, which separates out the platelets by weight in a spinning bowl and then shunts them into a collection bag. The remaining blood components are then returned to the donor via the IV line in her right arm. Approximately seven bowl-fillings are required to extract sufficient platelets for transfusion, and the procedure takes 2½ hours. Since most of the donor's blood is returned and the extracted platelets are replaced quickly, the procedure is harmless and can be done as often as once a week. *Photo courtesy of the New York Blood Center.*

centrifugal forces exerted by its rapid rotation separated out the various blood-cell types by weight into a series of discrete bands. The heavy, hemoglobin-packed red cells sank to the bottom, forming a thick red band that occupied nearly half of the total volume. On top of the red cells was a thin layer of white cells and platelets, appearing dark pink because of partial mixing with red cells, and then a fine white line of pure platelets. The top half of the bowl was filled with pale yellow plasma.

While the bowl was filling, Lisa chatted with Sally about Ellie and her other children. She tried hard to ease Sally's anxiety. The Hemophoresis Center relied on repeat performances by volunteer donors, and if too many of them found the procedure unbearable and failed to return, the center would not be able to continue functioning.

When the bowl had filled, the clear plasma began to flow out the tube at the top of the bowl and into a large plastic storage bag that hung down in front of the machine. Meanwhile fresh blood continued to be pumped into the bottom of the bowl so that it filled with packed red cells, raising the line of platelets slowly toward the top. As the platelets neared the valve, Lisa stopped talking and focused her concentration on the spinning bowl. Suddenly she punched a button on the console, instantly clamping off the plasma storage bag and directing the flow of pure platelets into a small collection bag. Collecting the platelets at just the right moment to obtain the maximum amount of product with the least amount of contamination was a matter of delicate timing. Next Lisa shunted the pinkish layer of platelets, mixed with some white cells and red cells, into a separate bag. This portion would later be spun in a small centrifuge to separate out its content of platelets, thereby increasing the yield obtained from each pass.

After the platelets had been extracted, Lisa stopped the bowl from spinning and pumped the red cells remaining in the bowl and the plasma in the storage bag up to a reinfusion bag hanging from a hook at the top of the processor. She then replaced the saline dripping into Sally's left arm with the mixture of plasma and red cells, which gravity-fed back into her vein. "As you can see, this is not a continuous process," Lisa explained. "After I've collected the platelets from each bowl-filling, I have to stop the bowl and empty it of red cells before I can begin another pass."

Because the blood had been mixed with anticoagulant and cooled during its passage through the machine, Sally's left arm suddenly felt cold as the reinfusion began. She soon became faint and queasy. Seeing her pallor, Lisa quickly removed the pillow beneath her head and told her to raise her knees so that the blood would flow to her brain. "Are you okay?" she asked, and Sally nodded.

Before the blood had fully reinfused, Lisa started up the centrifuge again and drew more blood from Sally's right arm. The entire bowl-filling and -emptying cycle would be repeated six more times.

For Sally, the first hour passed quickly. She was fascinated with the machine and enjoyed listening to Lisa explain how she had become involved in hemophoresis. A few other donors arrived for their appointments, keeping three or four machines busy at a time.

Sally felt foolish whenever she developed an itch on her face and had to ask Lisa to scratch it for her, but the technician was obviously used to this kind of thing. When Lisa had to concentrate on the bowl, the conversation dangled, and Sally watched a soap opera on the TV. Not wanting to bother with the headphones, she tried to guess the plot without the benefit of dialogue.

"How many passes left?" she asked after a while.

"Three more," Lisa replied. "We're more than halfway there."

Sally sighed. "Does it take this long to donate white cells?"

"Longer, actually—between three and a half and four hours. We have to add a chemical called Volex to the blood in order to get a better separation of the white cells from the red cells. Otherwise the polys—the white cells that fight infection—don't separate out from the red cells and we can't retrieve them. That procedure is a little more risky, because a few donors have a bad reaction to the Volex and get sick."

During the last hour, Sally was painfully bored. She had lost interest in deciphering the soap opera and felt washed out and uncomfortable, restlessly crossing and uncrossing her legs. The needles in her veins had begun to ache dully, the pain no doubt exacerbated by her rising anxiety. Ellie must have been wondering where she was all this time. What if something had happened while she was away?

Lisa noticed the furrows in Sally's brow and tried to distract her. "We're almost done," she said. "Just about fifteen minutes more."

Finally Sally managed to relax and doze. When Lisa woke her, the final pass was over. The technician held up the bag of pure platelets to show Sally how much she had given: the bag was two-thirds filled with a yellow-apricot solution. Combined with the platelets salvaged from the less pure portion, Lisa said, it would probably total about 8½ units.

"How much is a unit?" Sally asked.

"It's a standard measure that blood banking has been using for a long time. If you donate a pint of blood at a blood bank, they will spin the blood and extract the platelets. The quantity of platelets obtained from one pint of blood is called a unit; it's since been standardized to fifty-five billion platelets. With the blood processor, we can obtain six to nine units from one run, depending on the precount and how successful we are in the process of separation. It looks like you did really well."

Lisa told Sally that her platelets would first be irradiated in order to kill off any contaminating lymphocytes that might trigger or aggravate a patient's GVHD. Then the 8½ units would be administered to a marrow-transplant patient within twenty-four hours. No effort was made to match donors' platelets with their relatives, unless the patient's immune system began to recognize and destroy random-donor platelets and a close match therefore became necessary. Sally was disappointed to learn that because she was not a good HLA match with Ellie, her platelets would be given to someone else. According to Lisa, her platelets were very compatible with another needy patient on Three-South, although she would not reveal the name. Sally shrugged and said, "Well, if I can't give them to Ellie, I'm glad someone can use them."

When it was over and the needles had been removed, Sally felt drained but gratified, and amazed at what they had done to her blood.

28 Numbers

The course of methotrexate injections as prophylaxis against GVHD had been completed on Sunday, and over the next few days Ellie's white count gradually improved. Nonetheless, her high fever and rapid platelet consumption continued, in spite of an increased dosage of amikacin.

Ellie was increasingly irritable and dependent on her mother, behaving more like a child of three than one of six. Sally had to do everything for her: wash her face, clean her teeth with toothettes, scrub her down in the shower, and deal with her demands for drinks and toys. At the same time, Ellie struggled to assert herself, acting out her anger and frustration by refusing to cooperate with her bowel prep or procedures. The nurses were also targets of her moods. When Nancy tried to cheer her up by saying, "You look great today, Ellie," the child responded by making a face, growling, and hiding her head under the sheet.

On Tuesday, June 24, a bone-marrow aspiration was done, revealing immature blood cells growing in the marrow space. Krueger came in to tell Ellie and Sally the good news. "The marrow looks very good," he said. "It's still sparse, but there are encouraging signs of early engraftment, and there's definitely no problem with the leukemia."

Although Sally was elated by the news, Krueger remained cautious. The child still did not have polys to fight off the resistant bacteria that were causing her infections, and she continued to require frequent transfusions of white cells and platelets.

That afternoon, Lynn Schwartz came in to examine Ellie and noted that one of her old IV sites had become swollen and tender. Fearing that it had become the source of a *Staphylococcus aureus* infection, she consulted with Peters and decided to provide antistaph coverage by adding a third antibiotic, nafcillin, to Ellie's regimen. Much to Lynn's relief and satisfaction, her fever went down ten hours after infusion of the new drug. Lynn realized, however, that although Ellie had no fever, she was still harboring the bacteria; it was practically impossible to eradicate an infection in a patient without polys. All they were doing was keeping the infection subclinical, and as soon as the drugs were withdrawn it would most likely flare up again. They would therefore have to maintain Ellie on intravenous antibiotics until her white count recovered.

Ellie's temperature remained normal until early the next morning, Wednesday, June 25. The resident on call that night, Mark Dietrich, was sound asleep when he was paged by the night nurse at 4:00 A.M. and told that Ellen Murphy had spiked a fever of 102°. He went in and examined her, finding no obvious active sites of infection. The sores near her anus were dry and healing, and the swelling around her old IV site had gone down. Dietrich suspected that Ellie's rising temperature while on multiple antibiotics was most likely caused by a fungal superinfection with an organism such as *Candida*. Since the broad-spectrum antibiotics disrupted the normal balance of bacterial populations in various parts of the body, fungal overgrowth was a common side effect of antibiotic therapy.

Later on that morning, at the prerounds conference, Dietrich proposed adding the antifungal drug amphotericin B to Ellie's regimen. A discussion followed, with Peters pointing out that no fungi had been detected in blood cultures or the various surveillance cultures, although it was possible they had not yet had time to grow out. An alternate possibility, he contended, was that Ellie's *Pseudomonas* infection might be resistant to amikacin, in which case it would be preferable to switch to a newer antibiotic of the same type. Lynn Schwartz muddied the waters further by recalling that Ellie had been given a white-cell transfusion between 9:45 and 11:10 P.M. the previous evening, so that it was difficult to know whether the fever was anything more than a delayed allergic reaction to her transfusion. After some deliberation, the team finally decided to watch Ellie's fever for the next twenty-four hours. If it failed to improve, she would be presumed to have a fungal infection and would be started on amphotericin B. The suggestion to use amphotericin B had not been taken lightly because of the drug's considerable toxicity to the kidneys, especially in combination with other antibiotics.

Ellie's fever continued to rise over the next twenty-four hours, so the amphotericin B was started on the night of Thursday, June 26. Because the antibiotic was unstable in the light, the IV bottle had to be wrapped in foil during the four-hour infusions. Not long after the drug began to drip into Ellie's central line, she spiked a fever of 104.5° and was unable to sleep; she ached, her body shook with chills, and her teeth chattered uncontrollably. Between the once-daily infusions, however, her temperature fell as low as 100.4°, suggesting a possible response. On Friday, Krueger decided to continue the antibiotics and the amphotericin until Ellie's absolute poly count reached 500, paying close attention to possible kidney damage. In order to stop the high fevers associated with the drug infusions, he suggested that hydrocortisone be added to the IV bottle.

On Friday afternoon, Cindy Lewis drove down to Baltimore, bringing along a stuffed animal for Ellie and a book called *Healing from Within* for Sally. Long before the transplant, she had promised to come down and visit for a few days, doing whatever she could to help out. Sally had been touched, knowing what a sacrifice it would be for Cindy to leave her husband and two children, but she had gladly accepted.

Cindy had no idea what to expect, having gleaned only a few vague bits of information from phone conversations with Sally and Brian. Arriving on Three-South, she walked hesitantly down the corridor, reading the patients' names posted on the doors of their rooms in large construction-paper letters: Keith, Becky, Amanda . . . She stopped at the nurses' station and was directed to Ellie's room. Sure enough, taped to the door of 335, above the I & O sheets, was a large sign that Beth had made: WARNING: ONE WILD AND CRAZY GIRL AHEAD.

Cindy knocked, and Sally emerged, wearing a surgical mask. Her eyes lit up above an invisible smile, and the two friends embraced. "It's so good to see you!" Sally managed to say, swallowing her tears.

"Is she up?" Cindy asked, and Sally nodded, helping her friend tie on a disposable mask from the box outside the door and instructing her to scrub her hands thoroughly in the little sink inside before she approached the bed. Then they slipped into the room, shutting the door behind them. The light was so dim that it took Cindy's eyes a moment to adjust as she washed her hands. The walls were covered with humorous animal posters featuring kittens, puppies, and monkeys, along with dozens of get-well cards and crude, first-grade drawings. "Cindy's here to see you, Ellie," Sally said. "She's brought you a present."

Cindy barely recognized the child. She was chalky pale and bald again, with a few silky strands still clinging to her scalp. Three IV's flowed into her body: the hyperalimentation line, a bag of platelets feeding into her

Brobiac catheter, and a minibottle of antibiotics draining into a heparin lock in her left hand. There was a large cold sore near her mouth. Ellie looked up, her eyes dulled by fever.

"Wasn't it nice of Cindy to bring you something!" Sally said. "Shall I open it for you?" When Ellie nodded, she carefully undid the wrapping paper. "Look, Ellie, a monkey, your favorite!"

Ellie was too miserable to smile, but she accepted the stuffed animal. Cindy felt as if she were observing this scene through a thick pane of glass. She could not imagine how she would feel if Ellie were her own child—it would probably tear her apart. Yet Sally seemed to be coping reasonably well. Maybe you find the strength when you need it, Cindy thought. You have no choice; you just have to take it. There's no way out.

Cindy stayed in the room most of the afternoon, chatting with Sally while Ellie watched TV, played with her dolls, and received her antibiotics and transfusions. Cindy was very impressed by the cheerfulness and obvious concern of the nurses. If Ellie became withdrawn, Nancy would play and joke with her until she came out of it. Later on that afternoon, when it was time to change Ellie's central-line dressings, Cindy accompanied Sally to the lounge for a breather. "You've told me everything that Ellie's gone through this year and a half," Cindy said, "but until now I never realized what was involved. Nobody else will understand, either, unless they come down and see her here."

After hearing about hemophoresis, Cindy made an appointment to donate platelets the next morning. She stayed overnight in the trailer and the two friends caught up on all that had happened since the transplant. Cindy reported that Beth and Amy were doing fine, but that the Junior Women's Club was foundering in Sally's absence. By the time Cindy left for Menlo Park on Sunday, all the suffering she had witnessed had changed her outlook on life.

By Saturday Ellie's white count had reached 495, and over the next week it continued to climb slowly. As her counts improved, her spirits did also. Her mouth ulcers finally healed and the horrible scabs dropped off. Now it was physically possible for her to eat solid food, although she continued to refuse it, relying entirely on the hyperalimentation. Part of the problem was that she had not eaten for so long that her appetite had disappeared; the antibiotics also made her anorexic. Moreover, her refusals were an attempt to achieve some sense of control, however negative and self-defeating.

At the end of June, Lynn Schwartz rotated off Three-South, and Margo Barnes replaced her. Sally found it hard to adjust to the new resident; having started with one doctor, she felt they should finish with her. She was annoyed by the fact that she had to repeat explanations to Margo, but her complaints to Krueger were to no avail. The attending sympathized but said that there was no way to keep the residents longer than one month. The team approach to medical care involved certain trade-offs: while there was better coverage and sharing of responsibility among the various doctors, patients and families were forced to develop relationships with particular physicians knowing that they would rotate out in a month or two.

By Thursday, July 3, Ellie's white count had risen over 1,000 for the first time since the transplant, nearly three weeks before. Krueger said that if she remained without fever for another twenty-four hours, he would take her off isolation. No fever developed, and on the morning of July 4 the pink ISOLATION card was removed from Ellie's door and her amphotericin was discontinued. Krueger also took her off the bowel prep (which immediately boosted her morale), allowed Sally to enter the room without a mask, and encouraged them to walk laps around the nurses' station.

Although Ellie became chilled and shaky when she got out of bed, she insisted on escaping the confines of her room for the first time in nearly two weeks. As she walked slowly down the corridor with her mother, she paused to smile and wave at her fellow patients. She was very curious about how the others were doing. "Are they getting the same things I am?" she wanted to know. Asking about other patients seemed to be Ellie's way of finding out about her own prognosis. Although they walked slowly, she and Sally managed to do ten laps before they retired for the day.

That afternoon, Brian called Sally at the hospital to say that he would not be coming down the next morning because he needed to work overtime. Sally was angry and disappointed but not surprised. Increasingly, Brian had been withdrawing from her and Ellie. Although Sally spoke to him every day, their conversations were limited to a daily progress report: a summary of blood counts and symptoms. They no longer talked about themselves; all of their private hopes and plans as a couple had been set aside and both felt neglected, misunderstood, and often angry.

On the evening of the Fourth, the nurses took all of the patients who were not in protective isolation down to the covered walkway on the ground floor of the Oncology Center to watch the fireworks display over the Inner Harbor. The crowd of young patients, nearly all wearing surgical masks and hooked up to IV poles, walked through the hospital lobby like a strange pilgrimage. They were excited but also afraid; many of them had not been off the Unit in weeks. Sally held tightly to Ellie's hand as they watched the fireworks, enjoying her daughter's gasps of awe and running commentary on the explosions she liked best.

The next morning, Saturday, July 5, Ellie's temperature remained normal. Her white count was now 1,400 with 40 percent polys, which meant that her absolute poly count was sufficiently high for her to be taken off antibiotics. During morning rounds, Dr. Krueger noticed a rash developing on Ellie's thighs and a slight reddening of her ears. Although she had no other symptoms of graft-versus-host disease, such as diarrhea or a deterioration in her liver-function tests, Krueger decided to keep a careful watch and to alert the rest of the staff to the possibility of GVHD, however mild.

When Brian failed to arrive that morning, Ellie became upset. "Where's Daddy?" she asked. "It's Saturday. Why doesn't he come?"

Sally tightened her lips and replied, "Daddy has to work, so he can make enough money to pay the bills." Her answer just seemed to make Ellie more depressed; the child could not help feeling responsible for driving her father away. Sally understood by now that Brian loved Ellie so much that he could not bear to see her suffer, but the sad irony was that Ellie felt abandoned as if he did not love her anymore.

On Saturday afternoon, Sally saw Mrs. Willis in the lounge with her husband, who had flown in from South Carolina. She looked terrible: there were dark bags under her eyes and creases of worry in her brow. Something had snapped within her, and Sally understood why when she heard that Keith Willis was going rapidly downhill. The second marrow graft had taken, but soon afterward he had developed a severe case of GVHD that had caused a massive ulceration of his lower intestinal tract and opened him up to infection. When Sally went to visit Keith, she could tell that he was dying. He had a certain shakiness—a choppy, shallow, rapid breathing—and his eyes, gleaming out from his sallow face, betrayed his fear. He had fought and fought, but the disease was winning. The will to live was just not going to be enough.

Later that night, Keith went into septic shock and stopped breathing. Peters did cardiopulmonary resuscitation until he finally had to give up and pronounce the young man dead. Liz Ochs was present when it happened. Mr. Willis slammed the wall with his fist, and his wife broke down. "I'm so sorry we had to put him through so much," Mr. Willis murmured through clenched teeth.

"Keith was a fighter," Liz told him. "He fought the disease to the end. That's what he would have wanted."

Before they left, Mr. Willis told Liz to destroy all of his son's possessions remaining at the hospital. Liz decided to put them in storage, since she felt that Mr. Willis, in his acute grief, might have made a hasty decision that he would later regret. The Willises promised to come in the next morning to say good-bye to the other doctors, nurses, and parents, but they never did.

When Sally arrived on the floor the next morning, she passed Keith's room and was shocked to discover that it was empty, the bed made, the nameplate gone. It was surreal. The news did not take long to spread throughout the Unit. Although everyone had known that Keith was doing poorly, the finality and suddenness of his death hit hard and cast a shadow over the entire floor. The anxiety of the families rose: parents feared silently for their own child. Reluctant to antagonize the doctors, they took out their frustrations on the nurses. Parents complained about the nursing care, claiming that their child was not receiving optimal attention and treatments, that call lights were not being answered fast enough, and that routine procedures were done hastily and without enough attention to the patient's comfort. The more experienced nurses, accustomed to these reactions, understood that Keith's death also meant the loss of his entire family, which had been an integral part of the other parents' emotional support system.

That evening after Ellie had gone to sleep, Sally walked to the parking garage through the enclosed walkway from the Oncology Center so she would not have to leave the building alone. She carried a folded umbrella with her as a weapon and did not feel safe until she was inside her car with the doors locked. Her nerves were fragile and worn.

By the time she got to the campground it was after ten. She had become friendly with an older woman who lived in a trailer in the next lot, just twenty feet away. Mrs. Smith and her husband were both retired and had come to the campground for the entire summer. They were very kind and treated Sally like a daughter. Mrs. Smith would often watch for Sally's car at night and, if she looked as if she needed some boosting, would invite her in for a cup of coffee. The old woman was very cheerful and talkative and usually succeeded in taking Sally's mind off her troubles for a while. The Smiths also had a telephone in their trailer which they encouraged Sally to use for her convenience.

But tonight Mrs. Smith did not come out. Sally did not want to intrude, although she would have welcomed the company and the distraction. She had been strong all day, not letting Ellie know how frightened and depressed she was by Keith's death. Now that she was alone she could cry, releasing all the emotion bottled up inside.

Sally watched TV for a few hours in the trailer, feeling painfully alone, and finally crawled into bed. In the middle of the night, she was awakened by a scratching sound. At first she was terrified. "Oh, my God," she thought. "Someone's trying to break in." She tried looking out the window but it was pitch black outside. Her heart pounding, she put on her robe, got out a flashlight, and opened the front door a crack to peer out. The beam shone on a small animal chewing busily on the plastic garbage bag she had left outside. It was a skunk. For a moment Sally was relieved; then she realized with alarm that the creature might spray. She shut the door gently, locked it, and went back to bed, only to get up a few minutes later to make herself some tea.

29 Graft Versus Host

On Wednesday, July 9, the nutritionist came in to ask Sally about Ellie's preferred foods. The child's discharge would be contingent on a sufficient intake of protein and calories so that her hyperalimentation could be discontinued. Because intensive chemotherapy and radiation disrupted the normal function of the taste buds, Ellie might be disappointed and confused when she started eating again and discovered that the taste of foods did not meet expectations. Trial and error would therefore be needed to find foods that she would eat.

Nancy and some of the other nurses offered to bake Ellie anything she had a taste for, but all she wanted was some dry cereals, in particular Cap'n Crunch and Froot Loops. First Ellie ate the cereal dry and drank a lot of tea. Then she began to eat the cereal with milk, although she refused anything more substantial.

By Thursday, July 10, Ellie was in full hematological recovery: she had a white count of 2,900 with 60 percent polys and a platelet count of 290,000. A bone-marrow aspiration revealed a full complement of blood-forming cells. Nevertheless, the doctors continued to be worried by the reddening of Ellie's ears and face. Blood chemistries also revealed a rise in two liver enzymes—SGOT and SGPT—suggestive of early graft-versus-host disease.

Because Krueger suspected GVHD, he called in Tim Edwards, the physician's assistant responsible for protocol testing. Edwards took skin biopsies from two sites: the red plaque on Ellie's thigh and the mild rash on her arm. He sterilized each site with alcohol and numbed the area with an injection of xylocaine. Using a disposable punch, he removed a 3.5-millimeter-square piece of skin and dropped it into a small vial of formalin with a pair of forceps. After placing gelatin foam on the wounds to staunch the bleeding, he covered them with large Band-Aids. Then he took the specimens back to his office, made out a requisition form, and placed the two vials in a metal basket that would be hand-carried to the Dermopathology Lab that afternoon. Results would come through the following day.

By Friday morning, red blotches had appeared on Ellie's arms, face, and hands, accompanied by severe itching and burning sensations, and her skin had become dry and scaly. She was given an antihistamine and sent down to Physical Therapy for a cool whirlpool bath to soothe her rash and itching. That afternoon the report came back from Dermopathology: thin sections of the biopsy specimens, fixed, stained, and examined under a light microscope, had revealed changes in the structure of the skin that indicated GVHD. The epidermis (the outer layer of the skin) was shrunken, with abnormal cell architecture and a marked disruption of the normal pigmentary pattern. Even more striking was the infiltration of numerous lymphocytes into the junction between the epidermis and the underlying dermis. The dermis also contained numerous lesions produced by the dilation of small blood vessels packed with infiltrating lymphocytes. These lymphocytes—the mature white cells that had "contaminated" Beth's marrow—were now fiercely attacking the tissues of their new host.

Fortunately, Ellie's case was relatively mild. The intensity of GVHD was graded from I to IV-plus. Grade I described a lymphocyte infiltration into the skin that could be seen under the microscope but was not manifested by clinical symptoms. Grade II was associated with a skin rash, diarrhea, and mild liver damage, and Grade III had similar but more pronounced symptoms. Grade IV to IV-plus was what all the transplant doctors dreaded: a life-threatening breakdown of the skin, with severe blistering and scaling, massive diarrhea (sometimes choleralike in its intensity, with a loss of up to ten liters of fluid per day), extensive liver damage, and a profound impairment of immune function. Some degree of GVHD occurred in 70 percent of transplant patients with successful nontwin marrow grafts, but in only 20 percent of cases did the reaction warrant aggressive treatment. A graft-versus-host reaction thirty days or more after the transplant was considered to be the chronic form of the disease, which was generally milder but harder to eliminate.

Ellie had Grade II acute GVHD. When Dr. Krueger told Sally and Ellie the news that afternoon, it came as a devastating blow, particularly since Ellie's counts had recovered on schedule and they had been looking forward to an early discharge. Now she was covered from head to toe with a red, blotchy, itchy rash and had begun suffering from an uncontrollable liquid diarrhea that prevented her from leaving the room. Ellie cried often and became depressed. Sally was equally distraught. Having been traumatized by Keith Willis's death, she had prayed every night that Ellie would not develop GVHD. And now it had happened, just when Ellie seemed to have survived the hazardous first month in reasonably good shape.

Krueger sensed Sally's anxiety and made special efforts to be reassuring. "Chances are good that we can get it under control quickly," he said.

"We're going to start treating her immediately with high-dose steroids, which should be able to stop the disease in its tracks and keep it low grade until it eventually smolders out. Although GVHD is not something we like to see, there's some evidence that a mild case of it in leukemic patients may be beneficial in the long run."

Sally was startled. "What do you mean, beneficial?" she asked. "I thought GVHD was the worst thing that could happen."

"Well, there may be a positive side to it," the doctor replied. "Our colleagues in Seattle, who have done more transplants, feel that moderate to severe GVHD may have an antileukemic effect in some patients, reducing the risk that their leukemia will recur later on. As you know, identical twins have perfect immunological identity, so that a graft from one twin to the other never results in GVHD. The Seattle workers have found, though, that the rate of recurrence of leukemia in identical twins is higher than in HLA-matched recipients. This could mean that the GVHD may be partially directed against residual leukemic cells—the ones that are not destroyed by chemotherapy or radiation and might otherwise trigger a recurrence later on. This theory hasn't yet been proved, but it seems plausible, so a mild case of GVHD may not be all bad. The question is how to exploit the possible antileukemic effect of GVHD while trying to prevent its destructive effects on normal tissues."

Sally shook her head. "I don't know what to hope for anymore."

Krueger began the treatment of Ellie's GVHD with a short, tapering course of high-dose intravenous prednisolone, a steroid anti-inflammatory agent closely related to cortisone and prednisone, in the hope of killing off most of the lymphocytes that were responsible for the rejection reaction. The effectiveness of the drug varied from case to case. Krueger tried to get a response from steroids as quickly as possible, since prolonged high-dose treatments could weaken the patient's bones, cause diabetes, and seriously lower the white count, once again increasing susceptibility to infection. Prednisolone was also known to induce a state of physical dependence, so that it had to be withdrawn slowly after a reasonable improvement was achieved; too rapid withdrawal could cause serious physiological derangements.

When Ellie was told she had to get steroids again, she began to cry, remembering the terrible side effects of her maintenance chemotherapy. Twenty-four hours after the start of her intravenous prednisolone, however, both her rash and her itching improved markedly. Her diarrhea also eased, although her liver-function tests continued to deteriorate. Since Ellie was clearly responding to the treatments, Krueger decided to continue giving her high-dose intravenous infusions of the drug four times daily over four days. If she continued to do well, he would cut the dose in half and switch her to prednisolone pills, which would be tapered gradually. In the event that the disease flared up again after the tapering, he would have to increase her dose again. They would just have to wait and see.

By July 15, the fourth day of her therapy, Ellie's GVHD remained under control. The rash was mainly restricted to her inner thighs and arms, and her face was pink, with only mild itching. A skin biopsy revealed that the intensity of her GVHD had declined, and Krueger switched her to pills. Ellie's appetite had improved, perhaps in response to the steroids: she ate a doughnut and tea for breakfast, soup and crackers for lunch, and a large slice of watermelon for supper, although her sense of taste came and went unpredictably. Her spirits were good but she was bored and needed entertaining.

By Wednesday, July 16, Ellie's skin redness had gone down but the whites of her eyes had taken on a yellowish tint; in addition, her urine had turned dark and her stools were strangely pale. The following day, the skin of her chest and abdomen looked yellow when examined in daylight. Krueger concluded that Ellie had developed jaundice: an excessive accumulation in her blood and tissues of the yellow pigment bilirubin, a breakdown product of hemoglobin. Indeed, a blood test revealed that the child's bilirubin level was up to 6.4 milligrams per deciliter; the normal concentration in the blood was less than 1 milligram.

Jaundice appeared whenever bilirubin could not be excreted by the liver into the intestine in the bile; instead, the yellow pigment was recirculated into the blood, causing it to accumulate in body fluids and tissues. Krueger was unsure which of several possible mechanisms might be responsible, but two seemed most likely: damage to the liver cells due to a viral infection such as hepatitis, or obstruction of the bile ducts due to GVHD. Since either complication was potentially serious, Krueger decided to order a liver biopsy, which would reveal the cause and the extent of the damage.

A surgical resident performed the biopsy that evening in the operating room under light anesthesia. He inserted a needle through Ellie's abdominal wall and into her liver, extracting a small specimen of tissue that would be sent to Surgical Pathology for microscopic examination. When the results came back from the lab, they were unequivocal: Grade I GVHD, particularly in the bile ducts. Krueger decided to continue tapering Ellie's steroids gradually, waiting to see if her liver function improved.

Two days later, during morning rounds, Margo Barnes summarized Ellie's progress. "Ellen Murphy looks good," she began, as the medical team paused outside the child's room. "After her counts came back, she developed symptoms of GVHD with skin, liver, and GI tract involvement, although not life threatening. She's currently on 10 per kilo steroids every six hours and has responded well to the therapy. She has very little diarrhea now, her weight's up, her electrolytes are stable, her counts are good, and her bilirubin was down to 4.8 yesterday from 6.4 the day before. I hope to be getting more bilirubin levels today."

"How many days is she out now?" Krueger asked.

"Thirty-five," Peters replied.

"It seems a lot longer."

Peters nodded. "It does, doesn't it? She's had her share of problems. Of course, she still runs the risk of viral pneumonia later on."

Barnes closed the chart. "We're trying to push some alimentation on her now," she continued, "moving to semisoft foods, and she seems to be taking to that well. Her main problem now is dry mouth."

Krueger was all too familiar with that problem. One of the side effects of both TBI and GVHD was damage to the minor salivary glands of the mouth, which produced the saliva that facilitated digestion and bathed the teeth and gums, serving as a major aid in the prevention of tooth decay. When GVHD attacked and shut down the salivary glands, the child tended to get a tremendously dry mouth. Coupled with the fact that these kids often had mouth sores and low platelets already, severe dental and gum problems could develop. Krueger knew of a few cases in which children had developed huge cavities in every tooth. One little girl had required total replacement of her baby teeth with stainless-steel caps, and the doctors were unsure whether her permanent teeth had been damaged as well. Dry mouth was one of those seemingly minor complications of GVHD that could have a major, long-term impact. (The tear ducts were also affected by GVHD, so that children with the disease were often unable to cry.) Fortunately, Ellie had a mild case that was responding well to medication.

That day, Friday, July 18, Ellie's white count was 3,400. Her skin rashes were fading and she no longer complained of itching. She remained in bed until 11:30 A.M., when Sally took her down to Radiology for a chest X-ray. Later that afternoon Ellie went to Physical Therapy, where she was being given a general strengthening program to increase her endurance and muscle tone.

The weekend passed uneventfully, and by Monday Ellie's white count had jumped to 10,000. She was now managing to do laps without significant weakness. On Monday evening Nancy began discharge teaching, with special emphases on clinic routines and signs and symptoms to watch out for. "Ellie will be highly susceptible to infections for a long time, so she should avoid crowds," Nancy cautioned Sally. "To be safe, she should wear a mask whenever she's around people. Visitors should be limited to immediate family for a least a month, and then only one or two close friends until the first hundred days after the transplant have passed. She should be very careful about personal hygiene, and you should give her a shower or a pHisohex sponge bath daily to reduce her skin bacteria. Her temperature should be recorded at least twice a day. Any foods she can tolerate are fine with the exception of highly salted snacks, since they will only exacerbate the fluid retention caused by her steroid treatments. Ellie should remain as active as possible but must avoid the sun, since it might reactivate her GVHD. No swimming is allowed for another two months or so."

Ellie would be seen every weekday by the clinic P.A., Tim Edwards, who was on call twenty-four hours a day. She would have to continue taking her nystatin "swish-and-swallow" four times a day and Bactrim, an antibiotic, as prophylaxis against a form of pneumonia caused by *Pneumocystis carinii,* an amoeboid parasite. *Pneumocystis* was more common in some parts of the country than others, and fortunately the incidence of the infection in the Northeast was fairly low. The prednisolone tablets for GVHD would be tapered gradually. If Ellie developed any symptoms, including malaise, fever, cough, runny nose, bleeding, bruising, or undue fatigue, Sally was to inform Dr. Krueger immediately.

Krueger also came in to talk with Sally. He did not want Ellie to be too far from the hospital in the event of an emergency, and when Sally told him that the trailer park was a forty-five-minute drive away, he only reluctantly agreed. If any problems developed, he warned, they would have to move back to the Sheraton or to Reed Hall.

Sally worried about her ability to take care of Ellie outside of the hospital, without all the support staff available around the clock to intervene immediately if something went wrong. She feared that if a serious complication developed, she would be unable to catch it in time.

Over the next two days, Nancy tried to wean Ellie away from the constant attention of intensive care. In a sense, it was like growing up all over again, since Ellie had regressed to the level of a three-year-old, becoming dependent on her mother for washing her, feeding her, and cleaning her teeth. Although Ellie had regressed with relative ease, it was harder for her to resume the capacities of a six-year-old. Nancy had to discourage Sally from babying her, insisting that Ellie start washing and feeding herself and become more outgoing with strangers.

Ellie had been saying for weeks that she could not wait to leave the hospital, but as the day of her discharge approached she became apprehensive. She was afraid of emerging from the secure, womblike environment of the Unit and venturing out into the germ-laden world, where she might catch another infection. Nancy reassured her by saying that there were probably fewer nasty germs outside the hospital than inside, with so many sick people around.

On Tuesday, July 22, Ellie's central lines were discontinued. Removing the hyperalimentation catheter was a quick, painless procedure. Margo simply snipped the suture over the puncture site and slid the thin tubing out. The Brobiac catheter was more difficult to remove because of the Dacron cuff that anchored it beneath the skin, and a general surgeon had to come in and do the job. After infiltrating lidocaine anesthetic near the exit site in Ellie's chest, he made a small incision to free the Dacron cuff and then pulled the catheter out slowly and steadily. Sally distracted Ellie throughout the procedure, so that she was relatively cooperative. Afterward, the surgeon cultured the extracted catheter to test for bacteria, and Nancy applied a sterile dressing to the incision.

Since Ellie's liver-function tests and bilirubin levels continued to improve, indicating that her GVHD was now under control, Krueger said that she could leave the hospital Thursday morning if no new medical problems arose. On Wednesday Ellie developed some congestion and a cough, but nothing serious enough to delay her discharge.

Thursday morning, Sally filled out the discharge forms. Since Brian had told her he would be unable to leave work a day early to come down, she was alone. With Nancy's help, she packed Ellie's clothes into a suitcase and her dolls, toys, and stuffed animals into two large shopping bags. A few other nurses dropped in to say good-bye, adding that they hoped to see Ellie only as an outpatient. It was obvious that they were happy the child was leaving the hospital in relatively good shape after all she had been through.

The battles of the past weeks had left their mark on Ellie's body. She wore a surgical mask over her mouth and nose and a cotton scarf over her stubbly hair. The side effects of the steroid treatments—fluid retention with swelling of the face and belly—had already begun to appear, although her arms and legs remained thin. Few of Ellie's old clothes fit her, and Sally realized that she would have to buy the child a new wardrobe. Now, clinging shyly to her mother's arm, with her ill-fitting clothes and round face, Ellie looked like a tragic clown. At least she was no longer chalky pale; a red-cell transfusion early that morning had put some color in her cheeks.

Dr. Krueger came in to sign the discharge form and take a final look at her. He patted her on the shoulder and smiled. "I bet you're glad to be getting out of here, aren't you, Ellie?" he said. "I'm afraid you're going to have to come and see me at the clinic every day, but we'll give you the weekends off, okay?"

Ellie hid her face in her mother's dress, and Krueger turned to Sally. "In spite of all her problems, she's done remarkably well," he said. "Today is day forty-one since her transplant. The average release time is between thirty and sixty days, so she's right on schedule."

When all the formalities had been taken care of, Ellie and Sally rode the elevator down to the main floor of the Oncology Center. While Sally went to get the car, Ellie waited in one of the armchairs in the lobby, looking out through the picture window at the heat shimmering up off the asphalt. A few minutes later, Sally's battered white Volvo appeared in the circular driveway of the North Wolfe Street entrance. She got out, leaving the motor running, and came inside, taking Ellie by the hand. The child resisted, clearly frightened; she had not been outside the hospital building in seven weeks. "Come on, Ellie, I'll buy you a chocolate milkshake if you're good," Sally said.

The automatic doors swung open before them with a hydraulic hissing, and a wave of heat washed over Ellie's face. Her nostrils were suddenly assaulted by pungent odors of hot asphalt and exhaust, her eyes blinded by the midsummer sun, her ears buffeted by the deafening noise of the street and a nearby construction project. The very air seemed aswarm with invisible germs, menacing her on all sides. . . . She began to cry, and Sally picked her up and carried her to the car.

Sally climbed into the driver's seat, closed the doors, fastened both their seat belts, and put the car in gear. Ellie continued to whimper, holding tightly to her mother's arm as she turned the wheel. When the medical center disappeared from sight in the rearview mirror, Sally let out a great sigh of relief.

30 Reprieve

On their way to the campground, Ellie asked if they could stop for the milkshake she had been promised. Sally knew that they had to find a restaurant without a crowd of people. About twenty minutes from Woodbine, she saw a McDonald's sign and pulled into the parking lot. There were only a few people inside, so she sat Ellie down at a table in the corner, out of sight. Sally ordered a chocolate milkshake for Ellie and a hamburger and coffee for herself. She brought the food back to the table and untied the lower half of Ellie's mask so that the child would be able to sip through the straw. They talked about how nice it was to be out of that awful hospital and how Daddy, Beth, and Amy would all be coming down over the weekend, so that the family could be together again.

Ellie loved the trailer, which was like a big dollhouse on wheels. It was fun to be camping out in the woods with the birds and trees she had not seen for over a month and a half. The first evening they stayed inside and watched TV, enjoying ice cream and doughnuts. When it got dark they went out and looked at the sky. It was an unusually clear night and the stars seemed brighter and more numerous than Sally had ever remembered. Maybe it was just because she was so happy. She pointed out the Big Dipper and tried to remember how to find the North Star. "How many stars are there in the sky, Mommy?" Ellie asked. "More than a hundred?"

Sally laughed and said, "Oh, yes, Ellie, lots more than that."

They went back inside, and as Ellie got ready for bed, Sally began a goodnight story. The child fell asleep with no trouble at all.

The next morning Sally went over to the Smiths' trailer. Mrs. Smith was thrilled to hear that Ellie was now an outpatient. Sally explained that Ellie was still very vulnerable to infection, so that it would be important to know if there was a cold or anything contagious going around. The older woman nodded and said she understood.

At ten o'clock, they started out for the hospital. It was nearly eleven, Ellie's appointment time, when they arrived at the Outpatient Department in the basement of the Oncology Center. They checked in at the reception desk and sat down in one of the two rows of chairs. Two of the waiting patients had undergone transplants and were returning for their six-month checkups. The first was a boy of fifteen who sat quietly with his mother. Three months after his transplant, he had developed chronic GVHD; his face was covered with red blotches and the skin on his hands was dry and scaly, as if he were suffering from a bad case of sunburn. The boy's mother told Sally that he never went back up to visit Three-South because he was afraid of scaring the other patients. But he was alive, and his leukemia was apparently cured.

The other patient, a man of twenty-one, was by himself. Pale and thin but in relatively good condition, he sported a short growth of new hair. He seemed preoccupied and glanced around the room restlessly, ignoring the paperback edition of Camus essays he had brought along to read. While Ellie worked at her coloring book, Sally struck up a conversation with the young man, who told her that the transplant experience had caused him to do some serious philosophical thinking. He found it hard to relate to his peers, who were more concerned with sports and drinking beer than with deep reflections on the meaning of life. "I don't want to cut them off and appear to be a snob," he said, "but they can't understand what I'm feeling, and I'm not really interested in what they're doing."

As they began to talk about his plans for the future, Ellie's name was called. A nurse led them into a small examining room where she took Ellie's height, weight, and vital signs. Then, after a few minutes' wait, Tim Edwards came in and drew blood for counts and chemistries. Since it was Friday, he also did the weekly protocol tests, including urinalysis, throat culture, and blood gases. The blood-gas test was the worst since it required an arterial stick. Finally Ellie went for a chest X-ray and then to Dr. Krueger for a physical exam.

Exhausted and drained, Sally and Ellie returned to the campground a little after 3:00 P.M. After taking a two-hour nap, they drove to a department store fifteen minutes away and shopped for clothes to fit Ellie's new physique. Because the steroids had swollen her waist but left her legs as skinny as ever, it soon became clear that a perfect fit was impossible. They did the best they could and returned to the trailer for supper.

When the meal was over, they went for a short walk, stopping every few minutes to rest. Since Ellie's hematocrit was low, she became dizzy even after mild exercise. They reached a playground, where Sally gave Ellie gentle rides on the swing and the seesaw. Sally was acutely aware of the child's fragility, fearing that if Ellie so much as tripped and fell, she might bleed to death before they reached the hospital. They returned to the trailer as the sun was setting.

As the evening went on, Ellie became more relaxed and independent, although she still had her demanding and irritable moments. The prednisolone was at least partly responsible for her sudden changes in mood, since it usually took only a few minutes for her to return to her normal self. Although her skin biopsy showed no further evidence of GVHD, the steroids had to be withdrawn very slowly by cutting the dose in half every four or five days.

Saturday morning, Brian arrived with the other two children and Barbara, whom Sally had not seen in months, although they talked regularly on the phone. Now that Ellie was an outpatient, Brian had taken two weeks of vacation so that the family could be together. He seemed in very good spirits, although Sally disliked the way he treated Ellie, joking about her baggy pants and tossing her up in the air and catching her, while Sally cringed. Later on, Brian went for a solitary walk around the campground while Sally coddled Amy, trying desperately to make up for lost time. Aunt Barbara had brought down a craft box for Ellie. At first the child was possessive of her new gift, but when Beth complained, Sally told Ellie to share. After that, they played together with a minimum of squabbling.

Beth had mixed feelings toward her sister. She wanted very much for the transplant to be a success, since she felt personally responsible. Yet at the same time she resented Ellie for monopolizing their parents' attention. As the donor child, Beth had received a great deal of pampering on the days immediately before, during, and after the transplant. But since then her sense of being neglected had returned. In proportion to what she had done and the amount of discomfort she had sustained, she did not think that she had received sufficient gratitude from her parents. It seemed as if her only reward had been an increase in her chores: not only did she have to clean her own room but Ellie's room as well, and she also had to take care of her sister's pet gerbil.

That evening, the family drove to a nearby miniature-golf course and made it through the sixth hole before Ellie became tired and irritable, forcing them to return home. Sunday afternoon they all went out to see a Disney movie, and then Barbara left by train for New York.

On Monday morning, July 28, the daily visits to the Outpatient Department began again. Remembering the pain of the past Friday's tests, Ellie tried to avoid getting into the car. Sally had to reassure her that only blood would be drawn that day.

When the blood counts came back from the lab, Krueger noticed a disturbing decline in Ellie's counts from the previous Friday. Her white count had fallen from 15,400 to 11,500 and her platelet count had dropped from 173,000 to 118,000. He was concerned, but decided to wait and see if the trend continued.

Over the next two weeks, the situation worsened. Ellie's white count and platelet count continued to go down; only her hematocrit remained relatively stable:

	WHITE CELLS	PLATELETS	HEMATOCRIT
Wednesday, July 30	10,700	124,000	28.9
Thursday, July 31	9,300	127,000	30.2
Friday, August 1	7,600	104,000	28.8
Monday, August 4	4,700	92,000	28.8
Tuesday, August 5	4,500	69,000	30.0
Wednesday, August 6	4,100	50,000	28.7
Thursday, August 7	3,300	47,000	29.2
Friday, August 8	3,700	40,000	28.3

Sally and Brian watched this steady decline with increasing alarm. Dr. Krueger suspected that a viral infection might be causing the drop in Ellie's white count, but nothing had shown up in the surveillance cultures. He told Sally to take Ellie's temperature at least twice a day and to let him know if she developed a fever or any cold symptoms. On

Sunday, August 10, Brian and the other children left for Menlo Park, since his vacation time was up. That evening Ellie spiked a temperature of 103°, and she was still feverish when Krueger examined her the next morning in clinic. The doctor said that all he could do was wait until the cultures grew out. Without knowing the cause of Ellie's fever, they just had to hope that her weakened immune system would be effective.

Over the next week, Ellie's white count continued its ominous decline:

	WHITE CELLS	PLATELETS	HEMATOCRIT
Monday, August 11	2,800	38,000	28.1
Tuesday, August 12	2,300	23,000	28.3
Wednesday, August 13	2,200	23,000	27.1
Thursday, August 14	2,200	40,000	26.9
Friday, August 15	2,000	53,000	26.3

By Friday, the differential white count showed only 1 percent polys. Krueger had never before seen a selective loss of the ability to produce white cells; usually all of the precursor cell lines in the bone marrow acted as one. A bone-marrow aspiration revealed the seriousness of Ellie's predicament: she had normal red-cell precursors, occasional megakaryocytes, and absolutely no white-cell precursors. Although the cause of the problem remained mysterious, Ellie's situation was grave. Since no new white cells were being produced in the marrow, her white count would continue to fall rapidly over the next several days, rendering her dangerously vulnerable to bacterial and fungal infections.

Krueger reviewed Ellie's recent medical history. The child's fevers had spiked as high as 103° over the past week but had gone down in response to Tylenol. Except for a slow rise in the levels of liver enzymes in Ellie's blood, suggesting a mild deterioration in liver function, she had been completely asymptomatic, and her arterial blood gases and chest X-ray were normal. Krueger performed a thorough physical exam, the results of which were unremarkable, and took cultures of Ellie's throat, blood, urine, and marrow. The marrow would be cultured especially for viruses as a possible cause of her fever and liver abnormalities.

The crisis was ill timed; Krueger was about to leave for a scientific conference in Montreal and would not be around over the weekend to keep a close watch on Ellie. While the child and her mother sat out in the waiting room, Krueger paged Peters and discussed the case with him. Krueger's plan was to cut down Ellie's prednisolone immediately, since the drug had the side effect of further suppressing her immune system, and to institute intravenous antibiotics if her fever spiked over 101°. Although there was a bed available in one of the donor rooms, Krueger was reluctant to have Ellie readmitted right away, knowing what a crushing blow it would be to the child and her family to return to the hospital after a reprieve of only three weeks. Another reason was that if Ellie became an inpatient, she would no longer be in his care. Having finished his six-week rotation shortly after Ellie's discharge, Krueger had rotated off Three-South but continued to follow his outpatients in the clinic. Although he could still keep up with the status of the inpatients by attending the weekly census meetings, he was reluctant to abdicate his responsibility for Ellie.

Peters, on the other hand, strongly favored admitting Ellie because of the risk of infection, which could develop overnight and spread rapidly to her lungs. Krueger knew he had to give in; it was better to play it safe. Asking Peters to accompany him, he went out to the waiting room to tell Sally the bad news.

The two doctors sat down next to Sally, who deduced from Peters's presence that something was wrong. She braced herself for the worst. Ellie continued to flip through a storybook, seemingly oblivious to what was going on around her.

"Ellie's white count is down again today, to 2,000," Krueger began. "If it goes much lower we may have to put her back on intravenous antibiotics. The problem is that no new white cells are being made in her bone marrow, and we have to find out why that is. We think it's due to a viral infection of some kind, but so far nothing has shown up in our cultures. Since I'm going to be out of town this weekend, I feel the wisest course would be to have Ellie readmitted so that the staff can keep a close watch on her and do a thorough work-up of her low counts and fever."

"Readmitted?" Sally said vaguely, as if she had not understood. "For how long?"

"Probably another week or ten days, until her counts recover."

"Oh, God!" Sally moaned, covering her face with her hands. After all those days of holding the pain inside her, she was having trouble staying composed. Yet when she saw Ellie's look of alarm, she knew she had to be strong. "Ellie, come here a moment," she said gently. "The doctor says you have to come back to the hospital for a little while, so they can find out why your counts are so low. You'll just have to stay for a few days, and then we can go back to the trailer."

"No! I don't want to come back!" Ellie shouted. She looked up into the stern faces of the doctors and then back at her mother, as if awaiting a comforting response. When none came, she fell into Sally's arms and began to sob.

Krueger, looking grim, excused himself and went up to find Nancy, who

266

he hoped would be able to cheer Ellie up a little. But when Nancy came down, the child refused even to acknowledge her. She curled up on the chair next to her mother and covered her eyes with her hands. Sally had to drag her, struggling and crying, to a wheelchair to take her up to the floor. When Ellie was finally in bed and sedated, Sally sat down and called Brian, telling him what had happened and begging him to drive down to Woodbine that night. After some hesitation, he finally agreed to come, convinced by the real anguish in Sally's voice.

That night in New Jersey, before Brian left for Baltimore, he sat down with Beth and told her that Ellie's counts had dropped unexpectedly and that she was back in the hospital. Beth did not usually show much emotion—anger, yes, but rarely tears—yet she broke down and hugged her father, crying into his shirt. "Is Ellie going to die?" she asked.

Brian patted her gently, murmuring, "No, Beth, Ellie's going to be fine. I'm going down to see her tonight."

"Can I go with you?" Beth asked, wiping her eyes.

Brian shook his head. "You had better stay here and help take care of Amy. But you can come visit as soon as Ellie's feeling better."

Beth nodded. She felt painfully guilty, convinced it was her fault that the marrow was not growing well. She had thought some pretty bad things about Ellie during her fits of jealousy, and now it seemed that they were all coming true. To atone for her sins, she resolved to stop eating ice cream for a month. Maybe if she made herself suffer enough, the bone marrow she had given Ellie would start working again.

As Brian drove down to Woodbine, his tension changed into anger. The more he thought about what had happened, the more furious he became. He targeted his rancor at those smug, arrogant doctors who thought they knew what they were doing, and at Sally, whose total absorption in Ellie's care, at the expense of himself and the other children, was driving a wedge through the center of their marriage. He even found himself getting angry at Ellie, however irrationally. Why did she have to get sick again, just when he had thought that their long ordeal was finally ending?

With a strong pang of guilt, Brian wished that Ellie would die peacefully in her sleep, sparing the family any further agony. After Ellie's death, he fantasized, he would destroy all evidence of her existence: her clothes, her belongings, every photograph.

31 Crash

From Ellie's new room, there was no view of the busy nurses' station, only of an empty corridor. The view out the window had also changed: it was a panorama of Baltimore tenements. Sally noticed that the donor room was not kept as clean as the isolation room Ellie had been in before. The floor was particularly dirty and was overlooked when the woman from Housekeeping came in to wipe down the mirror and mop the bathroom.

Sally would have complained but for the fact that there had been a change of medical team on Three-South and she no longer had any direct contact with Krueger. When Krueger had first started attending on the Transplant Unit, he had tried to maintain contact with some of the families after completing his rotation, coming up to the floor to visit them and answer their questions whenever he found the time. He had soon discovered that he was undermining the authority and effectiveness of the attending who had replaced him, particularly when there were subtle differences of opinion between him and the new attending on how best to treat the child. As a result, he had decided to keep his distance in spite of guilt feelings about "abandoning" his patients.

The new attending, Dr. Charles Seymour, did not seem as warm and accessible as Krueger had been. He always sounded as if he were reading from a medical textbook. On the other hand, the new fellow, David Stern, seemed more considerate than Peters in his presentation of possible complications and side effects. But Sally still felt too insecure in her relationship with either doctor to complain about the dirtiness of the floor.

Ellie was without fever for her first twenty-four hours in the hospital, but she became extremely depressed and withdrawn. She would not smile or talk to anyone and stared fixedly into space. When a nurse came into the room, bright and cheery, Ellie refused even to make eye contact, and when the doctors came on rounds, she passively let them work on her but either did not answer their questions or murmured inaudibly. It embarrassed Sally to see her child behaving so rudely, and the doctors, too, seemed irritated. "We've just got to get her out of this depression," Seymour told Sally, but he offered no suggestions or encouragement.

Sally tried everything she could think of. She read to Ellie, brought her new games and stuffed animals, watched TV with her, and told her stories, but it was impossible to interest her in anything. The child lay still in bed with her eyes closed or pulled the sheet over her head. Brian found it very difficult to be with her when she was so withdrawn, and he came up with numerous excuses for going down to the hospital lobby or outside for a walk. Each time he returned to the room, Sally was continuing her vigil at Ellie's bedside, trying to coax the child out from under the sheets. Her endurance both awed and irritated him.

Ellie remained without fever until Sunday, August 17, when her 8:00 A.M. temperature was 101°. After blood and urine specimens and rectal and throat swabs had been sent to the Bacteriology Lab, Seymour decided to start her immediately on two broad-spectrum antibiotics, gentamicin and carbenicillin, while they awaited the results of the cultures. When the new resident, Phil Conrad, came in to start a heparin lock in Ellie's left forearm to administer the antibiotics, the child reacted with shouts and tears. She knew that if they were starting an IV it was very unlikely that she would be leaving the hospital soon.

Brian and Sally arrived at ten o'clock. To Sally, it looked as if Ellie was deteriorating rapidly. She had lost several pounds and was showing no interest in her toys or in watching TV. Her fever persisted in spite of the antibiotics, spiking to 102.2° in the early afternoon. Sally helped the nurse rub the child down with a cooling bath and then applied ice packs to Ellie's pulse points, which successfully lowered her temperature by two degrees. Later on, when Ellie's fever continued, a refrigeration blanket was placed under her.

During all this, Ellie alternated between crying and "hibernating" under the sheets for hours at a time. After two days of effort, Sally could not help letting out some of her anger and frustration: "If you're not going to talk, I'm not coming in here anymore to spend all these hours. You're being rude to the doctors and nurses by not answering them, and I did not bring you up to be a spoiled brat!"

She left the room and walked quickly to the lounge, where she sat by herself and wept for several minutes. Fortunately the lounge was empty; she did not feel capable of making small talk. After taking several deep, calming breaths, she returned to Ellie's room, expecting to find the child even more withdrawn. To her surprise, Ellie appeared more alert and responsive. It seemed as if, seeing how miserable she was making her mother, she had been able to pull herself out of her depression at least temporarily. Sally stroked the child's forehead lovingly.

That evening, Ellie became mildly delirious from her high fever, imagining horrible monsters lurking in the shadows of her room. She begged her parents not to leave her, convinced that if they went away something terrible would happen. When Sally assured her they would stay, the child's body and mind seemed to relax. Brian was impatient to leave, but Sally insisted on reading to Ellie until ten-thirty, when the child finally dozed off peacefully.

After stopping for a late, greasy supper at a diner on the highway, the Murphys finally arrived at the trailer around midnight, having said virtually nothing to each other during the long drive. As soon as they got into the bedroom, Brian turned on the TV while Sally undressed. "Brian, come to bed," she begged him. "We have to be back at the hospital early tomorrow morning, and I'm exhausted."

"I'm not going in tomorrow," Brian said.

"What?"

"I said I'm not going in. I need some relief from all this . . . tragedy."

"Brian, Ellie needs all the love and support we can give her. We can't just run away from this."

"What's the point of sitting there with her for hours on end? Do you really think she wants or needs us at her bedside ten hours a day? She spends most of her time under those damn sheets anyway."

"Brian, when you don't come down on a weekend, she misses you terribly. 'Where's Daddy?' she asks. 'Why doesn't he come?' I tell her that you have to work hard to pay the bills, but I think she feels abandoned."

"What about Amy and Beth?" Brian retorted angrily. "Aren't they our children, too? Little Amy hasn't stopped whining since you left. What am I supposed to say to her? That Mommy just loves Ellie more?"

"Brian, please!" Sally begged. "Ellie needs me here! Of course I feel terrible that I haven't been more of a mother to Amy. You knew what was involved when we decided to go ahead with the transplant, that it would mean a lot of sacrifices. But we thought it was worth it. You signed that consent form, too!"

"Yes, but only because you convinced me. Remember that night we agonized over the decision? 'We just have to have faith,' you said. Well, look where your damn faith has gotten us!"

"Brian, stop!" There was a shrill panic in Sally's voice. "We both knew that the transplant was a gamble, and we decided—together—to go for it. Nelson and Krueger said that it was her best hope, and that even if she didn't make it, at least we would have done everything possible. . . . I know you like everything to be fun and games, but let's face it: leukemia isn't fun, and neither is the transplant. We've all suffered and been plenty inconvenienced by it, but Ellie has suffered much, much more than any of us. I never forget that, no matter how much of a burden it sometimes seems, and I'm certainly not going to abandon her now!"

"Well, you can go to hell!" Brian shouted and stormed out of the trailer, slamming the door behind him. He stood for a moment outside in the night air, trembling with rage, and then seemed to collapse inwardly. Drawn and pale, he pressed one ear to the door, hearing the sound of sobbing within. He felt a twinge of guilt that was quickly overcome by pride and resentment. After wandering around in the moonlight for a few minutes, he went back inside to fix himself a double bourbon from the bottle he had brought with him. Then he sat down in the living room to sip the drink, his mind awhirl with tortured thoughts.

The ambivalence that had been haunting him for weeks had returned full force, and he deeply regretted their decision to go ahead with the transplant. If Ellie had died of her illness after a happy remission, they could have lived with that, however painfully. But now she might die from a complication of the procedure, having already endured weeks of suffering. She might die because of something they had chosen to do, making them directly responsible for her death.

He put down the empty glass and went into the bedroom. The lights were out and Sally was apparently asleep, her back turned to him. He undressed quietly and slid into the bed beside her; the six inches between them felt unbridgeable.

Brian apologized briefly the next morning, but a wall of tension separated them. At breakfast, they said little to each other and avoided making eye contact. Sally had hoped that Brian might go to the hospital alone on Monday so that she would have some time to relax and regain some of her physical and emotional strength, but she realized now that she had expected too much of him: it was all she could do to get him to accompany her.

When they arrived at the hospital, there was more bad news: Ellie's white count was down to 1,300 and she continued to run a fever in spite of her two antibiotics. The results of Friday's blood culture had come back from the Bacteriology Lab, and two types of bacteria had been found growing in Ellie's blood. Identification of the organisms and their sensitivities to antibiotics would come through in a couple of days, after which the appropriate changes in antibiotic coverage could be made.

After lunch, Brian drove back to New Jersey, leaving Sally numb and exhausted. Increasingly she resented his self-pitying silences, his lack of warmth or support, his unwillingness to understand or even tolerate the strength she derived from her faith. And yet she needed him. She was terrified by the prospect of going through a second long hospitalization alone, while trying to be a mother at long distance to her other children. At least as long as Ellie was still in danger she would do her best to keep the marriage together. When the crisis had passed, she and Brian could deal

271

with their problems more directly. But she definitely could not handle the emotional turmoil of a separation now, on top of everything else. Even the thought of it was overwhelming.

Later that afternoon, Gail Siegel came in to see Ellie, having been referred by Dr. Seymour because of the child's persistent depression. The social worker tried to get Ellie to verbalize her feelings. After much coaxing, the child finally talked: she was scared that she would have to stay in the hospital forever; she missed home and her friends at school, and she could not understand why Mommy and Daddy were letting the doctors do so many awful things to her again. "Nobody cares how much they hurt me," she complained.

Gail listened and empathized, trying to help the child redirect her anger in more constructive ways. She explained that the sickness was not anyone's fault, that Mommy and Daddy and the doctors were all doing their best to make her well, and that if she cooperated and told the doctors what she was feeling, she would get better that much faster. But it was hard to explain to a child that curing sickness often meant causing more pain and distress, and that her parents, whom she considered omnipotent and perfect, did not have the power to make her feel better instantly. After the interview, Gail wrote a note in Ellie's chart suggesting that the child be distracted from her obsessive fears with a combination of play therapy, craftware, and tutorial work. She concluded, "Patient requires support of staff centering on positive reinforcement for efforts, positive attitude, and understanding of emotional reactions."

Tuesday, August 19, was a difficult day on Three-South. It began with a serious setback for Neal Thomas, a ten-year-old boy with AML who had received a marrow transplant from his identical-twin brother. Neal was an intelligent and cooperative child who had won over the entire nursing staff. Perhaps because his donor was genetically identical and there was no risk of GVHD, his counts had come back unusually fast, enabling him to be discharged to outpatient status after only a month in the hospital. Tuesday was the ninety-first day after Neal's transplant, and that morning he came to the Outpatient Clinic for a final checkup, since he and his family were preparing to return home to Atlanta. Dr. Krueger did a routine bone-marrow exam in the clinic and, to his shock and dismay, discovered leukemic cells in the marrow smears. He had the painful task of informing the boy's family that although they could try to get Neal back into remission with chemotherapy, the odds of success of a second transplant were now so poor as to be unacceptable. Mrs. Thomas, enraged and bitter, accused Krueger of depriving her son of hope.

Ellie's situation was also grim. Dr. Seymour told Sally that the antibiotics were lagging about two days behind her infection, which was now progressing too fast for them to control. Part of the problem was that the source of the bacteria was still not known: the child's physical exam was unremarkable, with no active or identifiable sites of infection. Seymour was also mystified by Ellie's dropping white count, which had left her dangerously short of polys. He decided that if Ellie continued to have fevers all day he would start her that evening on a third antibiotic, nafcillin, to provide coverage for a possible staph infection.

The fevers did persist into the evening, and at 5:00 P.M. Ellie was given her first intravenous dose of nafcillin. She cried as the drug went in, complaining of a burning sensation above the IV site. The nurse slowed the flow rate as much as possible, but the child continued to whimper pitifully until she finally drifted off to sleep.

On Wednesday, August 20, Ellie awoke still feverish. By now all of her counts were down: her hematocrit was 21, her white count 891 with zero polys, and her platelet count 21,000. Since her white count had fallen below 1,000, Seymour put her back in protective isolation. Ellie was also receiving massive amounts of blood products, including transfusions of platelets every day, white cells every other day, and packed red cells twice a week.

Sally found it very hard to live with the uncertainty of why Ellie's counts were falling, particularly when it was clear that the doctors were equally mystified. If the child had developed a known complication with predictable risk, treatment, and outcome, that would have been easier. But they were all in unknown territory, and not even the experts were equipped with a map or a compass. Sally found herself more frightened now than she had been during the first month after the transplant.

Wednesday afternoon, a bone-marrow aspiration was done. Ellie's tolerance of procedures had markedly decreased and she now demanded heavy sedation. Dr. Stern gave her an injection of 10 milligrams of Valium to make her groggy and went ahead with the aspiration. He made smears of the aspirate, which he immediately stained and examined under a microscope in the small lab on Three-South. The marrow specimen was extremely sparse, with a decrease in the number of red-cell precursors and megakaryocytes and a total absence of white-cell precursors, indicating that Ellie's white count would continue its slow-motion crash. Notable was the large number of dead cells, still with no known cause. Stern put aside some marrow for viral cultures and another sample to culture for its proliferative ability, in an effort to understand the failure of the marrow to thrive.

The transplant team was not going to wait much longer before they considered a "booster": a second infusion of marrow from the same donor without additional preparative chemotherapy. (A second transplant—another course of Cytoxan followed by infusion of marrow from a different donor—was not an option since Beth was the only HLA-compatible sibling.) If they did go ahead with the booster, Beth would have to undergo another marrow harvest. Dr. Seymour asked Sally outright if she thought Beth would be willing, and Sally thought she would.

Seymour wanted to hold off for another week. He could observe Ellie and obtain results from at least two more bone-marrow exams before coming to a decision on the booster. In fact, that decision would not be made by Seymour alone. If he felt it was warranted, the case would be presented at a Special Therapeutic Session: an extraordinary meeting of all the transplant attendings that was called whenever there was an important decision to be made, requiring a cost-benefit analysis or the diffusion of responsibility among the members of the team. Since each attending had his own area of expertise within the field of marrow transplantation, together they could analyze the situation from a variety of perspectives. Nonetheless, Seymour knew that it was easier to give advice about someone else's patient when you were not personally involved. Until a decision was made, he would continue to give Ellie intensive supportive care, including antibiotics and blood products.

Sally prayed that a booster could be avoided. She was very reluctant to put Beth through the pain and trauma of another marrow harvest, and she dreaded the idea of starting the hundred days over from scratch. From what she had gleaned from conversations with other parents, the odds were slim that a booster or a second transplant would be successful. She had learned that Gregory Sikes, the boy whose optimism and many laps had inspired others, had failed to engraft the first time and had required a second transplant. He had subsequently died of infection while Ellie was an outpatient.

On Wednesday evening, the identifications of the bacteria growing in Ellie's blood cultures finally arrived: *Staphylococcus epidermidis*, a common skin bacterium that caused systemic infections only in patients with virtually no polys, and *Klebsiella pneumoniae*, an infection usually seen in alcoholics and other debilitated individuals. Seymour and Stern conferred about a change in antibiotic coverage and decided to replace Ellie's carbenicillin and nafcillin with cefamandole, while continuing her gentamicin.

Early Thursday morning, Neal Thomas died. Although he had responded initially to high-dose chemotherapy and rallied briefly, the drugs had devastated his bone marrow and lowered his white count, opening him up to massive infection. He had gone into septic shock and kidney failure, all within forty-eight hours of his relapse.

The suddenness of Neal's death affected everyone on the floor. Usually a dying patient went slowly downhill over a period of weeks, giving the staff and the other families a chance to adjust gradually to the impending loss. But Neal had been doing beautifully right up to the week he died, and with a twin donor his chances had seemed better than most. In spite of Krueger's own grief, he tried to improve staff morale by reminding them that Neal had never been in complete remission before the transplant, so that his prognosis had been less than excellent from the outset.

A second blow came that afternoon when Maria Gonzales, a fourteen-year-old transplant patient with chronic GVHD who had been out nearly a year, had to be readmitted because of her rapidly deteriorating liver function.

The parents on the Unit were hit hard by the crisis. Thursday evening, several mothers, including Sally, gathered in the lounge like a group of shell-shocked Londoners during the Blitz.

"I think the odds they give you are way off," one mother mused, shaking her head. "Since I've been here, I've seen more bad than good. It seems there's almost no one who doesn't get graft-versus-host disease, and the ones who don't get it relapse or the graft doesn't take."

"I don't agree," another said. "The ones that do well you don't see because they go home. I tried a hand count last night of the people I could remember, and the success rate was below fifty-fifty, but not by much."

"When we first came it was better," Sally said, "but now it's swung the other way. Dr. Krueger told me that the statistics they give out are averages taken over a four- or five-year period."

The first mother nodded grimly. "Well, I just hope the doctors learned something from Neal that will help other patients."

"Oh, yes," Sally said quickly. "Dr. Krueger told me that they learn an enormous amount from each transplant."

The others nodded. There was a small but significant consolation in that.

32 Double-Blind

When Sally came up to Three-South the next morning, Friday, August 22, she noticed that in addition to the pink ISOLATION card on Ellie's closed door, a new blue card reading NO PREGNANT WOMEN had been posted. She was puzzled, never before having seen this message taped on a patient's door.

Catching sight of Dr. Seymour, Dr. Stern, and two residents standing by the nurses' station, Sally walked over to ask them about it. As she approached, she could overhear Stern saying, "Oh, here she comes."

"What's that new sign on Ellie's door mean?" she asked. "The one about pregnant women."

Dr. Seymour cleared his throat. "One of Ellie's urine surveillance cultures grew out positive for CMV. The culture was taken August eleventh, when she first developed a fever, but it took ten days for the CMV to grow out. We only got the results this morning."

"That's nice," Sally said. "Now tell me what CMV is."

"Well, CMV is cytomegalovirus," Seymour replied.

"It's a fairly common viral infection," Stern added, assuming the task of explanation since it was obvious that Seymour was having trouble communicating on Sally's level. "About one in every hundred persons carries CMV in his white cells, although the virus usually remains latent because the immune system keeps it under control. Still, CMV is just waiting to flourish, and it often does in transplant patients because their immune defenses are suppressed. Ellie probably picked up the virus from one of her white-cell transfusions, since it's almost inevitable that they'll include some white cells infected with CMV. The fact that the virus is in her urine but not in her blood means that she has the infection, but it hasn't yet spread throughout her body."

"So what's it doing?" Sally asked.

"It's very possible that the virus has infected her bone marrow and is causing her low white count," Stern went on. "As long as the infection stays mild, Ellie's immune system should be able to keep it under control."

"And if it doesn't stay mild?" Sally heard herself asking.

"If the infection gets out of hand, she could develop viral pneumonia and there would not be much more we could do for her."

Sally started shaking. Unable to stand it any longer, she turned and walked away. Gail Siegel passed her in the hall and thought Sally looked so terrible that she arranged with one of the residents to give her a prescription of Valium to calm her nerves.

Meanwhile, Ellie's fever continued unabated in spite of her multiple antibiotics. Her white count was down to 250 with zero polys, and her blood cultures were positive for *Staph epidermidis* for the fourth consecutive day.

After lunch on Friday, Sally met with Dr. Seymour to discuss Ellie's prognosis and treatment plan. The attending told her that although it was still conjectural whether Ellie's CMV infection was responsible for her bone-marrow suppression, it seemed likely, and the fact that they had identified a probable cause was a major step forward. "Although there are no drugs proven effective against CMV," he went on, "we would like to put Ellie on a protocol study that will help us evaluate a new antiviral drug called acyclovir, which has been shown to reduce CMV proliferation in some test-tube and animal experiments. Acyclovir is an investigational drug, meaning that it has not yet been approved by the FDA for general use. The company that makes the drug has released it to us and a few other cancer centers around the country on the condition that we participate in a controlled study of its effectiveness in humans."

Seymour went on to explain that the patients enrolled in the study were randomized into two groups. One group received acyclovir by vein, and the other group received a placebo (a harmless intravenous solution) instead of the active drug. The randomization was "double-blind," meaning that neither the families nor the medical staff knew which patients were receiving the drug and which the placebo. The only individuals who had this information were the pharmacist and one of the investigators, so that he or she could break the code at a later date and analyze the results. Samples of urine and blood, along with routine surveillance cultures, were obtained periodically while a patient was on the study. If any adverse effects of the drug were suspected, the patient would be taken off the protocol.

"I don't think I understand," Sally said when he had finished. "Do you mean to say that Ellie could be assigned to a group of patients who will not receive the drug?"

"Yes, but that doesn't mean we would be depriving her of something we know is beneficial. The question we're trying to ask is: Does this new drug really make a difference, and if so, do its suspected benefits outweigh its side effects? The fact of the matter is that we don't know whether acyclovir will do more good than harm, precisely because it's never been studied before in a careful, rigorous manner. Studies of the drug in animals have been promising but inconclusive. For example, damage to the kidneys was seen in animals who received doses higher than those being used in this study. The only way we can really prove or disprove the effectiveness of acyclovir in human beings is by putting patients on this kind of double-blind protocol."

"Can't you get a good idea of its effectiveness by giving it to a few patients and seeing how they do?" Sally asked.

"That's old-fashioned, country-doctor medicine," Seymour replied scornfully. "The major problem in clinical research is that it's very easy to succumb to wishful thinking. If you give a patient a drug and he improves, there's a great temptation to conclude that the drug is effective, when in fact the reason may lie elsewhere. A double-blind study is by far the best way to avoid this subjective factor as much as possible. Put yourself in my shoes for a minute, Mrs. Murphy. If I have a patient who's severely ill, should I use a drug that I intuitively feel might work, or one that has been scientifically demonstrated to be effective?"

Sally shrugged. "The second one, I suppose. But I'm no scientist, Dr. Seymour. All I care about is what's best for Ellie, and I find it disturbing that there might be a new treatment that she would not be allowed to get because of the toss of a coin. It's a very strange business. Isn't there any way of making sure that Ellie is in the group that gets the drug?"

Dr. Seymour shook his head. "In good conscience I couldn't order the drug for her, because it would throw off the results of the study. I realize that this kind of protocol is hard for families, and it's also hard for me, but we don't have any better way of finding out what we need to know."

Seymour remembered that when he had first learned about double-blind studies as a medical student, he, too, had been appalled. Yet over the years he had come to learn that, more often than not, a new drug's side effects turned out to do more harm than the symptoms it was meant to alleviate or cure. As his expectation of new drugs had declined, he had become increasingly convinced that controlled studies were in the best interest of the patient population. Even so, Seymour understood the hardship involved for parents like Mrs. Murphy, who were naturally so caught up in the welfare of their own child that the idea of participating in a randomized study in the name of science seemed almost perverse.

As he had expected, Sally persisted in her questioning. "What if Ellie isn't on the drug and her CMV infection gets worse?" she asked. "Will you then be able to make sure she gets the drug?"

Seymour nodded. "If the infection becomes life threatening, we have what is known as a 'compassionate-plea' protocol, which gives us the opportunity to break the code and make sure the patient gets the study drug. We don't like to do that, of course, because then we will never know how effective the drug really is. But if Ellie's fever doesn't go down in a few days, I promise that we'll break the code."

A 50-percent chance of getting the drug was better than none at all, Sally thought, and the option of the compassionate-plea protocol relieved her worst fears. At least if things got really bad the doctors would compromise some of their experimental results for the chance that Ellie's life might be saved. Thank God for that.

After she had signed the consent forms, Seymour told her that Ellie would start receiving the infusion later on that afternoon and would continue getting it three times a day for a week.

At 4:00 P.M., Nancy started a heparin lock in Ellie's right forearm. The site was very fragile and tender, but Ellie put up little resistance except to moan softly. No adverse reaction was noted as the infusion began. Sally stared up at the small bottle of clear fluid dripping into Ellie's arm, wondering whether it was the active drug or merely saline solution. Despite Seymour's justifications for the double-blind study, she still could not understand why the doctors would consciously withhold something that might possibly be of help.

Ellie ate a third of her supper and then sat up for a while in the chair next to her bed, but she remained very lethargic. Her temperature at 6:00 P.M. was 102.2°; by 9:00 P.M. it had risen to 103° and the refrigeration blanket was turned on. Due to Ellie's persistent fever and the fact that her blood cultures had once more become positive for *Staph epidermidis*, nafcillin was again included in the antibiotic regimen. Beginning at nine-thirty, Ellie received hourly minibottles of antibiotics throughout the night. She cried during the nafcillin infusions because of the stinging at the IV site. The night nurse slowed the infusion as much as possible but the pain persisted, no doubt aggravated by the hourly awakenings to change the IV bottles and take vital signs.

Ellie's fever continued through the weekend, spiking to 103° in spite of her triple antibiotic therapy. Thorough surveillance cultures were done in an effort to determine the mysterious source of the infection. Stern had noticed a healing sore on Ellie's left inner thigh, which might have been the entry point for the bacteria, but the sore had scabbed over without any improvement in the child's fevers or positive blood cultures. In addition to the progressive and persistent decline in Ellie's poly count, she was experiencing a rise in liver-enzyme levels in her blood, which indicated a deterioration of her liver function.

On Monday, August 25, Ellie had to use the refrigeration blanket for most of the day. She was very weak and cried whenever she was asked to get out of bed. Her white count was still only 561 with zero polys, and Sally asked Seymour if it wasn't due time to resort to the compassionate-plea protocol. The attending replied that he was indeed concerned that Ellie's counts were not showing signs of recovery, and that he would wait only one more day before breaking the code.

Upset and depressed about Ellie's lack of improvement, Sally went to talk with Gail Siegel. She sat in Gail's cramped office, fighting back her tears. "I don't know how much longer I can keep pushing," she said. "It's been such a long, long ordeal, and a few weeks ago it seemed as if we were so close. . . . And then everything collapsed. Now it looks as if we're starting back at zero again. If Ellie has to have a booster . . ."

The tears overflowed and ran down Sally's cheeks. Once she had started, there seemed to be no end to them. Gail handed her a tissue and waited for Sally to speak again. "I'm really scared this time," Sally whispered. "I really think we might lose her. Sometimes I just want to run a million miles away. But of course that's ridiculous. The poor child is so helpless and needs me so much. It's not her fault she's so sick."

"I haven't noticed your husband around here much," Gail said. "Is that okay with you?"

"Well, I'm not very happy about the situation," Sally replied.

"Why isn't he here? What's happening?"

"Brian's never been able to handle the disease very well. When things are good he's fine, but as soon as things turn bad he withdraws, and I'm the one who ends up with all the hard times. It makes me so mad sometimes. I'm not saying that he doesn't love Ellie in his own way, it's just that he can't accept the idea of her not doing well." She added softly, "We hardly talk anymore."

"People deal with tragedy in different ways," Gail said. "Brian obviously needs to see things in an optimistic light, so he uses a lot of denial. By withdrawing, he may think that he's protecting Ellie from his anger and grief, when in fact he's hurting her—and you."

Sally nodded. "But what can I do about it?"

"I think you should ask him directly to come down. Tell him that you understand the way he feels but that you need him here, and Ellie needs him, too. It's very important that he come in and see her, if only for a little while—whatever he can tolerate is okay. But at least he should be here, physically."

"I've said all that. He just hates to come. Brian's very good at thinking up excuses."

"Maybe your asking him to come down isn't enough. Maybe if we both ask him, he'll come. But we can't accuse him of abandoning Ellie, because that will just make him pull away further. We can try to talk things out gradually. Sally, even the best relationships get challenged in this kind of situation. There are enormous stresses and feelings of anger and resentment. The trick is to deal with these problems up front, particularly the subtle tensions that can drive deep cracks in a marriage. What do you think?"

Sally sighed heavily, but managed to say, "I'll try." After thanking Gail she went back to Ellie's room, feeling drained but a little more optimistic. When she called Brian at his office that afternoon, he seemed distant and tense. He was clearly upset by the fact that Ellie's polys were still at zero, and when Sally brought up the subject of their talking to Gail together, Brian said defensively, "I don't need to talk to a shrink."

"Brian, she's not a psychiatrist, she's a social worker. Please come. I can't take this much longer."

"Oh, all right. But I'll only talk to her a few minutes."

The Murphys met with Gail Siegel on Tuesday morning; Brian had taken the day off from work. They began by talking about Brian's refusal to accept the seriousness of Ellie's condition.

"Part of the problem may be a fear of acknowledging the situation," Gail said. "Perhaps by denying the worst you may be trying to prevent it from happening. But just because you acknowledge your fears doesn't mean they will be realized."

"But I feel so totally helpless," Brian murmured.

"Well, even if you can't control the disease, one of the things you can do now is to participate in the living that's going on. You've been isolating yourself from your child and wife, partly because you want to save yourself some pain, but you're losing precious time. I'm a believer in insurance, and the best kind of emotional insurance is that of good feelings and memories later on. You may be withdrawing now from the situation to protect yourself, but later on you may look back and say: Why did I do that? Why didn't I just go in and sit with her and hold her hand? Why couldn't I face her? That will be a much worse feeling to live with later on. Nothing makes living with leukemia easy, but there are some things you can do in the present that will make it easier in the future. And by not participating now, you're missing out on some very important times."

Brian shook his head. "It's just so tough. She's so hard to look at, and when I go in to see her there's nothing for me to say. So I go and sit there for a few minutes until it becomes unbearable and I have to leave. I feel as if her eyes are accusing me of causing all her suffering. I feel as if I'm suffocating in there—I can hardly breathe. She never talks to me. She talks to Sally, but not to me."

Gail nodded gravely. "You must feel as if you're going to drown in those silences."

"Yes. They're so incredibly awkward."

"The fact is, though, Brian, that the silence is not empty. It's a loaded time. Just being there, sitting beside her bed, tells her something—that you love her and are not afraid to be with her, that her illness isn't so terrible that it's scared you away. Words don't have to be spoken in order to express your love; the action of being there is enough. And by being there, you're available in case there's something she wants."

"But I always feel as if I should come up with something to say."

"No, you don't have to. If she has a question, she'll ask you. One of the things kids sometimes don't like is to be constantly questioned. How do you feel? What do you want? Do you need something? That's artificial. If Ellie wants something, she'll ask you."

"What if I can't stand to stay in there very long?"

"You should go in anyway, for short periods of time. Stay for as long as you can tolerate, and if you have to leave, that's okay. While you're there, though, try to be giving. There are other ways of abandoning a child besides not going to the hospital. The person who walks into the room and says, 'Oh, what a lovely day it is,' and is totally out of touch with the patient's feelings is also abandoning the child. The patient thinks, 'He really can't tolerate what's happening to me, and I can't either.' The same is true of the parent who becomes profoundly depressed. Although he may sit in a corner of the room, he withdraws and is not really there. The child thinks: 'My illness is so terrible, look what I've done to my family.'"

Brian nodded. "All right," he said wearily but with conviction. "I'll give it a try."

He did try, spending more and more time with Ellie. The next morning he took his coffee and Danish into the room and had breakfast with her, and later on he sat in the room and read the paper. It was awkward and uncomfortable for him, but he was made to realize through working with Gail and Sally that it was okay to say nothing, and that the message was still clear to Ellie. He did it—not because it came naturally, but because he was being guided to understand that it was a helpful thing to do. Gradually it became more comfortable for him.

If Ellie ever asked him for anything, such as a cup of water or something to eat, he would jump up immediately and fetch it for her. He wanted to do anything tangible he could; the hardest thing was to do nothing. In the trailer Tuesday night, Brian discussed his feelings with Sally more openly than he had in a long time. He learned to his surprise that she was experiencing many of the same things—maybe at different times and in a slightly different way, but they shared the underlying pain and anxiety.

Thereafter, Sally still did most of the physical caring for Ellie, but Brian finally became a more active participant.

On Wednesday, August 27, Dr. Seymour noted an encouraging trend: none of Ellie's blood cultures had been positive for *Staph epidermidis* since August 24, suggesting that her infection might be resolving slowly. Seymour therefore discontinued Ellie's nafcillin, while maintaining her on cefamandole, gentamicin, and the acyclovir study drug.

Later that morning, Ellie experienced some pain on the right side of her face. Although she had felt pressure and discomfort in that area for nearly two weeks, she had tried to deny it, fearing that the admission of a new symptom would lead to more unpleasant testing. Finally the pain got so bad that she begged her mother for relief. Sally told the nurse, who called in Phil Conrad to do an examination. Suspecting a sinus infection, the resident sent Ellie down to Radiology for X-rays. The skull films supported his diagnosis: there was some cloudiness on the right side of her head, indicative of chronic sinusitis.

After a consultation with Stern, Conrad decided to work up Ellie's sinus problem as a possible source of her *Staph epidermidis* septicemia (blood infection), while having her treated at the Ear, Nose, and Throat Clinic. It was also agreed to leave the child's antibiotic regimen unchanged pending further studies, but to insert another Brobiac catheter for drawing blood and administering her intravenous medications, since by now nearly all the veins in Ellie's hands and arms had collapsed. Peripheral lines would last a few hours at the most or "blow" right away: the blood return would come partway and then stop, indicating that the vein was no longer viable. Although there was the danger that the central line would become infected, further use of her small, fragile veins to administer the irritating drugs would run the even greater risk of phlebitis (inflammation and scarring of the veins).

The central-line insertion was done in the operating room under short-acting anesthesia. Because Ellie's platelet count was less than 80,000, there was a significant risk of bleeding from the procedure. She was therefore given six units of platelets before the catheter was inserted and another six immediately after. Even so, the incision continued to ooze blood, and pressure had to be applied to the site for an hour and a half. The bleeding finally stopped at 5:30 P.M., and the line was redressed without further difficulty.

On Thursday, August 28, a bone-marrow aspiration was done. Much to Seymour's surprise and delight, the aspirate contained immature white-cell precursors for the first time in three weeks. Although there were still scanty megakaryocytes, which meant that Ellie would continue to require platelet support for some time, the presence of these very young white cells in the marrow was as fortunate as it was unexpected. Seymour much preferred the counts to come back on their own without the need for a booster, but he was mystified as to why the marrow had suddenly become functional again. He could not be sure if the change was due to the acyclovir study drug or to something entirely unrelated. Here was a clear opportunity to learn about a novel phenomenon.

Sally was afraid to get too excited about the results of the bone-marrow test; she did not want to become vulnerable to disappointment once again. It was better to expect nothing at all. Even so, she could not help hoping that things might be changing for the better.

That afternoon Ellie went to the Ear, Nose, and Throat Clinic, where her infected right sinus was drained, washed, and cultured. When she came back from the clinic at 5:00 P.M. her nose was oozing blood, and it continued to do so for hours. The nurse began an infusion of concentrated platelets and applied ice packs and pressure, with minimal relief. Finally Phil Conrad inserted a gauze nasal packing along with a drip pad, which stopped the oozing. During the night, however, Ellie inadvertently pulled out the nasal packing in her sleep. By the time the night nurse discovered the bloodstained sheets and replaced the packing, Ellie had lost quite a lot of blood. A complete blood count Friday morning revealed that her hematocrit had fallen to 24, well below the normal value of 44. Nevertheless, her white count had risen sharply to 957 with 5 percent polys, reversing direction for the first time in weeks, and her fever had declined to 100.4°.

Ellie's platelet count was still only 20,000 that morning, and after an infusion of six units of concentrated platelets it rose to 30,000—a minimal improvement. During rounds, the transplant team wondered where all her platelets were going. Since Ellie showed no signs of internal bleeding and her fever was going down, it seemed most likely that her immune system was starting to recognize and destroy the imperfectly matched platelets obtained from random donors, causing the incremental increase in her platelet count following transfusions to be small and short-lived. The team therefore decided that Ellie should start receiving transfusions of matched platelets.

The doctors knew that neither parent was a good HLA match and that Beth was too young to donate large quantities of platelets. Fortunately, the Hemophoresis Center had recently installed a computer system for matching platelet donors and recipients. A comparative-pool arrangement had also been set up with other blood centers in the Red Cross registry to provide matched platelets to patients with rare HLA types.

That afternoon, Ellie received her first transfusion of HLA-matched platelets. The resulting increment was excellent: her count was 21,000 before the transfusion and 80,000 afterward.

At 4:00 P.M., Ellie returned to the ENT Clinic for another sinus drainage and irrigation. Microscopic examination of the thick white mucus obtained from her right sinus the previous day had revealed gram-positive cocci in clumps—most likely *Staph epidermidis*. Most of these organisms appeared to be partially damaged by the antibiotics, which interfered with the formation of the bacterial cell wall. This observation strongly indicated that Ellie's sinus infection had been the source of her septicemia.

It was now possible to reconstruct a plausible scenario for Ellie's illness. She had apparently contracted CMV from her white-cell transfusions after the transplant. The virus had then infected and killed most of the white-cell precursors in her bone marrow, leading to the precipitous decline in her poly count. Next the *Staph epidermidis* had apparently entered her bloodstream from a chronic source in her right sinus. This organism caused systemic infections only when there were absolutely no polys present to fight it off, as was the case with Ellie. Under these conditions, antibiotics alone were not sufficient to eradicate the infection and white-cell transfusions were too short-lived to make a significant impact. Now that Ellie's marrow was recovering and her poly count was beginning to rise, however, it seemed likely that the infection would be eliminated soon.

That evening the final dose of the acyclovir study drug was given, for a total of twenty-one doses. Since Ellie had done so well, Sally was convinced that she had received the active drug (a speculation that later proved to be true). Seymour now started Ellie on hyperalimentation through her central line, mostly with amino acids and vitamins, as a nonspecific aid to her regenerating marrow.

By Saturday, August 30, Ellie was without fever and her white count had risen to 1,300 with 52 percent polys. From then on, her white count climbed amazingly fast. On Sunday it was 3,650, more than double what it had been the day before, and on Monday it was 4,800. The rise was so rapid that at first Seymour was afraid that Ellie's leukemia had returned and that her high white count was due to blasts. He went down to the Hematology Lab and double-checked the blood smears himself to make sure that the cells were normal. The blood levels of Ellie's liver enzymes had also fallen back into the healthy range. Whether her liver abnormalities had also resulted from her CMV infection was a matter for conjecture.

Sally finally let herself be elated by the rising counts, and Ellie's spirits also improved, particularly when she was taken off the bowel prep and allowed to do laps again. Seymour said that if she maintained her current white count and remained without fever and culture-negative, she could be discharged to the Outpatient Department by the end of the week. The only other concern was that she eat more protein.

On Wednesday, September 3, Ellie's white count was 7,400 with more than 65 percent polys. She spent much of the morning doing laps with her mother and then ate a bowl of chicken soup and her favorite treat—a chocolate milkshake—for lunch. Dr. Seymour told Sally that he planned to do a bone-marrow aspiration Thursday morning to make sure that the marrow was recovering well. If there were no hitches, he would switch Ellie from IV to oral antibiotics and discharge her on Friday.

Ellie had yet to begin the final phase of her treatment, which would be

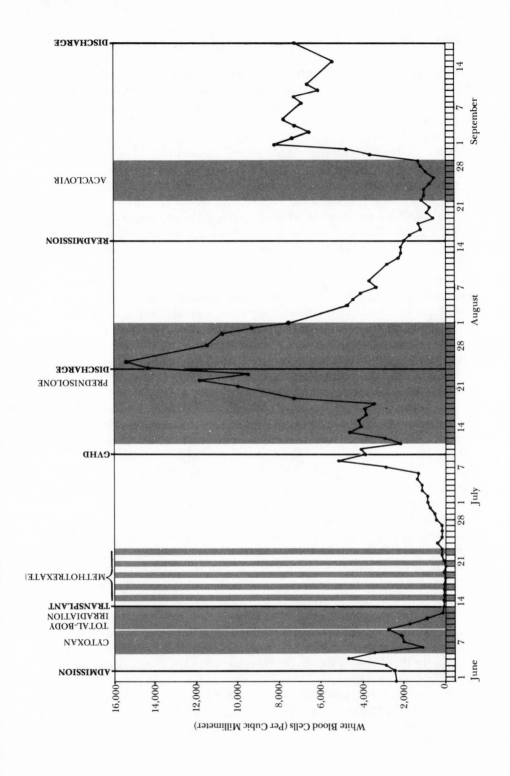

Graph of white-blood-cell count throughout Ellen Murphy's bone-marrow transplant documents the various stages of treatment, her complications, and her final recovery. During the two weeks prior to the transplant on June 13, 1980, Cytoxan chemotherapy and total-body irradiation (TBI) were used to destroy Ellie's own bone marrow, causing a rapid decline in her blood count. Her count continued to fall for a week after the transplant, approaching zero on June 18. As the graft began to take, her count rose rapidly, only to be stalled by the development of graft-versus-host disease on July 9, the twenty-sixth day post-transplant. Treatment of her GVHD with the steroid drug prednisolone caused her count to drop initially, but as her GVHD came under control, her count rose dramatically, more than doubling each day. She was discharged to outpatient care on July 24. Soon thereafter her counts of both white cells and platelets began to fall for unknown reasons, forcing a readmission on August 15. When CMV (cytomegalovirus) was discovered in her urine, the medical team suspected a viral infection of the marrow as the cause for its failure to thrive, and placed her on an experimental antiviral drug, acyclovir. The drug apparently worked, since within a week, her white count began to recover, returning to normal by September 1. She was once again discharged to outpatient status on September 18, but was still required to make daily visits to the hospital. *Graph by Sarah and Steven Black.*

done when she was an outpatient. Because leukemic recurrences after the transplant usually originated in a protected site such as the central nervous system or the testes, where systemic chemotherapy could not penetrate, additional therapy was given to these areas in order to kill off any remaining leukemic cells. Ellie would have to receive a series of five injections of methotrexate into her spinal fluid to reduce the risk of relapse from residual blasts in her brain and spinal cord. According to the transplant protocol, this procedure was supposed to begin on day seventy, but because of Ellie's low white count and infection it had been delayed until her full recovery. The therapy had some risks associated with it, but the transplant team felt they were more than counterbalanced by the potentially disastrous consequences of a leukemic relapse. Seymour told Sally that the spinal injections would prolong their stay in Baltimore by another two or three weeks, after which they would be allowed to go home. Sally was weary at the thought of yet another delay, but she accepted it as she had everything else.

Ellie's central line was removed Wednesday afternoon, and for the first time in weeks she had no IV's or catheters. The bone-marrow aspiration the next morning revealed the presence of all cell lines, although they were still somewhat sparse. Ellie's sinus film also showed improvement. She was out of bed most of the day and in good spirits, looking forward to her discharge Friday following a final ENT Clinic appointment.

On the morning of Friday, September 5, the eighty-fourth day after the transplant, Sally signed the discharge papers and packed up Ellie's things. Nancy and Gail came in to say good-bye and presented Ellie with a cupcake, complete with a candle for good luck. "Make a wish, Ellie," Sally urged. The child clapped her hands and blew out the candle. "Her pulmonary function looks good to me," Nancy said with a laugh. "She did it on the first try!"

Ellie was excited about leaving the hospital and less apprehensive than she had been the first time. Wearing the child's wig Sally had bought for her, she sat in the lobby and waited for her mother to bring the car around. As mother and daughter walked out into the sunlight together, Sally became aware for the first time of how the illness had changed Ellie: she had become quite shy and there was a noticeable stutter in her speech. Still, Sally could not help feeling a surge of real joy as they climbed into the car and drove off toward Woodbine. Ellie's setback and recovery had been so sudden and unpredictable that it would take a few days to fully absorb the events of the past few weeks. As a special treat, they stopped for a chocolate milkshake on their way back to the campground. When they arrived at the trailer, a box of flowers was propped up against the front door. The card was signed "From Brian, with love."

33 Badge of Courage

When Ellie had been rehospitalized, word had spread rapidly through the families at the trailer park, some of whom the Murphys had met only once or twice. A group of these people organized a drawing that raised a substantial amount of money, which Mrs. Smith presented to Sally on Ellie's return. Sally was very touched by this spontaneous outpouring of generosity from people she hardly knew.

The week following Ellie's discharge passed fairly routinely; they went to the hospital every day for tests and came back to Woodbine in the afternoon. The requirements for leaving the Baltimore area included an excellent physical exam, normal blood counts and blood gases, a fully cellular marrow, and normal X-rays. Ellie's white count stabilized near 7,000 and she continued to do well except for a mild case of pleurisy, an inflammation of the membrane surrounding the lungs. After the first week, Sally began to pressure Dr. Krueger—whom Ellie continued to see as an outpatient—to let them go home. Although Ellie was scheduled to get her methotrexate injections at Hopkins, Krueger called Dr. Nelson and they agreed that it would be possible for her to receive the treatments in New York. Krueger therefore informed Sally that they would be allowed to go home on Thursday, September 18—the ninety-seventh day after the transplant, just short of the hundred-day mark.

Sally asked Krueger what he felt Ellie's chances were now of living a normal life. He answered that although the child had survived the most hazardous phase of the transplant process, it would still be another year or two before she was out of danger. "You don't have to worry about her losing her counts again," he said, "and it's unlikely that she'll have any more trouble with her GVHD since it tends to burn out after a while. If it was going to convert to the chronic form, we probably would have seen some evidence of that by now."

Sally nodded. She had learned that between 15 and 25 percent of patients who survive the transplant later develop the chronic form of GVHD, which is generally less severe than the acute form but can linger for months or even years. It is characterized by red, scaling rashes on the arms, hands, and feet, mild liver abnormalities, and lowered resistance to infection. The incidence of late infections in patients with chronic GVHD is 75 percent, compared to 15 percent in transplant patients who do not develop the complication. Sally could not imagine the endless nightmare of having a child with chronic GVHD.

"Remember," Krueger continued, "that Ellie's immune system is still weak in spite of the fact that she now has plenty of polys. Since her lymphocytes are few in number and only partially mature, her immunity cannot be built up fast enough when an infection occurs. As her lymphocytes gradually mature and take on their appropriate functions, she will become progressively more resistant to infections. Until then, she must be very careful."

Sally nodded, trying to understand. "So there are different parts of the immune system that come back at different times after the transplant?"

"Precisely," Krueger replied. "I like to make the analogy that the immune system is like an orchestra, since it is made up of different types of cells with specialized functions that interact in complex ways to defend the body against infection. After a marrow transplant the entire immune orchestra must be reconstituted from scratch, and it can take up to a year before all the members are present and playing in harmony. The regeneration of the immune system after a transplant is a fascinating process to watch, since it recapitulates the original formation of the system in the fetus and the newborn child. If you were an evangelist, you might say that Ellie's immune system is being literally 'born again.'"

Because of Ellie's impaired immune function, Krueger went on, several precautions would have to be taken on her return home. She would have to continue wearing the mask, even inside the house, avoiding crowds and exposure to people with colds or contagious illnesses. Visitors would be limited to one or two close friends or relatives per day, with the number increasing by two people per week. Ellie would not be allowed to share a bedroom with either of her sisters or to visit another home for three months. She could not return to school until spring at the earliest and would have to be tutored at home.

Krueger also mentioned that because Ellie's immune system was being "reborn" she would fail to retain any immunity to viral infections, including common childhood diseases such as measles and chicken pox. The Hopkins team now recommended reimmunizing transplant recipients to the various childhood diseases a year or so after the transplant, when the ability to manufacture antibodies had returned. At that time, she would receive vaccinations for diphtheria, tetanus toxoid, mumps, measles, chicken pox, and polio. Current hospital policy was to use killed-virus vaccines for immunization, waiting until two or more years after the transplant to use live-virus vaccines because they were more effective but potentially more dangerous.

"But for now," Krueger continued, "other than infection, Ellie's biggest problem is her leukemia. Where is it, and where do we stand with it?" He explained that for patients transplanted in remission like Ellie, the rate of recurrence was much lower than for patients transplanted in relapse. The reason for a recurrence was either that the pretransplant chemotherapy and radiation had failed to kill every last leukemic cell, or that the disease had arisen in the *donor's* formerly healthy marrow. This latter phenomenon was very rare but had been proved conclusively in a few cases in which donor and recipient were of the opposite sex, so that the transplanted marrow cells and the original leukemic cells could be distinguished by their different sex chromosomes. (The discovery of cases in which the donor's healthy marrow had become leukemic in its new host had provoked endless speculation about the presence of some "transforming factor" in the recipient, capable of reinducing the disease.)

"Most leukemic recurrences occur in the first six or seven months after the transplant," Krueger said. "As simplistic as it sounds, the longer Ellie does well, the better her chances of staying well. If she survives for a year, I'll start to feel optimistic, and if she survives for two years, I'll cautiously say that she's cured."

There were also some long-term effects to watch out for, Krueger went on. One day, perhaps three or four years out, Ellie might develop some early cataracts—a clouding of the lens of the eye—as a result of her total-body irradiation; eye surgery might eventually be necessary. She would most likely remain permanently sterile, but even if she turned out to be fertile, having children would be strongly discouraged because of the risk of genetic damage. There would probably be a certain amount of growth retardation due to the effects of TBI on the pituitary gland, but the long-term impact of radiation on cognitive development and learning ability was still a matter of controversy. Ellie's lung problems were apparently minor and hence unlikely to develop into restrictive lung disease, and her liver function was also stable.

Finally, there was a very small risk that the high doses of chemotherapy and radiation Ellie had received might induce another malignancy in the future. In five hundred bone-marrow transplants done at Seattle, there had been three or four patients who had later developed other cancers, a rate of less than one percent. Krueger apologized to Sally for the long list of possible complications and reassured her that, in all probability, the worst was over.

On September 18, Brian drove down to Baltimore with Beth and Amy in preparation for Ellie's final discharge. Sally took her in that morning for her last clinic visit, which included blood work and a physical. At its conclusion, Krueger gave Sally a copy of Ellie's medical chart to give to Dr. Nelson, along with several large manila envelopes containing X-rays and a box of bone-marrow slides. Then, while Sally waited, he dictated a letter to Nelson:

Dear Dr. Nelson,

We very happily send Ellen Murphy back to her home environs and your care. She has done quite well, and we are pleased with her marrow engraftment and antileukemic response. I would like to see Ellie again on January 5, 1981, for her six-month checkup.

We appreciate your referral of this child and her family; they have been a pleasure for us to know. Thank you also for your help in her post-transplant management, including her CNS consolidation.

I will be serving as Ellie's primary physician here and am available by phone, day or night, at the numbers listed below.

Sincerely yours,
James Krueger, MD

Ellie's discharge medications were dicloxacillin (an oral antibiotic) for her sinusitis and Bactrim as prophylaxis against a variety of other infections. She would also be getting K-lyte, a potassium supplement, and a low dose of methylprednisone for her GVHD, to be gradually tapered to zero.

That night the family celebrated by going out to a restaurant at the Inner Harbor. They went early, so as to avoid the crowds at the dinner hour, and sat in a booth in the corner. The party was a joyful one. Brian had become his jovial self again, cracking jokes and making inane puns to amuse the children. In Sally's euphoria she was convinced that their problems were finally over: now that Ellie was well again, Brian would become a true husband and father. Although she knew that Ellie's lease on life was still tenuous, she felt only optimism; just the fact that maintenance chemotherapy would no longer be needed was something to be thankful for.

Beth, too, was in good spirits. She was receiving a great deal of attention now that the transplant had worked after all. "Look how wonderful it is that you helped your sister," her mother said, giving her a hug. Beth was grateful that her private atonement had allowed the bone marrow to grow back. Her only regret was that the scars from the operation were already fading from her hips; she had felt proud looking at them in the mirror or showing them off to her girl friends.

That night the Murphys stayed at the Sheraton; Brian's uncle and aunt had also driven down that afternoon and were sleeping overnight at the trailer, with the intention of towing it back to New Jersey the following morning.

Friday afternoon, the Murphys returned to Menlo Park. Sally felt her excitement rise as they drove through the center of town and turned onto their street. Ellie was disoriented; everything looked new and yet strangely familiar, like the landscape of a dream. As they neared the house, Sally saw to her surprise that an old sheet had been hung from the jutting eaves; painted on it in large red letters were the words WELCOME HOME, ELLIE AND SALLY! Thrilled, Sally rushed to the front door and into the house, which was elaborately decorated with balloons and streamers. The kitchen table was arranged with party settings and placemats, along with a chocolate cake, a can of Hawaiian Punch, and a large bottle of wine. There was also a brief note, signed by Cindy Lewis. "Have a party!" it said, and the Murphys proceeded to do just that.

Over the next few days, however, Sally's euphoria faded. She had been building up Ellie's discharge in her mind as the great day when all would be well, and it was sobering to realize that the transplant had been merely a hurdle; they were not yet out of the woods. She could find no particular comfort in the remission, not until the doctors could say with complete certainty that it was a cure. Until then the transplant had merely reinstated the fragile status quo that had existed before the relapse, only now their lives were even more restricted than before. For at least a year she would have to watch carefully over Ellie, having to cope with the constant fear of infection or relapse, and the hospital would remain a dominating presence in their lives.

Sally recalled the lists of possible complications that had been presented in great detail. Back then she had listened to that seemingly endless litany of horrors and assured herself that there was no real choice. "That may be the price we'll have to pay," she had rationalized, "but at least she'll be alive." The idea of life at any cost had sustained her for a long time. Now that Ellie was home and the intensity of the hospital stay was behind them, however, Sally resented the child's disabilities. Ellie walked with a perpetual stoop and a slight limp, coughing incessantly and sleeping much of the day. The low doses of steroids she was getting made her moody and gave her cravings for pickles and candy bars. Sally desperately wanted her whole child back again—wanted her fine.

On Wednesday, September 24, the day of Ellie's checkup at Memorial, Sally took the bus into the city with her. As they found their way to the last two empty seats together in the back of the bus, other passengers stared openly at the surgical mask covering the lower half of the child's face. Sally overheard someone saying, "Did you see that little girl with the mask on? I wonder if she's catching." The fear and ignorance reflected in that remark saddened Sally; she could only imagine the emotional strains Ellie would soon confront in the reactions of other children and their families and the intrusive stares and comments of strangers. Thank God the child was still young and not particularly self-conscious; it would be much worse for a teenager. Sally remembered what Nancy had told them on the day of Ellie's discharge: "That mask is nothing to be ashamed of; it's a badge of courage." But she wondered whether Ellie could really learn to feel that way.

From the Port Authority Bus Terminal in Manhattan, they took a cab across town to Memorial Sloan-Kettering. The waiting room of the Children's Day Hospital had changed little since their first visit there, two years before. Sally looked around her at the drawn faces of the parents and the smiles of the children playing nearby, those on chemotherapy immediately recognizable by their sparse hair and steroid-swollen cheeks. These were new faces to Sally, but she felt compassion for all of them. She remembered how terrified she had been during Ellie's first hospitalization and wished these parents well, hoping for their sake that they would not have to go through the same ordeal. If she had learned anything from the whole experience, it was the ability to care genuinely about relative strangers. She was now more able to empathize with the sufferings of others, and she knew which words comforted and which did not.

Ellie weighed in and then went for a finger-stick. After a fifteen-minute wait, the receptionist called her name and Dr. Nelson came out to greet them. Sally was happy to see him, and he seemed equally pleased. Ellie cowered from him shyly, clinging to her mother's leg. He crouched down and stroked the short growth of fine, curly hair on the child's head. "Hello, Ellie," he said. "It seems like they did a wonderful job with you down in Baltimore, though I bet you're glad to be home. Let's have a look at how you're doing."

They went into the examining room, and Sally gave him the chart, X-rays, and bone-marrow slides from Hopkins, which he looked over quickly. He then proceeded to do a complete physical exam, which was normal except for Ellie's cough and mild pleurisy. Nelson said that he wanted to wait a month before starting the methotrexate injections in order to allow the lung problem to clear up and Ellie's hematocrit to recover fully. According to the transplant protocol, Ellie would receive five spinal injections of methotrexate over a seventeen-day period. For the twenty-four hours after each dose, she would be given frequent tablets of Leucovorin (folinic acid), an antidote to methotrexate. The tablets were required because methotrexate injected into the spinal fluid could diffuse out into the general circulation, raising the concentration of the drug in the bloodstream to toxic levels.

Between clinic visits, the Murphy family tried to adjust to their new constrained life-style. Ellie had assumed that once she was back home her life would begin again as it had before. She wanted desperately to be like other children and to forget all her terrible experiences; she even refused to talk about the hospital when asked. Yet there were many limitations placed on her. She was not supposed to associate with many other children at first, and she could not spend more than a few minutes outdoors for fear the sunlight would reactivate her GVHD. The surgical mask was supposed to be worn at all times around the house, yet whenever Sally looked it was dangling from the child's neck or off completely. Sally would scold her, and Ellie would reply, "I forgot it," or "It just fell off." As a result, Sally was particularly careful about whom she let into the house. No one came in with the slightest cold, a rule that Beth resented because her friends were often excluded.

Every weekday morning a tutor came from the school to work with Ellie. When Beth returned from school in the afternoons, she and Ellie would play indoor games together and watch TV, but inevitably Beth got bored and wanted to play outside, and Ellie would not be able to join her.

It did not take long for Ellie to become irritable from being cooped up inside. She had always been a demanding and assertive child, and now she was making Sally's life miserable. The topic came up during a clinic visit a few weeks later.

"How are things at home?" Nelson asked, after completing Ellie's physical exam. "Since Ellie isn't in school, how does she amuse herself all day?"

"She's driving me nuts, let me tell you," Sally said. "She's gotten irritable again and throws temper tantrums if she doesn't get her own way, which she hasn't pulled in a long time."

"Ellie, how come?" Nelson asked the child, who became embarrassed and hid her face in her hands.

"You can talk, it's all right," Sally told her. "I'm not hollering at you." She turned back to Nelson. "Last week I sent her to her grandmother's house for a few days because I just couldn't take it anymore. Ellie took chocolate syrup and put it in the dishwasher, with clean dishes! I didn't realize what had happened until I got home from food shopping and went to take the dishes out. I had so much to do that day and I was exhausted. When I saw the chocolate syrup over everything, that was the last straw. 'I don't believe this is happening,' I kept saying and just cried and cried. Lord, it really wasn't my day. If Ellie's immune function doesn't improve soon, so she can go somewhere and do something . . ."

"She's been indoors for a long time," Nelson said. "I bet that's part of the problem. Right, Ellie?"

"Yes," Sally answered. "We just have to get her out of the house. There's not enough to do at home, so she gets into trouble. She has to be with other kids. Her grandmother let her outside a little bit in the backyard last week, but I hate to leave her out—I'm always afraid that something's going to happen."

"It's not the germs floating around in the air that we worry about so much," Nelson assured her. "It's what people carry that can cause problems. As long as she wears her mask, I don't see any problem with her playing outside with a limited number of children, so long as she doesn't overexert herself."

Sally breathed a sigh of relief. "Thanks, doctor. You just saved my sanity."

Although Ellie was delighted with her new freedom, her lung capacity was not up to par with that of her neighborhood friends and she was often left behind, exhausted after a few minutes of exertion. Stubborn, she struggled hard to keep up even as her pleurisy grew progressively worse. When part of her lung collapsed a week later and she had to be rushed to the hospital, Sally could not help feeling that whatever there was to get, Ellie got.

The doctors at Memorial admitted that they were not sure what had caused Ellie's latest problem. For a while Sally debated taking her back to Baltimore, but the pleurisy slowly resolved itself and Ellie seemed to be building up her strength once more.

Sally felt she had come to a crossroads. She urgently wanted to get on with her life, having become so acutely aware of its preciousness and fragility. Yet she was burdened by a persistent sadness. She was not ungrateful, because she knew of so many families at Memorial and Hopkins who had not been as lucky as theirs, but she refused to accept at face value what they had gone through; she could not put her bitterness behind her and say, "Well, it happened, but look at what we still have."

Instead she found herself dwelling on the unfairness of it, mulling over the different possibilities of why it happened and what might have caused it. The disease seemed so incredibly arbitrary the way it hit one family and not another. Whenever she heard about other people's children or saw happy families in the street, she could not help feeling a twinge of envy and then anger that her own family's life had been so disrupted.

Her marriage to Brian was still intact, but she was not sure how much longer it would last. Ironically, her newfound sense of self had subjected the relationship to new strains. Forced to become independent and self-reliant because of Brian's failure to confront the realities of the illness, she had become aware of her own hidden strengths. Now she wanted to be something more than just a wife and mother. After years of boredom and frustration as a housewife, with few creative outlets other than her unpaid work on behalf of the Junior Women's Club, she was beginning to think seriously about getting a part-time job. She and Cindy Lewis had discussed the possibility and decided to go job hunting together for mutual support.

When Sally brought up this idea with Brian he acquiesced, but she could tell that he was threatened by the changes in their relationship that the illness had brought about. He was mercurial in his moods, sometimes bringing her unexpected gifts and flowers but just as often coming home from work without even a greeting and spending the evening in somber silence.

Now that Ellie was doing well, Brian had doubtless assumed that their lives would revert to the old status quo, with Sally happily returning to her former role. But in fact everything had changed. Sally could not forget how Brian had repeatedly let her down, and as a result there had been a major power shift in the relationship. She wondered if he was capable of adjusting to her new needs and desires, knowing that she was willing to compromise only so far.

Barbara Murphy came to visit the family fairly often these days. Ever since the chicken-pox crisis, Barbara had remained closer to Sally and the children than to her brother. She seemed much happier of late, having recently quit her job at New York Hospital to work as a nurse for a large corporation. Relieved of the enormous responsibility and tension that burdened a floor nurse in a large urban hospital, she was enjoying the relaxed pace, regular hours, and lack of hassles in her new environment. In retrospect, she concluded that hospital nursing had never really fit her personality. Brian's parents also kept in close touch with the family, and the children spent a few days with them every few weeks so that Sally could have some time to herself for job hunting.

In mid-November, the day that the methotrexate injections were to begin, Dr. Nelson took a sample of Ellie's spinal fluid for analysis. Microscopic examination revealed the presence of some suspicious-looking cells—atypical lymphocytes that might possibly have been blasts. Concerned, Nelson started the spinal treatments immediately. After the five doses had been administered, however, Ellie's spinal fluid was clear. Either the questionable cells had been destroyed or they had merely gone into hiding; there was no way of knowing for sure. Since no evidence of the cells remained, Nelson deemed it unnecessary to inform Sally. The diagnosis had not been clear in any case and there was no need to alarm her further. It was almost certain that the chemotherapy had done its job.

34 Epilogue

After a long, frustrating search, Sally finally found a low-paying trainee position with a real-estate chain, with good opportunities for advancement, and two days later Cindy Lewis took a part-time retail-sales job in a nearby shopping center. In early December, Sally and Brian decided to live apart for a few months. They had begun seeing a marriage counselor and the temporary separation was not done in anger but was rather part of a plan, approved by the counselor, to save the marriage. They both needed time to think things through and let their resentments cool down, so that the marriage would not continue to deteriorate.

It was Sally who had first suggested that they live apart for a while. She had struggled with the relationship a lot longer than Brian had, primarily out of fear; she had not been sure she could manage alone with the children. It had taken her a long time to realize that nobody was going to relieve her of her sick child and her failing marriage; she had to take responsibility for her own life. She felt that she had grown enormously from the experience of caring for Ellie and wanted Brian to do some growing of his own, so that he could feel comfortable accepting her as the equal she had become. She no longer needed him the way she once had, but she was willing to work at the marriage as long as he was, too. Of course it was better for the children to have their father at home, but not if that meant being surrounded by an atmosphere of tension.

Brian did not like the way Sally had changed—her abrasive self-assertiveness angered him—but he did not like the way he was acting, either. He needed time to himself to sort things out and to see whether he could find a role that would make him happier and be better for the family. The way things were going, with his current confusion and moodiness, he wasn't doing anyone a favor by staying.

On December 15, a Saturday, Brian moved out. He packed up his station wagon and drove to the one-bedroom apartment he had rented in a large building in Park Slope, Brooklyn, a short commute from Manhattan. Having been passed over for promotion in his old job because of his preoccupation with the illness, he had found a new position selling advertising space for a national magazine so that he could work full time in the city.

According to the informal agreement, Brian spent time with the children every weekend and continued to support them. Besides the weekly sessions with the marriage counselor, he and Sally had dinner together every Sunday evening after he brought the children back. The hope was that they might have an easier time getting along after Sally had the weekend to unwind.

Inevitably, Sally found it very difficult to live alone with the three girls during the week. She liked her new job, but her entry-level responsibilities were tedious and she was painfully insecure about making mistakes. A third of her meager salary went to baby-sitters, who stayed with Ellie and Amy during the day whenever Brian's parents (who remained very involved with the children despite the separation) were unavailable. Beth would get off the school bus at the Lewises' and stay there until four-thirty, when Sally returned home from work.

Sally discovered that she had proved her independence and strength to the point where it made her unhappy. Could she adjust to a relationship with Brian and still be her new self? Although the sessions with the marriage counselor were slow and painful, she did feel that they were gradually making progress to a new understanding of each other. The hope of starting over in the marriage, with a new set of assumptions and expectations, remained alive.

As the date of Ellie's six-month checkup neared, Sally became increasingly anxious. On Sunday, January 4, 1981, Sally dropped Beth and Amy off with Brian's parents and drove down to Baltimore with Ellie. The two of them stayed overnight at the Sheraton and then went to the Outpatient Department the next morning for a nine o'clock appointment. Over the next two days Ellie underwent a battery of tests: blood was drawn for cell counts, chemistries, bacterial and viral cultures, hormone studies, and a complete immunological work-up; a bone-marrow aspiration and a spinal tap were performed under heavy sedation; an electrocardiogram was done to check her heart for long-term damage from the chemotherapy; plus X-rays, urinalysis, and throat cultures. Tuesday morning she went from one appointment to another: a dentist inspected her teeth, a dermatologist did a skin biopsy, and a respiratory therapist gave her a pulmonary-function test.

Finally she saw Dr. Krueger for a complete physical exam. He was impressed with her progress: she had grown taller, her hair was coming in nicely, and some of her steroid-induced swelling had gone down now that she was off the drug. He told Sally that Ellie was doing much better than expected; she had passed all her tests with flying colors.

The weight that had been pressing on Sally's chest for weeks lifted immediately. "Oh, thank God," she whispered.

"I'd like to see Ellie in another two weeks for a complete evaluation of her immune status," Krueger went on. "If things look good, she'll be able to stop wearing the mask and might be able to return to school in the spring."

"That would be wonderful!" Sally said with a sigh. "Here's hoping."

Even Ellie seemed to perk up at the possibility.

"See you in two weeks, then. The receptionist will give you an appointment."

Driving back home from Baltimore after the checkup, Sally felt a sense of peace come over her for the first time in months. Knowing that Ellie was doing well made her grateful, although she doubted that she would ever be able to relax completely. The disease would remain unpredictable; they would have to take it one day at a time. She did look forward to the spring, when Ellie might go back to school, and the summer. Next September would be the third anniversary of the illness, and if Ellie was still in remission . . . But she did not look any further than that. It was just too frightening.

Her thoughts were interrupted by a tug from Ellie. "Mommy, can we stop for a chocolate milkshake?"

Appendix
The Varieties of Leukemia,
Their Classification,
and Incidence

According to statistics compiled by the American Cancer Society, leukemia strikes some 21,500 persons in the United States annually and is responsible for approximately 15,000 deaths each year. Although leukemia is the most common cancer of childhood and the second leading cause of death between the ages of two and fifteen (exceeded only by accidents), the disease actually occurs considerably more often in adults: some 19,000 adults develop leukemia annually, compared with about 2,500 children.

There are several varieties of leukemia. They are classified according to two criteria: the source and type of the leukemic cells, and the rate of the disease process. About 90 percent of all cases of leukemia involve either the lymphocytes, formed in the lymph glands (spleen, thymus, and lymph nodes), or the polys or granulocytes, formed in the myeloid tissue (bone marrow). Thus leukemias are classified as being either lymphocytic or myelocytic.

In addition, physicians have long distinguished clinically between acute leukemias, which in the absence of treatment have a rapidly fatal course, and chronic leukemias, which can smolder on for years without killing the patient. The proliferating cells in the acute leukemias are blasts: immature white cells that have been arrested early in their developmental sequence and hence are nonfunctional and unable to fight off infection. In the chronic leukemias, on the other hand, the white cells are mature and seem capable of combating infection; there are simply too many of them. Patients with chronic leukemia therefore tend to suffer fewer infections than those with acute leukemia, but their leukemic cells often infiltrate into vital organs and tissues, leading to serious complications. Ironically,

301

in recent years the terms "acute" and "chronic" have become misleading because there are now effective and sometimes curative treatments for the acute leukemias but not for the chronic ones. As a result, a child with acute leukemia may far outlive a child with chronic leukemia.

The two types of leukemic cells and the two clinical categories can therefore be combined to yield four major forms of human leukemia: acute lymphoblastic (ALL), chronic lymphocytic (CLL), acute myeloblastic (AML), and chronic myelocytic (CML). In addition, there are rare leukemias affecting other types of white blood cells (such as monocytic leukemia, involving the large amoeboid scavenger cells of the immune system) or the red-blood-cell precursors in the bone marrow (erythroleukemia). But 90 percent of patients with leukemia have one of the four major types listed above.

Although leukemia can strike at any age, including just after birth or even in the womb, the four major types of leukemia generally affect different age groups. ALL accounts for about 80 percent of childhood cases and has a peak incidence in three-to-four-year-olds. For unknown reasons, the incidence of ALL is also slightly higher among boys than girls (1.3 to 1) and much higher among whites than nonwhites (2 to 1), although nonwhites do not respond as well to therapy. AML occurs at all ages but is primarily a disease of young adults. It accounts for less than 20 percent of childhood cases, although it is more common than ALL during the first year of life. The incidence of AML in whites and nonwhites is approximately the same. Children with Down's syndrome (mongolism), a cluster of birth defects that results from an extra chromosome, are fifteen times more likely to contract ALL or AML than normal children are.

The chronic leukemias are exceedingly rare in childhood, accounting for only about 2 percent of cases. CML tends to affect adults between the ages of thirty and fifty, whereas CLL occurs primarily in older people between fifty and seventy.

This book describes in detail the treatment of ALL, the most common form of childhood leukemia. Since the less common varieties of childhood leukemia— AML and CML—differ significantly in their symptoms, prognoses, and treatments, a description follows. (CLL is hardly ever seen in children and hence will not be discussed here.)

Acute Myeloblastic Leukemia (AML)

The presenting clinical symptoms of AML are very similar to those of ALL: anemia, infection, bruising and petechiae, a history of unexplained fevers, and bone tenderness, particularly in the ribs or sternum. Nevertheless, there are major therapeutic and prognostic differences between the two types of acute leukemia.

Diagnosis of AML is made on the basis of characteristic changes in the peripheral blood and marrow. The presence of leukemic cells with typical blue-black granules helps distinguish AML from ALL, as does the presence in the cells of Auer rods, distinctive red-purple rod-shaped inclusions.

While the complications of AML are generally similar to those of ALL, an important difference is that in AML the risk of central-nervous-system involvement is considerably less, so that prophylactic radiation to the brain and the injection of chemotherapy into the spinal fluid is not an important component of therapy.

Unfortunately, the treatment of AML has not yet approached the dramatic success story of childhood ALL. Vincristine and prednisone, so effective in inducing remission in ALL with relatively low toxicity, have little effect on AML. Because the drugs that do work are less effective and highly toxic, complications of AML therapy are more common.

As with ALL, combination-chemotherapy regimens for AML consist of four phases: (1) remission induction, in which drugs are chosen that will quickly destroy large numbers of leukemic cells and produce a clinical remission; (2) consolidation or intensification, in which the patient is given repeating cycles of the same or different drugs in an attempt to destroy as many hidden leukemic cells as possible; (3) maintenance therapy, consisting of repeating cycles of various antileukemic drugs to maintain the remission; and (4) reinduction, in which patients who fail to obtain a complete remission, or who subsequently relapse, are subjected to second or even third drug combinations in an effort to obtain a complete remission.

In AML, induction is usually attempted with a combination of three drugs: cytosine arabinoside (Ara-C), daunomycin, and 6-thioguanine. These drugs all interfere with the synthesis of the long, spiraling DNA molecules that encode the information of the genes. Since the continually dividing leukemic cells absorb the drugs more readily than do the intermittently dividing normal cells, they are killed off faster.

Ara-C is given as a continuous infusion or an intravenous injection; its major toxic side effects include severe suppression of the bone marrow, nausea and vomiting, and liver dysfunction. Daunomycin (also called daunorubicin) is an antibiotic derived from a fungus; it is given intravenously or as an infusion over several hours. Its major toxic side effects include severe bone-marrow depression, ulcerations of the mouth and throat, hair loss, and irreversible cardiac toxicity. Thioguanine, given orally, also suppresses the bone marrow.

About 60 percent of patients with AML achieve a complete remission; those who fail to go into remission usually die in a matter of months. The duration of the first remission averages from nine to eighteen months. There has been a steady increase in the number of patients surviving one year, from 8 percent in the 1950s to about 25 percent today, but it is still unusual for the first remission to last for more than a year and a half. (In contrast, remissions of childhood ALL usually last two or three years and, in 50 percent of cases, five years or more.) Second remissions of AML are rare, and with each relapse the remission rate following reinduction declines and the duration of the remission is shorter. Thus, the major way to prolong survival is to increase the duration of the first remission.

To accomplish this, one approach has been late intensification therapy, consisting of a combination-chemotherapy regimen, different from the one used in induction, that is administered after the patient has been in remission for a year. This protocol has been associated with a more favorable duration of the first remission. Virtually all recurrences take place within the first two years following discontinuation of therapy, and the risk of relapse declines progressively the longer a patient remains in first remission. Although the duration of remission has not improved a great deal for the average patient, 4 percent of patients with AML are alive after five years, and a small but detectable proportion now appear to have been rendered free of any signs of their disease.

Further improvements in therapy for AML will require better methods of supportive care for the patient. There is unfortunately a very thin line between the amount of chemotherapy that will destroy the leukemic cells and that which will destroy the normal marrow, making it difficult for healthy blood counts to recover. Because of the nature of the disease and the intensity of the treatment, about 15 percent of AML patients develop blood infections, 27 percent get pneumonia, and a significant fraction (about 25 percent) die during the first two weeks of attempted remission induction. The major infectious threats to patients with AML are bacteria such as *Pseudomonas* and *Staphylococcus aureus*, viruses such as hepatitis and chicken pox, and fungal infections.

To reduce the probability of infection, chemotherapy is increasingly being administered in a laminar-airflow room, or "life island," in which filtered air flows in only one direction across the patient's bed to minimize the risk of bacterial contamination. The patient's skin, mouth, and gastrointestinal tract may also be sterilized with antibiotic "cocktails" and lotions.

A second approach has been to do bone-marrow transplants on patients with AML in first remission (for those fortunate enough to have a compatible donor). Since such patients are in good clinical condition before the transplant, about 50 percent achieve a long-term remission or apparent cure.

Chronic Myelocytic Leukemia (CML)

The typical patient with CML is middle aged, although the disease also strikes infants, children, and young adults. Before the symptoms of CML become apparent, the patient may be asymptomatic for a period ranging from a few months to a year; even so, telltale signs of incipient trouble include a slightly elevated white count or a reduced number of lymphocytes. As the number of leukemic cells increases, generalized metabolic symptoms appear, including low-grade fever, fatigue, weight loss, and night sweats. On physical exam, the spleen is often massively enlarged, although the lymph nodes are rarely swollen. Blood tests reveal a white count ranging from 20,000 to 50,000 per cubic millimeter, slight to moderate anemia, and an increased platelet count that declines over time. The course of the disease is complicated by low blood counts and the massive enlargement of the spleen. Nevertheless, patients with CML usually survive, even without treatment, for three years or more from the time of diagnosis.

In approximately 90 percent of patients with CML, the disease is associated with the appearance of a chromosomal abnormality in the leukemic cells: one of the chromosomes in pair 22 loses some of its genetic material, which is transferred to another chromosome. This defect is known as the Philadelphia chromosome because it was discovered by Peter C. Nowell of the University of Pennsylvania

School of Medicine, located in West Philadelphia. A study of pairs of identical twins (who are born with exactly the same chromosomes), one of whom had CML, revealed that only the twin having the disease carried the Philadelphia chromosome. This finding indicates that the Philadelphia chromosome is an acquired defect rather than an inherited trait. It is not known, however, what causes the defective chromosome to appear or how it influences the course of CML.

The massive enlargement of the spleen characteristic of CML is due to the infiltration of leukemic cells and can become very painful. In addition, the patient may suffer from overactivity of the spleen, or hypersplenism. Normally the spleen acts as a filter for the blood, screening out senescent red cells and platelets. When the spleen becomes enlarged, it starts doing its job too well, removing perfectly healthy red cells and platelets and thereby causing anemia and low platelet counts. To treat the pain and hypersplenism caused by CML, small pulses of radiation (about 100 rads) to the spleen or courses of chemotherapy can be administered, resulting in a temporary shrinkage of the organ. Chemotherapy is considered superior because it is continual rather than episodic, but neither therapy actually increases survival time; it merely reduces the discomfort associated with the symptom.

Some authorities recommend removing the enlarged spleen surgically—a procedure called a splenectomy—early in the course of CML, but no evidence suggests that this approach prolongs life or improves symptoms better than chemotherapy. In fact, there is a high risk associated with the operation due to the increased chances of infection, and in some cases the white-cell and platelet counts rise precipitously after the spleen has been removed.

In about 80 percent of cases of CML, the disease eventually converts to an acute phase in which the leukemic cells become progressively less mature. When this happens, the bone marrow suddenly unloads hundreds of billions of blasts into the bloodstream, causing what is known as a "blast crisis" in which the patient's white count may rise to over 100,000 in a short time. In the majority of patients undergoing this acute phase, it is indistinguishable from AML, but unfortunately blast crisis is much more aggressive and resistant to treatment than even AML. (A minority of patients in blast crisis have leukemic cells that resemble lymphoblasts, respond to ALL-type therapy, and have an enzyme marker characteristic of ALL.) Patients in blast crisis seldom live more than several months, and remissions, if obtained at all, are partial and of short duration. As in all forms of acute leukemia, the primary causes of death are infection and internal bleeding.

A disturbing feature of CML is that it is almost impossible to predict when blast crisis will occur, although the terminal phase of the illness may be announced by an unexplained fever, sudden enlargement of the liver or spleen, or a low platelet count and anemia. Some unfortunate patients develop blast crisis within six months of diagnosis, whereas others enjoy very prolonged periods of survival—up to twenty years—before the disease suddenly accelerates and kills them. It is known, for example, that patients who lack the Philadelphia chromosome respond less well to therapy and have earlier blast crises. Their median survival is approximately one year, compared to three or four years for patients with the Philadelphia chromosome.

In marked contrast to ALL, little progress has been made in the treatment of CML over the past twenty-five years. Since at present no drugs or drug combinations exist that can eliminate all or even most of the chronic leukemia cells, cure is not possible and treatment is aimed at palliation: relieving symptoms or preventing their onset. Although complete remissions can be achieved with chemotherapy, the Philadelphia chromosome persists in marrow cells even during remissions, suggesting that the disease has not been cured. Even so, while the length of survival is variable, 20 to 25 percent of patients achieve remissions lasting from five to ten years.

CML is treated intermittently in the chronic phase with chemotherapy to reduce enlargement of the spleen or to control excessively elevated or rapidly rising white-cell counts. The drugs employed are known as alkylating agents and work by cross-linking the complementary strands of the DNA double helix so as to block cell division; the two drugs used most often for CML are busulfan and phenylalanine mustard. Busulfan's major side effects include bone-marrow depression, which may persist for weeks after administration, fibrosis (the formation of fibrous tissue) in the marrow and other organs, and an unexplained darkening of the skin. Phenylalanine mustard also has a prolonged suppressant effect on the marrow and, more rarely, can cause gastrointestinal upsets. Hydroxyurea is employed when patients no longer respond to the alkylating agents.

Another approach to controlling the chronic phase of the disease has been the use of a continuous-flow blood processor to remove large numbers of leukemic white cells from the blood before returning it to the patient. This process, known as leukophoresis, must be done daily for a week or two in order to reduce significantly enlargement of the spleen, and it is most effective in conjunction with chemotherapy.

The treatment of blast crisis with chemotherapy employed for AML has been singularly ineffective. A newer approach has been to treat blast crisis with vincristine and prednisone for two or three weeks, and if remission is not induced, to shift to a combination of cyclophosphamide (another alkylating agent), vincristine, cytosine arabinoside, and prednisone. Relatively long partial remissions have been obtained with this regimen without severe toxicity.

Bone-marrow transplantation is just beginning to be applied to the treatment of CML. The initial approach was to freeze a sample of the patient's marrow during the chronic phase and then, when he went into blast crisis, to give him a transplant of his own marrow in an effort to restore the chronic phase of the disease. Unfortunately, the remissions achieved were invariably short-lived because it was impossible to eradicate the acute disease once the patient was in blast crisis. As a result, this approach has been abandoned. Nevertheless, transplants are now being attempted between identical twins or HLA-identical siblings in the chronic phase, before the disease has undergone blastic transformation, in an effort to achieve long-term remissions.

Glossary

Acyclovir: an antiviral drug shown to be particularly effective against viruses of the herpes type.

ALL: acute lymphoblastic leukemia, the most common form of childhood leukemia.

AML: acute myeloblastic leukemia, which accounts for about 18 percent of childhood cases. It is primarily a disease of adolescents and young adults.

Anemia: low red-cell count, associated with a decreased oxygen-carrying capacity of the blood. It has several causes, ranging from iron deficiency to leukemia. Symptoms include pallor, weakness, headache, shortness of breath, and rapid heartbeat.

Antibody: a protein molecule that helps fight infection by attaching to the surface of invading bacteria or viruses and clumping them together so that they can be more easily engulfed and destroyed by white blood cells.

Antigen: any substance that, when injected into the body, stimulates the production of antibodies.

Antiserum (also, immune serum): blood serum from animals or humans containing specific antibodies to a virus or bacterium. When introduced into a patient's body, an antiserum can produce passive immunity against the original infectious agent.

Aplasia: a severe deficiency of normal blood cells of all types, due to the suppressant effect of leukemia or chemotherapy on the bone marrow.

Aplastic anemia: a severe shortage of blood cells of all types, due to the failure of the bone marrow to produce new cells. It has been treated successfully with bone-marrow transplantation.

Attending: an attending physician; a member of the senior hospital staff who is ultimately responsible for the patients in his or her care, and directs their treatment by the house officers.

Atypical lymphocyte: a lymphocyte that, when examined under the microscope, shows abnormal features such as vacuoles (air bubbles) in the cytoplasm, a distorted or lobulated nucleus, or nucleoli—bluish spots within the cell nucleus reflecting intense gene activity.

Babinski's sign: a neurological test that reveals the presence or absence of damage to the central nervous system. A pointed object, such as a key or a pen, is drawn across the bottom of the patient's foot; if the patient's toes curl up instead of down, this response suggests a lesion in the brain.

Benadryl: trade name for a preparation of diphenhydramine, an antihistamine that can be administered orally or by injection to prevent or to treat severe allergic reactions, such as those sometimes associated with drugs or multiple transfusions of blood products.

Betadine: trade name for preparations of povidone-iodine, a yellow-brown antiseptic solution applied to a patient's skin before surgery.

Bilirubin: a yellow pigment formed when the hemoglobin in red blood cells is broken down. Bilirubin is normally excreted from the body in urine and feces; in various disease states it can accumulate, causing jaundice.

Biopsy: removal of a small sample of living tissue for examination, e.g., from the liver or the skin.

Blast: an immature blood cell found in the bone marrow. In leukemia, a line of white blood cells stops maturing at this early stage and continues to proliferate, flooding the body with useless cells.

Blood-brain barrier: a functional barrier that permits some substances to pass freely between the blood and the brain, but severely hinders the passage of others. Most antileukemic drugs are unable to cross the blood-brain barrier into the central nervous system.

Blood gases: a blood test in which newly oxygenated blood is drawn from an artery in the wrist so as to determine how much oxygen and carbon dioxide are in the bloodstream—an index of lung function. The test also reveals the acid-base balance of the blood.

Blood plasma: the clear yellowish fluid portion of the blood and lymph in which the various blood cells are suspended.

Blood serum: the clear fluid, enriched in antibodies, remaining after the blood has clotted.

Blood type: the chemical identity of red blood cells, defined by several systems of marker molecules (antigens) on the surface of the cells that are specified by genes, and hence differing among individuals.

Bone-marrow aspiration: removal of a small amount of bone marrow from the hip or sternum by suction through a needle; the sample is then either smeared on glass slides and examined under a microscope or sent off for chemical analysis. The procedure is done using a local anesthetic or a short-acting general anesthetic.

Bone-marrow biopsy: similar to a bone-marrow aspiration, but done with a larger needle. A small core of bone and marrow is cut out and removed for fixation and sectioning. The biopsy reveals the intact cellular architecture of the marrow, as well as the number and types of cells present.

Bone-marrow booster: an additional transplant of marrow, done when the first transplant has failed to engraft or to thrive, taken from the original donor.

308

Bowel prep: a mixture of oral antibiotics, taken every four hours in either pill or liquid form, which kills the bacteria and fungi normally found in the throat, stomach, and intestines that could cause serious infections in a patient with severely impaired immune defenses.

Broad-spectrum antibiotic: a chemical substance capable of killing or inhibiting the growth of a wide range of bacteria.

Bronchitis: inflammation of one or more of the bronchi, the large passages conveying air to and within the lungs.

Capillaries: the minute blood vessels that connect the arteries and the veins.

Caries: tooth decay; cavities.

Cataract: a clouding of the lens of the eye, obscuring vision; it can be a long-term side effect of total-body irradiation.

Catheter: a length of hollow tubing made of metal, rubber, or plastic that can be passed through body channels, such as arteries, veins, or the urinary system.

CAT scan (computerized axial tomography): a cross-sectional X-ray, reconstructed by computer.

CCSG: see Children's Cancer Study Group.

Central line: a catheter inserted into a large vein in the chest for the delivery of nutrients, medications, or blood products, or for the sampling of the patient's blood.

Cerebrospinal fluid: the fluid that bathes the brain and spinal cord, cushioning them from traumatic injury.

Chemotherapy: treatment of cancer or leukemia with drugs (chemical agents). Some of the side effects of these medications are nausea, vomiting, increased body temperature, and loss of hair.

Chemzyme series: a set of twelve different chemical analyses of the blood, also known as "blood chemistries."

Children's Cancer Study Group (CCSG): a nationwide cooperative group in the United States that does clinical research on childhood leukemia and other cancers.

Chromosomes: elongated bodies within the cell nucleus incorporating the DNA molecules that encode the genes, and involved in the transmission of inherited characteristics. Chromosomal defects have been associated with some forms of leukemia.

Clinical Investigation Committee: a group of doctors, lawyers, clergymen, and other laypeople who meet a few times a year to evaluate all new clinical research projects planned by a teaching hospital to ensure that the proposed studies involving patients or human volunteers are well designed, worth doing, and ethically sound.

CML: chronic myelocytic leukemia, accounting for some 2 percent of childhood cases. This form of leukemia strikes people primarily between the ages of thirty and fifty.

CMV: see cytomegalovirus.

CNS: central nervous system.

CNS leukemia: infiltration of leukemic cells into the CNS, specifically the three membranes (meninges) surrounding the brain and spinal cord. Since most antileukemic drugs cannot cross into the brain from the circulation, the meninges provide a protected site where the leukemic cells can multiply unimpeded. CNS leukemia is a common complication of ALL, occurring in about 75 percent of cases in the absence of prophylactic therapy, but it is rare in other forms of leukemia.

CNS prophylaxis: use of radiation to the brain and the injection of methotrexate into the spinal fluid to prevent CNS leukemia, a frequent complication of ALL. As a result of this therapy, the incidence of leukemic relapse beginning in the brain or spinal cord in children with ALL has declined from a rate of 50 percent before the therapy was devised to less than 10 percent subsequently. Still, there is concern that CNS prophylaxis may cause long-term intellectual deficits and learning problems in young children.

Colony-forming assay: a culture of isolated bone-marrow cells used to measure their ability to multiply in a transplant recipient.

Combination chemotherapy: the use of several drugs, each with distinct mechanisms and side effects, to kill off leukemic cells. With multiple drugs, those cells that become resistant to one drug may still be vulnerable to another.

Compassionate-plea protocol: a special protocol that a patient who develops life-threatening complications can invoke if, during a clinical trial of an experimental new drug (which is being compared with an established drug or a placebo), it is thought that it could possibly be of help in treating the illness.

Consolidation therapy (also called intensification therapy): continued treatment of leukemia after a complete remission has been obtained. Drugs are administered in an effort to eliminate any hidden leukemic cells that could eventually trigger a relapse.

Cooperative group: a national consortium of cancer-research groups that draws up standard treatment regimens (protocols) so that patients at participating hospitals across the country will receive the same therapy. As a result, the effectiveness of different regimens can be compared and evaluated at the national level.

Coulter counter: an electronic device that automatically measures the number of white cells, red cells, and platelets in a sample of blood.

Counts: numbers of the various types of blood cells per cubic millimeter of blood, representing a patient's hematological status.

CPK: creatine phosphokinase, an enzyme. When the concentration of CPK in the blood is elevated, it indicates tissue damage, particularly injury to the heart muscle.

Cross-matching: determination of the compatibility of the blood of a donor and that of a recipient before transfusion by placing the donor's red cells in the recipient's blood serum, and vice versa; the absence of a reaction indicates compatibility.

Culture: an attempt to grow a disease-causing microorganism on a nutrient medium in a glass dish or test tube so that it can be identified and its sensitivity to antibiotics ascertained. The goal is to make the treatment of an infection as specific as possible.

Cytomegalovirus (CMV): a common virus, present asymptomatically in the white blood cells of one out of every hundred people, that can cause serious infections and pneumonia in patients with an impaired immune response. CMV infections are often transmitted through transfusions of concentrated white cells.

Cytoxan: trade name for cyclophosphamide, an anticancer drug that is extremely toxic to the bone marrow. It is used to destroy a patient's existing marrow and suppress the immune response in preparation for bone-marrow transplantation.

Deep-tendon reflex: sudden contraction of a muscle elicited by a sharp tap on the connecting tendon; e.g., the knee-jerk reflex.

Differential count: the relative numbers of the various types of white blood cells in a patient's blood as a percentage of the total. A normal differential count has about 65 percent polys, 25 percent lymphocytes, and 10 percent all other cell types (with less than 5 percent blasts).

Differential diagnosis: the determination of which of several diseases may be producing a patient's symptoms.

Diuretic: a drug that enhances the flow of urine from the kidneys, causing the patient to urinate more frequently and hence lose excess body fluid. A common diuretic drug is furosemide.

Double-blind study: a clinical-research study of the effectiveness of a new drug in which neither the subjects nor the investigators know who is getting the active drug and who a placebo. The purpose of this approach is to eliminate any subtle bias on the part of the investigators from influencing the results of the experiment.

Drug sanctuaries: body sites such as the testes or the central nervous system in which there is restricted blood flow or limited passage of drugs from the bloodstream into the tissue, thereby reducing the effectiveness of chemotherapy and providing a "sheltered" site for leukemic cells to multiply. Specific therapies must be given to these sites to eliminate the sequestered leukemic cells.

Dry mouth: lack of saliva in the mouth due to the toxic effects of total-body irradiation and graft-versus-host disease, a complication of bone-marrow transplantation. Since the normal saliva participates in the prevention of tooth decay, patients with dry mouth often develop serious dental problems, such as massive cavities and gum irritation.

Echocardiogram: recording of the position and motion of the heart walls or of internal structures of the heart by the echo obtained from beams of ultrasonic waves directed through the chest wall.

Edema: accumulation of excessive fluid in a tissue or tissues; e.g., pulmonary edema, which involves a diffuse accumulation of fluid in the lungs and air spaces.

EEG: see electroencephalogram.

EKG: see electrocardiogram.

Electrocardiogram (EKG): a recording of electrical impulses from the heart.

Electroencephalogram (EEG): a recording of "brain waves," made with electrodes placed on the scalp, which is indicative of abnormal brain function.

Electrolytes: salts that regulate the body's fluid balance, including sodium and potassium. These salts are also essential for the electrical activity of nerves and brain cells.

Encephalitis: an inflammation of the brain, usually caused by a viral infection.

Endotracheal tube: a plastic cylinder inserted into the trachea (windpipe) of an anesthetized patient to keep the breathing passages open and free of obstructions.

Enzymes: protein substances made by cells; they serve as catalysts in biochemical reactions.

Exudate: fluid with a high content of protein and cellular debris that oozes from blood vessels onto tissue surfaces, usually as the result of inflammation.

Fellow: a young physician who, having completed his or her residency, is doing a two-year fellowship to obtain additional training in a medical specialty, such as cardiology or oncology.

Femoral: pertaining to the thigh.

Finger-stick: jabbing of a sterilized metal tine into a patient's fingertip in order to obtain a few drops of blood for blood smears and counts.

Flora: the normal bacteria that colonize the gut, mouth, and skin, living in delicately balanced ecological harmony. In healthy people these bacteria are harmless and even helpful, assisting in digestion and producing an essential vitamin. But in patients with a severely impaired immune system, the flora can multiply out of control and cause serious infections.

Flow-sheet: a standardized form put out by the cooperative groups on which the attending physician transcribes a patient's lab values, clinical signs and symptoms, therapies, complications, side effects, and supportive treatments while on a standard protocol study. These sheets are mailed four times a year to a central operations office, where patient files are computerized and continually updated. In this way, it is possible to evaluate the effects of different treatment regimens on large numbers of patients across the country.

Fluid overload: a state of surplus fluids in the body, which can be caused by excessive intravenous infusion of liquids and can result in high blood pressure and edema.

Forced vital capacity (FVC): a lung-function test that measures the amount of air that a patient can force out of the lungs at one time. This test is done every day during a bone-marrow transplant.

FVC: see forced vital capacity.

Gastrointestinal tract: the digestive system, including the mouth, esophagus, stomach, large and small intestines, and rectum.

GI: gastrointestinal.

Graft-versus-host disease (GVHD): a complication of bone-marrow transplantation, consisting of an immunological reaction of the transplanted marrow cells directed against certain tissues of the transplant recipient. It is very common after marrow transplantation and is usually mild, but can be serious and even life threatening unless treated appropriately. The disease affects primarily the skin (rash, blisters, thickening, itching), the liver (swelling, inflammation of liver cells), and the gastrointestinal tract (diarrhea, belly pain, inability to absorb food).

Granulocyte: same as a poly; a white blood cell with characteristic blue-black granules seen in the cytoplasm when the cell is stained.

GVHD: see graft-versus-host disease.

Hematocrit: a measure of the number of red cells in the blood in terms of the percentage of the total fluid volume they occupy; also called the packed cell volume (PCV). Normally the hematocrit is between 40 and 45 percent.

Hematology: the medical specialty encompassing the function, anatomy, physiology, pathology, and therapeutics of the blood.

Hematoma: a localized collection of blood that has escaped from a blood vessel and remained, usually clotted, in an organ, space, or tissue.

Hemoglobin: an iron-containing protein in red blood cells that carries oxygen from the lungs to the tissues. The normal hemoglobin content of the blood is greater than 12 grams per deciliter (100 milliliters).

Hemophoresis: a procedure in which several pints of blood from a healthy donor are passed through a continuous-flow blood processor; the platelets or white cells are extracted from the blood and the remaining blood components are returned to the donor. This process takes around three hours.

Hemorrhagic cystitis: inflammation of the bladder lining resulting in bleeding into the urine. It is a common side effect of chemotherapy with Cytoxan (cyclophosphamide).

Heparin: a drug that prevents blood clotting.

Heparin lock: a special type of IV that can be turned off and reused at a later time without the need for continual infusion of fluids to keep the line open. Between infusions, the needle must be flushed with heparin solution every six hours to prevent it from becoming clogged with clotted blood.

Hepatitis: inflammation of the liver, usually caused by a virus.

Herpes zoster: shingles; an acute, self-limited inflammatory disease of the peripheral nerves in adults, associated with neuralgic pain. It is caused by the same virus that causes chicken pox in children. Indeed, herpes zoster may result from reactivation of the virus, which has lain dormant in spinal nerves since a childhood episode of chicken pox.

Histocompatibility testing: identification of the genetically determined chemical markers on the tissue cells of prospective transplant donors and recipients, in order to make sure that the graft will be accepted and remain functional. Nonhistocompatible grafts will be recognized and destroyed by the host's immune system.

HLA: human leukocyte antigens; the set of major histocompatibility antigens present on the surface of all nucleated human cells and determined by a single set of genes called the HLA locus. These molecular markers, designated A, B, C, and D, are important in the matching of tissues for organ transplantation.

House staff (also called house officers): the MDs who are responsible for the hour-to-hour management of patients in a teaching hospital. The house staff includes interns, in their first year of hospital training; junior residents, in their second year; and senior residents, in their third year. The house staff is supervised by the senior medical staff, including fellows and attendings.

Hydration: the administration of intravenous fluids.

Hyperalimentation solution: an intravenous solution, infused through a central line, that provides all of the nutrients and calories needed when a patient is unable to eat solid food.

I & O: intake and output; a record kept by the nursing staff to chart a patient's daily consumption and excretion of fluids, in order that the body's fluid balance be maintained.

Imed: a battery-powered infusion pump attached to an IV pole that regulates the hourly rate of an intravenous infusion. When the flow is obstructed by a kink or bubble in the line, a beeping alarm goes off.

Immunosuppression: the inability of the body to form antibodies or to react normally to invading microorganisms or other foreign substances. This state may be the result of the leukemic disease process, or of its treatment with chemotherapy and radiation.

Incentive spirometer: a small, portable, hand-held device used to "exercise" (expand) the lungs. Following a bone-marrow transplant, patients often blow into it to help strengthen their lungs and prevent pneumonia.

Increment: a rise in blood counts achieved by a specialized transfusion, such as of packed red cells, white cells, or platelets. If the increment is poor, an immunological rejection may be responsible.

Induction chemotherapy: the initial treatment of acute leukemia with a battery of three drugs or more, designed to obtain a remission of the disease.

Infection: invasion of the body by microorganisms such as viruses, bacteria, fungi, and parasites; or excessive multiplication of "normal" microbes such as intestinal flora due to lowered body resistance.

Inflammation: the reaction of the body to an irritating substance or infecting agent. Symptoms include heat, redness, swelling, and pain.

Informed consent: detailed information about a planned procedure or treatment, as well as possible alternatives, given by the medical staff to a patient and the family prior to securing their consent to proceed with the proposed therapy. Consent may take the form of a written waiver that the patient or parent signs, indicating a willingness to participate. Informed consent is considered essential, for ethical reasons, when patients are being offered unproved or experimental therapies.

Interstitial pneumonitis: a serious, chronic form of pneumonia resulting from inflammation of the nonfunctional tissues of the lungs, and leading to a decline in lung volume. It is a fairly common complication of bone-marrow transplantation, since total-body irradiation can cause lung damage and increase vulnerability to infection.

Intramuscular: an injection directly into the muscle.

Intrathecal methotrexate: methotrexate injected into the fluid-containing sheath (theca) surrounding the spinal cord. This is done in order to prevent the multiplication of leukemic cells within the central nervous system (see CNS prophylaxis).

Intravenous: an injection or infusion of medication or fluids directly into a vein.

IV: intravenous line; inserted into a superficial vein and used for the administration of fluids, blood products, or medications.

Jaundice: a yellow discoloration of the skin and eyes, due to an excessive accumulation of bilirubin in the body.

Ketamine: a short-acting general anesthetic used in young children during painful procedures such as bone-marrow aspiration and spinal taps. Its major side effect is that it can cause nightmares. (It is unusable in adults because it gives rise to frightening hallucinations.)

Laminar-airflow room: a special environment designed to minimize the risk of microbial contamination in patients with severely impaired immune systems. Highly filtered air flows in one direction across the patient's bed, preventing microbes from settling and providing a protective screen from germs brought in by staff and visitors, who must wear sterile gloves and masks (and sometimes gowns, hats, and shoe covers, as well).

Leukemia: a cancerous condition of the blood brought about by the uncontrolled multiplication of one type of white blood cell in the blood-forming tissues.

Leukophoresis: removal of excessive numbers of white cells from the blood of patients with chronic leukemia using a continuous-flow blood processor.

Liver-function tests: a variety of biochemical tests done to evaluate liver function, usually by measuring the concentration of liver enzymes or metabolic end-products in the blood. Examples include serum bilirubin, alkaline phosphatase, transaminases (SGOT, SGPT), serum albumin, blood lipids, etc.

Lumbar area: the base of the spine, extending between the lowest ribs and the pelvis.

Lumbar puncture: see spinal tap.

Lymphatic system: a secondary system for the circulation of body fluid. The lymph nodes detect invading microorganisms and turn out large numbers of white cells that produce antibodies and attack the foreign agents.

"Magic bullet": the ideal antileukemic drug—one that has yet to be invented. It would selectively kill leukemic cells without harming normal tissues.

Maintenance chemotherapy: repeating cycles of two drugs or more, designed to maintain a complete remission by killing off (or at least inhibiting the multiplication of) any residual leukemic cells hidden away in body tissues.

Mannitol: a sugar alcohol used as a potent diuretic, particularly to clear the kidneys rapidly of red-cell breakdown products following a transfusion reaction.

Megakaryocytes: giant cells in the bone marrow that are the progenitors of platelets.

Microorganism (also microbe): an infecting agent such as a bacterium, virus, fungus, or parasite.

Minibottles: small IV bottles, such as those used to administer intravenous antibiotics.

Mixed-lymphocyte culture: a test done to determine whether the bone marrow of a prospective donor is compatible with the immune system of the recipient, so as to predict whether there is potential risk of graft rejection or of graft-versus-host disease.

Myocardiopathy: damage to the heart muscle.

Nurse-anesthetist: a registered nurse who has completed an additional two-year course and is thereby qualified to administer anesthesia for routine operations.

Nystatin: an antifungal drug in solution that is "swished and swallowed" by patients on intensive antibiotic therapy to prevent fungal infections of the mouth and gut.

Oncology: the branch of medical science dealing with tumors.

Ophthalmoscope: a diagnostic instrument with an illuminating light and a magnifying lens, used to peer through the pupil at the interior of the eye.

Optic disk: a part of the optic nerve inside the eyeball, appearing as a pink or white disk at the back of the eye, that is formed by nerve fibers converging from the retina.

Orally: taken by mouth.

Oriented times three: mentally aware of person, place, and time; a basic indicator of normal consciousness obtained at the start of a neurological or psychiatric examination.

Papilledema: swelling of the optic disks with fluid, due to increased pressure of the cerebrospinal fluid bathing the brain and spinal cord. This sign can be indicative of a brain tumor, a hematoma (large blood clot) within the skull, or leukemic infiltrates in the central nervous system.

Para: a woman who has produced one or more viable offspring.

Pathogen: a microorganism that causes disease.

Peripheral line: an IV placed in the patient's hand or arm, or very rarely in the foot or leg.

Petechiae: tiny red spots or blood blisters on the skin, caused by spontaneous bleeding from capillaries due to an excessively low platelet count; also called splinter hemorrhages.

Physician's assistant (P.A.): a graduate of a two-year training program who performs paramedical duties.

Physician's Desk Reference: a guide to prescription drugs, which contains detailed descriptions of all proprietary drugs currently available, including information on drug activity, side effects, manufacturers, and available forms and dosages.

Pituitary gland: the peanut-sized gland at the base of the brain that secretes a variety of hormones, including one that controls growth. The adverse effects of total-body irradiation on the pituitary include stunted growth in young children.

Placebo: a harmless solution or pill, lacking in active ingredients, that is given deceptively to a patient who believes he or she is getting a real drug. It is used in studies of drug effectiveness to control for psychosomatic effects produced by the patient's expectation of improvement.

Platelet: a small, flat, platelike cell in the blood that aids in clotting and seals off leaks in capillaries to prevent hemorrhaging.

Platelet consumption: rapid disappearance of platelets that can occur when serious bacterial infections of the blood release toxins that damage the walls of blood vessels, causing platelets to adhere to them and form blood clots. Clotting factors in the blood are also consumed, and the resulting clots obstruct capillaries. The outcome is a lowered platelet count and increased risk of bleeding, along with tissue and organ damage due to widespread coagulation. A more technical term for this serious complication of blood infections is disseminated intravascular coagulation (DIC).

Pleurisy: inflammation of the membranous sacs that enclose the lungs.

Pneumocystis carinii: an amoeboid parasite that causes a serious form of pneumonia in debilitated individuals, including leukemic patients on chemotherapy or following bone-marrow transplantation. *Pneumocystis* infections can be prevented with prophylactic administration of the antibiotic combination trimethoprim-sulfamethoxazole (trade names Bactrim or Septra).

Poly: abbreviation for polymorphonuclear leukocyte; a type of white cell that engulfs invading bacteria and fungi. These cells are easily identifiable by the characteristic shape of their cell nucleus, which is divided into a series of lobes connected by thin strands. Polys, also known as granulocytes, are essential for combating bacterial infections.

Prognosis: anticipated outcome of a disease, often predicted at diagnosis.

Prognostic groups: ALL can be divided into at least three subcategories with different prognoses on the basis of clinical and laboratory tests done at diagnosis. These three types of the disease are identified on the basis of the patient's age, sex, and white count, and are designated low risk, average risk, and high risk. Special treatment protocols have been devised for each prognostic group, in an effort to tailor the intensity of treatment to the aggressiveness of the disease.

Protective isolation: isolation of a child with very low white counts in a special room with reduced bacterial contamination, so as to lower the risk of infection.

Protocol: a standard treatment procedure followed so that the results achieved by different hospitals can be compared accurately. Most childhood-leukemia protocols are drawn up by nationwide cooperative groups made up of dozens of pediatric cancer centers.

Pseudomonas aeruginosa: a motile, rod-shaped bacterium that is gram-negative (it does not retain the violet dye when stained by Gram's method). Serious infections with *Pseudomonas* are almost always a consequence of damage to local tissue or diminished host resistance. Localized infections do not present a threat to life unless the bacteria invade the bloodstream, in which case the mortality rate is 75 percent.

Pulmonary: pertaining to the lungs.

Purpura: large, weltlike black-and-blue marks caused by spontaneous bleeding under the skin and associated with a low platelet count.

Rad: radiation absorbed dose; a unit of radiation exposure in living systems.

Radiation chimera: an animal whose body contains grafted bone marrow from a genetically nonidentical donor. This is done by irradiating the transplant recipient to inhibit its immune response before grafting the marrow; the resulting chimera comprises two different cell populations that are genetically distinct.

Rale: an abnormal respiratory sound heard through a stethoscope, indicating some pathological condition of the lungs.

Randomization: chance assignment of patients to different treatment regimens for research purposes, when the ideal treatment for their disease is not yet known.

Red blood cell: also called an erythrocyte; a cell that carries oxygen from the lungs to all areas of the body. Lacking a nucleus, shaped like a biconcave disk, and packed with hemoglobin, red blood cells are made in the bone marrow.

Remission: healthy state of the body in which all leukemic blasts have vanished from the blood and the bone marrow. Since some leukemic cells can linger on in the testes, the central nervous system, or other protected sites, however, a remission is not necessarily a cure.

Respirator: a machine that forces air into the lungs, thereby keeping alive patients who are no longer able to breathe on their own.

Reticulocyte count: the number of immature red blood cells in circulation. Normally only a small percentage of the red cells are immature, but if the bone marrow is making more blood (e.g., after a bone-marrow transplant), the number of reticulocytes in circulation will increase.

Reverse isolation: isolation of a patient who has a contagious disease, so that other patients are not exposed to the infectious agent.

Sclerosis: hardening or scarring of a blood vessel, often due to inflammation.

Septicemia: also called sepsis or blood poisoning; systemic disease associated with the presence and persistence of pathogenic microorganisms or their toxins (poisons) in the blood.

SGOT: serum glutamic oxaloacetic transaminase, an enzyme. When present in increased concentrations in the blood, tissue damage is indicated, particularly of the liver.

SGPT: serum glutamic pyruvic transaminase, an enzyme. High blood levels of it are associated with liver damage.

Sitz bath: a plastic tub filled with warm water that fits into the commode and is used to clean and soothe the perianal and rectal areas.

Spiking fever: a fever characterized over a span of several hours by recurring peaks of very high body temperature, separated by valleys of near-normal temperature.

Spinal tap: passage of a needle between the lumbar vertebrae of the lower spine and into the reservoir of cerebrospinal fluid surrounding the spinal cord. A sample of spinal fluid is removed for analysis of its sugar and protein content and examined microscopically for the presence of blood cells, leukemic blasts, or bacteria.

Spleen: an organ in the left side of the abdomen that filters the blood, removing senescent red cells and platelets. Since the spleen also produces white cells, it may enlarge in response to infection or as a result of the infiltration of leukemic cells into the blood-forming tissues.

Staphylococcus epidermidis: a common skin bacterium that causes systemic infections only in those patients who have virtually no polys or other immune defenses.

Sterile: uncontaminated by bacteria, viruses, or other pathogens.

Sternum: breastbone.

Steroids: chemical agents, sharing a common basic structure, that are produced within the body as well as artificially. This class of compounds includes many hormones, such as the corticosteroids, which suppress inflammation and the immune response.

Stylet: a thin metal rod that fits snugly inside the bore of an aspiration needle so that it does not bend or become clogged when penetrating muscle or bone. Once the needle is in place, the stylet is removed and a sample of fluid or tissue is sucked out through the hollow needle.

Superinfection: a new infection complicating the course of antibiotic therapy for an existing infection, due to invasion of the body by bacteria or fungi resistant to the drug or drugs in use.

Surveillance cultures: routine specimens of urine, throat secretions, and stool that are periodically sent to the microbiology lab to be cultured for bacterial, viral, and fungal pathogens, allowing infections to be detected early, before they become life threatening.

TBI: see total-body irradiation.

T-cell leukemia: also called T-lymphoblastic leukemia; a subcategory of ALL that affects a minority of patients with the disease, most of them over age ten. T-cell leukemia runs a more aggressive course than ordinary ("null-cell") ALL and is often associated with a mediastinal mass (a tumorlike aggregation of leukemic cells in the chest cavity). The disease is relatively resistant to treatment.

Thrombocytopenia: a low platelet count (less than the normal minimum of 250,000 per cubic millimeter), associated with increased risk of spontaneous or prolonged bleeding, especially from the gums, nose, urinary tract, or into the skin, causing bruising, purpura, and petechiae.

Thrush: an infection of the mouth by the fungus *Candida albicans* in patients with a suppressed immune response; often associated with mouth ulcers produced by chemotherapy. The major symptom is a white-coated tongue.

Toothettes: small sponges on a stick used instead of a toothbrush by leukemic patients with very low platelet counts, to prevent bleeding from the gums.

Total-body irradiation (TBI): exposure of the entire body to ionizing radiation from a linear accelerator in order to destroy the patient's bone marrow and suppress the immune system in preparation for bone-marrow transplantation. Total-body irradiation is usually given in several small doses rather than a single large one so that its toxic side effects on healthy tissues, particularly the lungs, can be minimized.

Transfusion reaction: a serious immunological reaction due to the accidental infusion of incompatible red cells. Rapid destruction of large numbers of red cells occurs immediately, releasing excessive amounts of hemoglobin into the blood and urine. Immediate symptoms include fever, abdominal pain, and possibly shock, followed later on by low blood pressure and kidney failure. Transfusion reactions can be treated with an intravenous infusion of mannitol or kidney dialysis to clear the toxic substances from the blood.

Triage nurse: an emergency-ward nurse who, on the basis of the acuteness of the medical problem, decides which patients need treatment first.

Tympanic membranes: eardrums.

Ulcer: an inflammatory lesion or sore on the skin or an internal body cavity, resulting in an excavation of the surface due to the sloughing of dead tissue.

Uric acid: the end product of the degradation of nucleic acids, which is excreted in the urine.

Vaccine: a weakened sample of disease-producing microorganisms that induces the formation of antibodies but does not produce overt symptoms of infection; the resulting antibodies then protect against future infections by the same agent.

Varicella: chicken pox, an infectious disease characterized by fever and widespread skin eruptions. It is highly contagious, with attack rates of 70 percent or more among susceptible persons exposed to a patient with the disease. In children with impaired immune function, the varicella virus can invade internal organs such as the lungs, liver, and brain, causing life-threatening complications.

Vital signs: basic indicators of body function, recorded by the nursing staff at regular intervals. Routine vital signs include body temperature, respirations per minute, pulse rate, and blood pressure.

White blood cell: also called a leukocyte; a nucleated cell necessary to combat infection. There are several types of white blood cells, each with a specialized function, including polys, lymphocytes, and monocytes.

Work-up: a thorough physical exam and battery of laboratory tests designed to arrive at a differential diagnosis for a set of symptoms.

Wright-Giemsa stain: a dark blue stain used to render bone-marrow cells visible under the microscope.

ZIG: see zoster immune globulin.

Zoster immune globulin (ZIG): an antiserum, enriched in specific antibodies to the chicken pox virus (varicella-zoster), derived from the blood serum of adult patients recovering from shingles (herpes zoster). If administered to a child with an impaired immune response within ninety-six hours of exposure, it can prevent the infection or at least reduce its severity. Since ZIG is in very short supply, it is not normally used for healthy children who are exposed to the disease.

Bibliography

NONTECHNICAL BOOKS

Baker, Lynn S. *You and Leukemia: A Day at a Time.* Philadelphia: W.B. Saunders Company, 1978.

Glasser, Ronald J. *Ward 402.* New York: George Braziller, Inc., 1973.

Gunther, John. *Death Be Not Proud.* New York: Harper and Brothers, 1949.

Jampolsky, Gerald G. *There Is a Rainbow Behind Every Dark Cloud.* Millbrae, Calif.: Celestial Arts, 1978.

Lund, Doris. *Eric.* New York: Dell Publishing Company, 1974.

Roach, Nancy. *The Last Day of April.* New York: American Cancer Society, 1974.

Rosenberg, Mark L. *Patients: The Experience of Illness.* Philadelphia: W.B. Saunders Company, 1980.

Sherman, Mikie. *The Leukemic Child.* Bethesda, Md.: NIH Publications No. 79-863, 1979.

TECHNICAL BOOKS

Ackerknecht, Erwin H. *Rudolph Virchow: Doctor, Statesman, Anthropologist.* Madison, Wisc.: University of Wisconsin Press, 1953.

Altman, Arnold J., and Schwartz, Allan D. *Malignant Diseases of Infancy, Childhood and Adolescence.* Philadelphia: W.B. Saunders Company, 1978.

American Cancer Society. *Proceedings of the National Conference on the Care of the Child with Cancer.* New York: American Cancer Society, 1979.

American Cancer Society and the National Cancer Institute. *Proceedings of the National Conference on the Lymphomas and the Leukemias.* New York: American Cancer Society, 1978.

Forkner, Claude E. *Leukemia and Allied Disorders.* New York: The Macmillan Company, 1938.

Gunz, Frederick, and Baikie, Albert G. *Leukemia.* 3rd ed. New York: Grune & Stratton, Inc., 1974.

Kagan, Benjamin M. *Antimicrobial Therapy.* 2nd ed. Philadelphia: W.B. Saunders Company, 1974.

Neth, Rolf; Gallo, Robert C.; Spiegelman, Sol; and Stohlman, Frederick, Jr.; eds. *Modern Trends in Human Leukemia.* New York: Grune & Stratton, Inc., 1974.

Plumer, Ada Lawrence. *Principles and Practice of Intravenous Therapy.* 2nd ed. Boston: Little, Brown & Company, 1978.

Pochedly, Carl. *The Child with Leukemia.* Springfield, Ill.: Thomas Publishers, 1973.

Reich, Paul R. *Hematology: Physiopathologic Basis for Clinical Practice.* Boston: Little, Brown & Company, 1978.

Scipien, Gladys M., et al. *Comprehensive Pediatric Nursing.* New York: McGraw-Hill Book Company, 1975.

Smith, Carl H. *Blood Diseases of Infancy and Childhood.* 3rd ed. St. Louis: C.V. Mosby Company, 1972.

Sutow, Wataru Walter. *Clinical Pediatric Oncology.* 2nd ed. St. Louis: C.V. Mosby Company, 1977.

NONTECHNICAL ARTICLES

Cohen, Edward P. "His Brother's Healthy Bone Marrow Saved Phil Smith's Life." *Today's Health,* July–August 1975.

Drake, Donald C. "A Rare Disease, a Rare Boy: Bone Marrow Transplant Saves an Anemia Victim." *Philadelphia Inquirer,* October 19, 1980.

———. "Putting Death in Its Place." *Philadelphia Inquirer,* December 14–December 21, 1980 (eight-part series).

Folster, David, and Padmore, Tim. "An Act of Brotherly Love." *Macleans,* April 23, 1979.

Johnson, Jeanette. "The Case of Carol Tam." *Cancer Center* (Memorial Sloan-Kettering Cancer Center), Winter 1980.

Rabkin, B. "Childhood Leukemia: A Stalemate in a Long War." *Macleans,* April 23, 1979.

Ross, Walter S. "They're Gaining on Leukemia." *Today's Health.* October 1970.

Wheelright, Jeff. "Saving the Children: Turning the Tide Against Cancer in the Young." *Life,* December 1980.

TECHNICAL ARTICLES

Adams, Margaret A. "Helping the Parents of Children with Malignancy." *The Journal of Pediatrics* 93: 734–38.

August, Charles S.; Serota, Frederic T.; and Koch, Penelope A. "Donor Consent for Participation in Bone Marrow Transplantation at the Children's Hospital of Philadelphia." Mimeographed. 1981.

Fefer, Alexander. "Bone Marrow Transplants in Leukemia Patients in Remission [interview]." *CA: A Cancer Journal for Clinicians* 30: 45–52.

Ford, C.E.; Hamerton, J.L.; Barnes, D. W. H.; et al. "Cytological Identification of Radiation-Chimaeras." *Nature* 177: 452–54.

Frei, Emil, III, and Freireich, Emil J. "Leukemia." *Scientific American,* May 1964, pp.88–96.

Gardner, G. Gail; August, Charles S.; and Githens, John. "Psychological Issues in Bone Marrow Transplantation." *Pediatrics* 60: 625–31 (supplement).

Geist, Richard A. "Onset of Chronic Illness in Children and Adolescents: Psychotherapeutic and Consultative Intervention." *American Journal of Orthopsychiatry* 49: 4–23.

Jacobson, L.O.; Simmons, E.L.; Marks, E.K.; et al. "The Role of the Spleen in Radiation Injury and Recovery." *Journal of the Laboratory of Clinical Medicine* 35: 746–70.

Kagen-Goodheart, Lynn. "Reentry: Living with Childhood Cancer." *American Journal of Orthopsychiatry* 47: 651–58.

Bibliography

Lorenz, E.; Uphoff, D.; Reid, T.R.; et al. "Modification of Irradiation Injury in Mice and Guinea Pigs by Bone Marrow Injections." *Journal of the National Cancer Institute* 12: 197-201.

Nowell, P.C.; Cole, I.J.; Habermeyer, J.G.; et al. "Growth and Continued Function of Rat Marrow Cells in X-Radiated Mice." *Cancer Research* 16: 258-61.

O'Mally, John E.; Koocher, Gerald; Foster, Diana; et al. "Psychiatric Sequelae of Surviving Childhood Cancer." *American Journal of Orthopsychiatry* 49: 608-16.

Pinkel, D. "The Ninth Annual David Karnovsky Lecture: Treatment of Acute Lymphocytic Leukemia." *Cancer* 43: 1128-37.

Ross, Judith W. "Coping with Childhood Cancer: Group Intervention as an Aid to Parents in Crisis." *Social Work in Health Care* 4: 381-91.

Santos, George W. "Bone Marrow Transplantation: Present Status." *Transplantation Proceedings* 11: 182.

Santos, George W.; Tutschka, Peter J.; Elfenbein, Gerald J.; et al. "Allogenic and Syngenic Marrow Transplantation in Patients with Acute Lymphocytic Leukemia and Acute Myelogenous Leukemia with CNS Disease: Protocol JH-79-15." Mimeographed. Johns Hopkins Bone Marrow Transplant Program, March 1979.

Taylor, C. Inga; De Antonio, Miriam; Draffin, Nancy C.; et al. "A Group Experience for Parents of Children with Malignancy." *The Journal of the South Carolina Medical Association*, June 1978, pp. 290-92.

Thomas, E.D. "Current Status of Marrow Transplantation for Aplastic Anemia and Acute Leukemia: The Philip Levine Award Lecture." *American Journal of Clinical Pathology* 72: 887-92.

Thomas, E.D.; Buckner, C.D.; Fefer, A.; et al. "Marrow Transplantation in the Treatment of Acute Leukemia." *Advances in Cancer Research* 27: 269-79.

Thomas, E.D.; Clift, R.A.; Fefer, A.; et al. "Bone Marrow Transplantations: Risks Involved, Successes Achieved." *Resident and Staff Physician*, June 1976, pp. 53-63.

Thomas, E.D.; Lochte, H.L.; Lu, W.C.; et al. "Intravenous Infusion of Bone Marrow in Patients Receiving Radiation and Chemotherapy." *The New England Journal of Medicine* 257: 491-96.

Thomas, E.D., and Storb, R. "Technique for Human Marrow Grafting." *Blood* 36: 507-15.

Thomas, E.D.; Storb, R.; Clift, R.A.; et al. "Bone Marrow Transplantation." *The New England Journal of Medicine* 292: 832-43, 895-902.

Vernick, Joel, and Karon, Myron. "Who's Afraid of Death on a Leukemia Ward?" *American Journal of Diseases of Children* 109: 393-97.

Index